THE PROFESSION OF NURSING

SECOND EDITION

THE PROFESSION OF NURSING

A Foundation for Caring in Technology-Driven Settings

MARIA A. REVELL

Middle Tennessee State University

cognella

SAN DIEGO

Bassim Hamadeh, CEO and Publisher
Amanda Martin, Executive Publisher
Amy Smith, Associate Editorial Manager
Samantha Hansen, Production Editor
Jana Jarvis, Project Editor
Monica O'Keefe, Editorial Associate
Jess Estrella, Senior Graphic Designer
Alexa Lucido, Senior Licensing Manager
Natalie Piccotti, Director of Marketing
Kassie Graves, Senior Vice President, Editorial
Alia Bales, Director, Project Editorial and Production

Printed in the United States of America.

cognella® ACADEMIC PUBLISHING
320 South Cedros Ave., Ste. 400, Solana Beach, CA 92075

Brief Contents

Detailed Contents

Preface

This new edition, formerly titled *Professionalism in Nursing: A Foundation for Practice*, was developed from a deep commitment to guiding aspiring and current nurses toward a professional identity that upholds the highest standards. Over my 50-year journey in nursing, I have witnessed the profession evolve in remarkable ways. It has been shaped by advancements in knowledge, shifting healthcare policies, and the ever-expanding scope of nursing roles. Yet, through all these transformations, one element has remained unwavering: the trust that patients and communities place in nurses. This trust is built on the very essence of nursing, which is caring. Professionalism in nursing is not merely about competence in clinical skills; it is about integrity, respect, accountability, and an unwavering dedication to the well-being of others.

This book is designed to help readers reimagine what nursing is and what it can be for them. It goes beyond defining professionalism, guiding individuals through some of the roles, responsibilities, and specialties that make up nursing. By exploring the core values and behaviors that define a professional nurse, this book encourages readers to cultivate their own sense of purpose within the profession. It offers a roadmap for personal and professional development, helping nurses and nursing students align their career aspirations with the fundamental principles of nursing practice.

Key features of this book revision include new chapters on nursing professionalism; core nursing concepts, including Caritas; and advocacy and leadership. Chapter revisions incorporate effective communication, nursing leadership, current technological innovations in nursing, and the ever-important role of continuing education in maintaining nursing excellence. Each chapter provides insights that encourage self-reflection, allowing readers to consider what professionalism means to them personally and how they can integrate it into their daily practice. The book also highlights the impact of professionalism on patient outcomes, interdisciplinary teamwork, and the broader healthcare system. By embracing these principles, nurses can not only enhance their own careers but also contribute to the overall advancement of the nursing profession.

The book incorporates pedagogical aids designed to enhance student learning and engagement, ensuring that key concepts of professionalism in nursing are both accessible and applicable. These aids include chapter objectives and key terms highlighted when first mentioned in each chapter. Summaries with key takeaways help reinforce chapter essential concepts, making it easier for students to retain and integrate knowledge into their clinical experiences. Chapter references offer additional sources for student investigation. These aids promote structured guidance to support the development of essential professional skills, encouraging students to cultivate ethical reasoning, effective communication, and leadership qualities that are fundamental to nursing excellence.

Ultimately, *The Profession of Nursing: A Foundation for Caring in Technology Driven Settings* serves as a guide to help both new and experienced nurses refine their approach to patient care and professional interactions. It is my hope that this book inspires a renewed sense of dedication to the art and science of nursing, one that fosters a deep commitment to lifelong learning, ethical practice, and compassionate care.

I view nursing as more than just a career—it is a true calling. As a nurse, your commitment to professionalism strengthens the caring, integrity, and trust that are the foundation of this honorable profession.

Maria A. Revell, PhD, MSN, RN, COI
2025

CHAPTER 1

Introduction to Nursing Professionalism

Objectives

Upon completion of this chapter, the learner will be able to do the following:

1. Define key elements of professionalism within the nursing field.
2. Analyze how professionalism in nursing contributes to improved patient outcomes, safety, and satisfaction.
3. Identify strategies and behaviors that can be adopted to promote and maintain professionalism throughout one's nursing career.

Key Chapter Terms

- Professionalism
- Competence
- Integrity
- Accountability
- Empathy
- Communication skills
- Teamwork and collaboration
- Cultural competence
- Time management and organization
- Altruism

Professionalism as a Foundation

Professionalism is not just a buzzword. It is a real term that serves as a foundation for nursing care delivery. It is a critical pillar that supports the entire nursing professional structure. It represents a set of values, behaviors, and relationships that establish nurse trustworthiness. The professionalism concept ensures delivery of the highest standards of patient care. The nursing code of conduct is an imperative to displaying professionalism, but it is not just about adherence to this code of conduct. The concept extends to a commitment to continued education, ethical practice, and the development of a caring relationship with patients. It ensures quality patient care delivery and development of patient trust and contributes to nursing's professional growth.

Professionalism Elements

Professionalism is a multidimensional and dynamic process that is complex, varied, and ever changing. The concept is instilled through a process of socialization. This process includes elements that influence nursing actions and performances. Professionalism elements promote a commitment to providing the highest standard of patient care. These involve a combination of **competence**, **integrity**, **accountability**, and **empathy** (see Figure 1.1; Cao et al., 2023; Cornett, 2006; Hintistan & Topcuoglu, 2017).

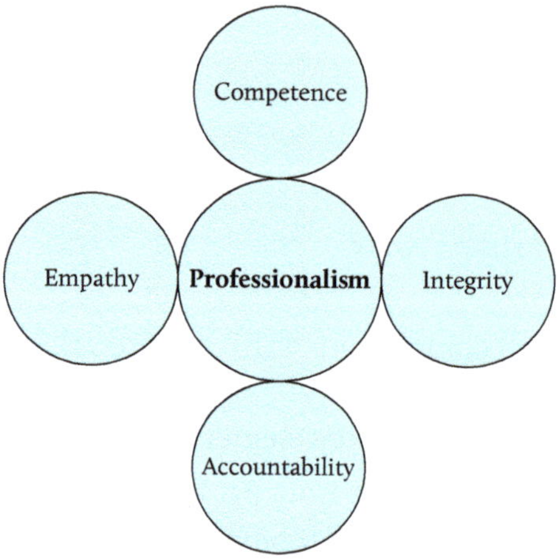

FIGURE 1.1 Some Key Professionalism Elements

Competence

Competence is a safe and effective patient care cornerstone. It is reflected in the nurses' ability to apply evidence based clinical knowledge and skills to ensure that patients receive the best health care possible. *Nurse competence* refers to the knowledge, skills, and abilities that nurses possess. These promote the provision of safe and effective patient care by enabling nurses to adapt to numerous dynamic health environments. Competence includes the theoretical and practical knowledge of the clinical setting, the organization, and one's own abilities. Clinical guidelines and organizational knowledge are required to be competent in administering care within a professionalism framework. Competence in one's own abilities maintains self-awareness and allows an understanding of personal attributes that promote effective use of clinical and organizational information.

Providing care based on knowledge and skills allows nurses to be autonomous while delivering care within their scope of practice level. This facilitates self-awareness of one's own limitations and promotes a sense of lifelong learning to maintain up-to-date abilities. Knowledge and skill refinement and updating facilitates collaborative interactions to both learn and provide care that is safe and current. Competence promotes a patient safety culture that improves safe practice and professional development. These minimize errors and thus adverse events (Zaitoun et al., 2023).

Competence extends to critical thinking, which allows nurses to assess complex situations, prioritize tasks, and make quick decisions that affect patient outcomes. Critical thinking allows nurses to adapt to ever-changing patient situations. The combination of knowledge, skills, and experience allows nurses to deliver high-quality, patient-centered care.

Integrity

Integrity involves adhering to moral and ethical principles in patient care delivery. This requires nurses to maintain honesty in professional interactions and uphold patient dignity and privacy. Integrity is the moral compass that guides nurses in professional practice and requires them to be not only honest in their patient, family, and colleague interactions but also transparent. Truth is a requirement, based on this professional element, even when it is difficult to give realistic information that one knows will result in life-altering situations for patients and their family. It is also reflected in nurses' commitment to patient confidentiality, which involves protecting patient personal health information and disclosing it to only those who are approved (patients or legal representatives) or who have a legitimate need to know (other healthcare providers directly involved in patients' care).

Nurses are often faced with ethical decisions in which integrity is specifically important. When nurses are faced with an ethical dilemma, integrity requires that they adhere to ethical guidelines or seek advice from an experienced nurse, a supervisor, a hospital ethics committee, or another person or committee that serves to facilitate ethical decision-making. Using the American Nurses Association code of ethics can serve as a foundation for ethical decision-making. Using these resources ensures that ethical nursing decisions are aligned with the highest standards of care delivery.

Integrity requires a commitment to personal and professional growth based on self-reflection and the desire for continuous improvement. Using self-reflection allows nurses to recognize their limitations, seek feedback from others, and learn from their mistakes. A commitment to self-growth ensures up-to-date nursing knowledge that promotes the delivery of current, high-quality care. This knowledge gives nurses the confidence to advocate for what is right regarding patient safety and practices in order to promote the best outcomes. A commitment to ethical practice, honesty, and personal growth gives nurses with integrity the overall strength and credibility to deliver the best care possible.

Accountability

Accountability is a fundamental aspect of nursing professionalism that involves nurses taking responsibility for their decisions and actions. Nurses must be answerable to patients, colleagues, employers, and all of those in the healthcare system. Nurses must ensure that their decisions are based on sound clinical judgment, evidence-based practice, and ethical considerations. This can be accomplished in nursing by ensuring that decisions adhere to established protocols, standards, and guidelines. Nurses who hold themselves accountable for their actions contribute to a culture of patient safety and the delivery of high-quality care. In this way, errors are reduced, and patient outcomes are optimized in all settings.

No nurse is without errors at some point in their career. Being accountable means that these errors are acknowledged and that steps are taken to reduce the potential for them to be repeated. Accountable nurses do not shy away from admitting when something has not gone as planned and an error has occurred. They take the opportunity as a learning moment, report the issue, and actively participate in efforts to prevent future occurrences. Presenting this attitude of openness fosters a culture of continuous improvement in which errors are situations to learn from rather than a situation for pure punishment. Accountability contributes to the advancement of nursing practice and improvement of patient care delivery.

Empathy

Empathy is the ability to sense the emotions of others vicariously and experience another's feelings, perceptions, and thoughts. Nurses understand people from the individual's frame of reference and not their own. This allows nurses to connect with patients and understand their concerns and fears. Through experiencing empathy, nurses are able to provide comfort and support. Empathy requires the skill of active listening, in which nurses pay close attention to what patients are saying about their concerns and feelings. It helps create an environment in which patients feel that they are understood, valued, and cared for. These feelings can go a long way toward making patients feel safe and perceive that their health care experience was a positive one.

Empathy is important in establishing a trusting patient relationship. It facilitates rapport or a more harmonious relationship between patients and nurses. A genuine display of nurse empathy gives patients a more secure environment in which to share their fears, concerns, and underlying thoughts about their specific situation. Open communication allows for a more effective health history retrieval, which, in turn, allows nurses to develop a more accurate and holistic care plan. This holistic approach addresses the total patient, which includes physical, emotional, and psychological well-being. An empathetic relationship allows nurses to better support their patients and therefore offer them the potential for a more positive health outcome.

Empathy is foundational to nurse emotional resilience. *Resilience* is the ability to positively adapt to difficult and stressful situations, which are often met by nurses in their healthcare setting and can include pain and suffering, traumatic situations, deaths, and the necessity for difficult ethical decisions (Badu et al., 2020; Earvolino-Ramirez, 2007; Han et al., 2023; Kim & Chang, 2022). Exhibiting empathy allows nurses to engage with their patients while maintaining a healthy balance between personal involvement and professional detachment. This does not mean that nurses do not exhibit emotions, but this balance allows them to provide compassionate patient care without getting burned out. *Burnout* is a state of emotional, physical, and mental exhaustion that reduces nurse satisfaction and subsequently patient satisfaction. Reducing the potential for burnout can promote a more positive nursing career. Maintaining a healthy work-life balance also extends to colleagues (Shah et al., 2021). By having a healthy relationship with colleagues, not only can nurses offer peer support, but this relationship can serve to contribute to overall well-being for one's self and the health care team as a whole.

Strategies and Behaviors to Promote Professionalism

Professionalism is a multifaceted concept that is demonstrated through nurse behaviors. It includes a wide range of strategies and behaviors that nurses must consistently demonstrate in their practice to promote professionalism. Nurses can use specific strategies used to ensure that professionalism is relayed to others through **communication skills, teamwork and collaboration**, awareness of **cultural competence**, and promotion of **time management and organization** (Rhodes et al., 2012). These elements enhance nurses' ability to provide quality patient care and contribute to a more supportive and efficient healthcare environment in which they work. Integrating these strategies ensures that patients in their care have the best possible outcomes. Table 1.1 identifies key strategies and behaviors as well as how they are exhibited, their impact on professionalism, and which outcome specifically correlates to the strategy or behavior.

TABLE 1.1 Strategies and Behaviors That Promote Professionalism

Strategy/ Behavior (Name)	How They Are Exhibited and Their Impact on Professionalism	Strategy/Behavior (Outcome)
Communication Skills	• Clear, concise, and respectful communication (a) fosters trust and (b) ensures that information is accurately conveyed. • The communication approach used should meet the needs of diverse patients and clinical situations. • Promote active listening to fully demonstrate understanding of patient concerns for correct actions and response generation. • Prioritization of communication skills reduces misunderstandings and promotes patient satisfaction.	Effective verbal, nonverbal, and written communication
Teamwork and Collaboration	• Work as part of multidisciplinary team to collaborate on care delivery strategies for the best patient outcomes. • Demonstrate mutual respect, shared goals, and open communication among team members. • Actively participating in team huddles and discussions, offering support to colleagues, and being open to feedback for improvement. • Foster a teamwork culture.	Working effectively and efficiently with inter-professional and intra-professional healthcare members and teams
Cultural Competence	• Display understanding and respect for the diverse backgrounds and needs of patients. • Exhibit an awareness of cultural differences that may impact patient care, such as beliefs about health, communication styles, and family dynamics. • Be open-minded, avoid assumptions, and adapt holistic care to meet the unique needs of each individual patient. • Promote inclusivity and equity within the healthcare system.	Understanding and a cultivated respect for individuals from diverse backgrounds
Time Management and Organization	• Demonstrate the ability to prioritize tasks, manage workloads, and allocate time efficiently to meet patient needs, complete documentation, and reduce potential for errors. • Dedicate the time to collaborate with health care colleagues and engage in the delivery of culturally competent patient care. • Facilitate maintaining nurses' work-life balance.	• Ability to balance responsibilities and set priorities in the care environment • Successful promotion of work-life balance

Strategy Integration for a Comprehensive Approach to Professionalism

A comprehensive approach to integrating communication skills, teamwork and collaboration, cultural competence, and time management and organization promotes professionalism in nursing. Each strategy supports the other. Communication enhances teamwork, and cultural competence improves the quality of communication with diverse patient populations (Červený et al., 2022). Having good time management and organizational skills allows nurses to dedicate time necessary not only to strategize with colleagues but also engage in culturally competent patient care delivery. Consistently integrating applicable strategies contributes to a positive and ethical healthcare environment.

Altruism in Nursing Professionalism

Altruism means helping others without the expectation of a direct or an indirect reward. It drives nurses' caring behavior and is the foundation for a choice of a nursing career. Altruism is a fundamental principle in nursing professionalism. It mirrors the essence of nursing where the primary focus of care is on the patient and addressing their specific need with compassion and dedication (Chen et al., 2022). Many individuals identify that their choice of nursing as a career was driven by a genuine desire to make a positive difference in the lives of others.

Patient-centered care is rooted in altruism. When nurses use an altruistic mindset as a basis to approach holistic care delivery, they are better able to address the unique needs and concerns of each patient. Using altruism allows nurses to attentively listen to patient needs, be true patient advocates, and provide comfort and support even during the most challenging times, such as during disasters and pandemics. An altruistic foundation fosters a therapeutic environment in which patients feel understood and, most important of all, valued (Slettmyr et al., 2019).

Difficulties in providing altruistic care can extend to managing difficult patients. In these situations, positive coping measures and a structured intervention such as *BREATHE* may be beneficial. The *BREATHE* pneumonic stands for:

> "(1) **B**ias/assumption you have about this patient; (2) **RE**flect on why you identify this patient as "difficult"; (3) list 1 thing you'd like to Accomplish today; (4) **TH**ink about 1 question you'd like to address today that would enable you to further explore your assumptions;

> and (5) stop before you **E**nter the examination room and take 3 deep breaths, in through your nose and out through your mouth" (Edgoose et al., 2015, p. 15).

In this intervention, the provider is able to use active reflection on biases, an agenda, and context; mindful breathing; and maintain an openness to surprise. Using positive methods can provide an opportunity to maintain and even improve the use of altruistic methods for successful patient-centered nursing interactions.

Altruism shapes professional behavior and ethical practice. It encourages nurses to act with integrity. This commitment is reflected in behaviors such as serving as patient advocates, providing care without prejudice, and maintaining patient confidentiality. Altruism is the driving force for many nurses to expand their knowledge base through continuing education or formal academic programs of study. This allows nurses to better serve their communities.

Altruism Challenges and Sustainability in Nursing Professionalism

Altruism is a powerful nursing motivator, but it is not without its challenges. The nursing perception of altruism has experienced some ambiguity over the past few years. The nursing shortage at times necessitates nurses to be more task-oriented and technical in their attitude toward patient care. This can be in direct conflict to the intent of altruism. Although nursing can be a rewarding career, it can be difficult to maintain altruism throughout the lifespan of the career, which can be long and demanding. Individuals in a nursing career can experience high levels of stress with resulting emotional exhaustion. Altruism can be threatened by the reduction of empathy over time and an increasing rate of nurse burnout. Fostering a supportive and positive work environment and a collegial relationship with one's peers can serve to maintain nursing altruism. Promoting self-care and work-life balance is also critical to sustaining an altruistic spirit in one's professional life. Addressing challenges before they arise allows nurses to remain in the profession and continue to deliver high-quality care to those in need.

Summary

Professionalism in nursing is a multifaceted concept. It is essential to the delivery of high-quality, holistic care delivery. It includes several strategies and behaviors that nurses should consistently demonstrate in various settings.

Fostering a supportive and positive work environment and a collegial relationship with one's peers can serve to maintain nursing altruism. Promoting self-care and work-life balance is also critical to sustaining an altruistic spirit in one's professional life. Integration of these strategies enhances nurses' ability to provide care for patients and address self-care and work-life balance. Integrating positive strategies into one's daily personal life and professional nursing practice allows nurses to uphold the nursing professionalism elements and ensure the best possible patient outcomes in various healthcare settings.

References

Badu, E., O'Brien, A. P., Mitchell, R., Rubin, M., James, C., McNeil, K., Nguyen, K., & Giles, M. (2020). Workplace stress and resilience in the Australian nursing workforce: A comprehensive integrative review. *International Journal of Mental Health Nursing*, *29*(1), 5–34. https://doi.org/10.1111/inm.12662

Cao, H., Song, Y., Wu, Y., Du, Y., He, X., Chen, Y., Wang, Q., & Yang. (2023). What is nursing professionalism? A concept analysis. *BMC Nursing*, *22*, 34. https://doi.org/10.1186/s12912-022-01161-0

Červený, M., Kratochvílová, I., Hellerová, V., & Tóthová, V. (2022). Methods of increasing cultural competence in nurses working in clinical practice: A scoping review of literature 2011-2021. *Frontiers in Psychology*, *13*, 936181. https://doi.org/10.3389/fpsyg.2022.936181

Chen, Y., Xie, C., Zheng, P., & Zeng, Y. (2022). Altruism in nursing from 2012 to 2022: A scoping review. *Frontiers in Psychiatry*, *13*, 1046991. https://doi.org/10.3389/fpsyt.2022.1046991

Cornett, B. S. (2006). A principal calling: Professionalism and health care services. *Journal of Communication Disorders*, *39*(4), 301–309. https://doi.org/10.1016/j.jcomdis.2006.02.005

Earvolino-Ramirez, M. (2007). Resilience: A concept analysis. *Nursing Forum*, *42*(2), 73–82. https://doi.org/10.1111/j.1744-6198.2007.00070.x

Edgoose, J. Y. C., Regner, C. J., & Zakletskaia, L. I. (2015). BREATHE OUT: A randomized controlled trial of a structured intervention to improve clinician satisfaction with "difficult" visits. *Journal of the American Board of Family Medicine*, *28*(1), 13–20. https://doi.org/10.3122/jabfm.2015.01.130323

Han, P., Duan, X., Jiang, J., Zeng, L., Zhang, P., & Zhao, S. (2023). Experience in the development of nurses' personal resilience: A meta-synthesis. *Nursing Open*, *10*(5), 2780–2792. https://doi.org/10.1002/nop2.1556

Hintistan, S., & Topcuoglu, B. (2017). Professionalism characteristics of nurses working in internal medicine clinics continuing education. *Universal Journal of Public Health*, *5*(1), 46–53.

Kim, E. Y., & Chang, S. O. (2022). Exploring nurse perceptions and experiences of resilience: A meta-synthesis study. *BMC Nursing*, *21*, 26. https://doi.org/10.1186/s12912-021-00803-z

Rhodes, M. K., Schutt, M. S., Langham, G. W., & Bilotta, D. E. (2012). The journey to nursing professionalism: A learner-centered approach. *Nursing Education Perspectives*, *33*(1), 27–29.

Shah, M. K., Gandrakota, N., Cimiotti, J. P., Ghose, N., Moore, M., & Ali, M. K. (2021). Prevalence of and factors associated with nurse burnout in the US. *JAMA Network Open*, *4*(2), e2036469. https://doi.org/10.1001/jamanetworkopen.2020.36469

Slettmyr, A., Schandl, A., & Arman, M. (2019). The ambiguity of altruism in nursing: A qualitative study. *Nursing Ethics*, *26*(2), 368–377. https://doi.org/10.1177/0969733017709336

Zaitoun, R. A., Said, N. B., & de Tantillo, L. (2023). Clinical nurse competence and its effect on patient safety culture: A systematic review. *BMC Nursing*, *22*, 173. https://doi.org/10.1186/s12912-023-01305-w

CHAPTER 2

Nursing's History

The Road Traveled

Marcia A. Pugh, DNP, MBA, HCM, RN

Objectives

Upon completion of this chapter, the learner will be able to do the following:

1. Trace nursing's development from its roots to establishment as a profession.
2. Describe the contributions of influential figures who served to shape nursing.
3. Analyze how major historical events, such as wars, pandemics, and social movements, influenced the evolution of nursing roles and responsibilities.
4. Explore how the history of nursing influences current nursing practice.

Key Chapter Terms

- Florence Nightingale
- Hannah Anderson Ropes
- Dorothea Lynde Dix
- Susie King Taylor
- Mary Ann Bickerdyke
- Clarissa Harlowe Barton
- Linda Anne Judson Richards
- Mary Eliza Mahoney
- Isabel Adams Hampton Robb
- Lavinia Lloyd Dock
- Mary Adelaide Nutting
- Anne Warburton Goodrich
- Lillian Wald
- Mary Breckinridge
- Margaret Sanger
- Licensure

Care: The Beginning Focus

Nursing care was provided by individuals in society long before nursing was identified as an occupation and subsequent profession. The first known documents that mention nursing were written in approximately 300 A.D., relating to the Roman Empire. In medieval times, men provided care for the ill as part of their daily-life activities. During the Victorian era, care was provided by female paupers from workhouses. Women were the primary care providers for the injured and ill in the early Americas. In 1873, formal teaching and learning were implemented based on the British model of education. There was no conceptual base for nursing education, so foundationally, this education was managed by administrators and medical entities. Nursing has evolved through the centuries to focus on evidence that supports its specific patient care activities. This chapter will take you through nursing's evolution and introduce you to key individuals in its progression from occupation to profession.

Before nurses evolved to establish a formal structure for helping the sick, illness and suffering were a part of everyday life. Since the beginning of time, there have been afflictions and illnesses. Those with the misfortune to experience such were cared for by family. With the nuclear and extended family all under the same roof, there was no lack of available hands. This, however, did not guarantee health. With thatched roof houses, water from any source available, lack of indoor plumbing and refrigeration, and all manner of insects and animals ever present in the home, illness was a norm. Treatment sometimes meant a concoction of herbs and animal entrails. Caring for the sick only meant palliative care until the person succumbed to their illness or "miraculously" returned to health.

A History of Tending the Sick

The nursing profession is linked to **Florence Nightingale**. But long before Nightingale, there were people who tended the sick. During the Crusades, those who cared for the wounded and ill were called *hospitallers* (Gandet, 1907). These individuals performed this work not only out of duty but also out of personal preference. During the Middle Ages, nursing care activities were provided by male-dominated religious, military, and secular orders. The Knights of Saint John was one such religious order who performed these activities. One predominant principle of this order was devotion to duty in care for the sick. This became a standard in nursing across the ages and continues to be a standard in nursing today.

Many Catholic orders cared for the sick in the Middle Ages. These individuals did so using information passed down from person to person through apprenticeships. These caring and humane activities lacked hygienic measures and were administered under primitive conditions. Institutional primordial provisions, coupled with overcrowding, also made it necessary to go into the communities to care for the sick.

During the Reformation, Catholic support for the monasteries and institutions designed to care for the sick severely waned, thus allowing abolition by the Protestants. Many Catholic hospitals of the time were replaced by workhouses and almshouses. These were aimed primarily at the poor and destitute. Care in these new institutions was provided by pardoned criminals, alcoholics, and older prostitutes. Nurses in these times were depicted by Charles Dickens in the portrayal of his character Sairey Gamp. This "nurse" was more concerned with her own comforts than those of her patients. This was an attitude distinctly different from prior care providers.

The Reformation brought a new wave of thinkers and philosophers. These individuals began to view values and ideals from a different perspective. The evolution of nursing took on a new dimension with the onset of the Industrial Revolution, when capitalism, individualism, and freedom of thought formed the foundation for a more democratic view of government. This view took several years to evolve an accepting attitude, in which women worked outside the home. It was also unthinkable that women from upstanding families worked to tend the sick and dying. This was the era into which Florence Nightingale was born.

Florence Nightingale

Nightingale was the second daughter born to an upstanding aristocratic family in Victorian England in 1820. She had a carefree life and was well educated in languages that includes Latin, German, French, and Greek as well as mathematics, science, and politics, to name a few. These laid the foundation for her future innovations in nursing.

While Nightingale was young, she often visited the sick as part of her aristocratic custom. This work suited her and gave her a sense of purpose. When Nightingale was age 30 years (Figure 2.1), she entered a training program for nurses in Kaiserworth, Germany. This three-year program preceded her continued training in Paris under the Sisters of Charity. By the age 33, Nightingale had become superintendent of an "Establishment for gentle women during illness" (Garofalo & Fee, 2010).

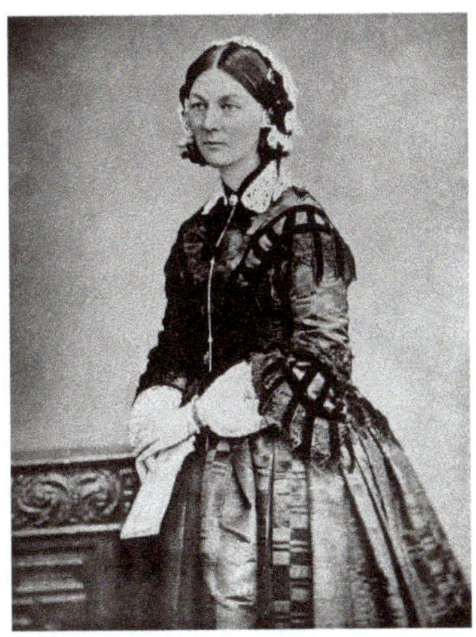

FIGURE 2.1 Florence Nightingale (1820–1910)

The Crimean War paved the way for Nightingale to exhibit the exceptional administrative and organizational abilities that she learned as a child. Responding to an appeal by the minister of war, Nightingale and several nurses went to care for British soldiers injured in the war effort. When she arrived at the Scutari Barracks Hospital, the conditions were unbelievably horrible. The 1,500-patient facility had soldiers crowded into dirty, poorly ventilated wards. The area was filled with filth and vermin. Poorly cooked food was served to the sick and injured at irregularly long intervals. Soldiers were covered with dirt, and some lay on straw floor mats. Many were still in their uniforms stained with their own blood. Death in this facility occurred not related to battlefield injuries but rather due to cholera and disease.

Upon seeing these horrible conditions, Nightingale set about making life better for these sick and wounded soldiers. Despite military officer opposition, she achieved order in the healthcare facilities. She established care based on cleanliness requirements for patients and their surroundings and managed to achieve total reorganization of these facilities. This development resulted from statistical information she retrieved and analyzed. She kept detailed data on Scutari soldier morbidity and mortality during the Crimean War. Nightingale monitored and gathered data through nightly rounds in the dark halls and rooms of soldiers in the facility. She was thus known as "Lady with the Lamp" (Stanley, 2007) These analyses served to change not only military perspectives but also those of society regarding care of the sick. These analyses resulted in the idea that sick and wounded soldiers had the right to adequate nutrition, suitable living quarters, and appropriate health care. These interventions, built on evidence-based results, achieved a significant reduction in mortality from 43% to 2% during the Crimean War. Nightingale established a correlation between environmental conditions and health status (Johnson & Webber, 2009).

From the war years, Nightingale moved toward working to improve the education of nurses. In 1860, the Nightingale School and Home for Nurses, established at St. Thomas' Hospital, improved public perception and promoted discipline in nursing. Due to her own illness, Nightingale was unable to take an administrative position in the school. Despite this, she was involved and offered advice based on her Crimean War experience. In 1860, she published *Notes on Nursing: What It Is and What It Is Not*. In this document, she called nursing an art that encompassed activities that promoted good health and healing activities. Nightingale stated that education was imperative to promote the nursing profession. She was a proficient writer and author during her lifetime. She was the keystone for mastering a body of knowledge specific to nursing.

The Influence of War on Nursing in America

Women of War Who Nurse the Sick

War has been an important impetus for nursing. Just as it was foundational to nursing in England, war served to promote nursing in America. The Civil War served as the stimulus for nursing's foundation in America. During the Civil War, there were many wounded on both sides of the fighting. Union and Confederate soldiers suffered as a result of poor sanitation and improper nutrition and care activities. Approximately 2,000 women served as volunteer nurses in North and South military hospitals during the American Civil War. These women served under some of the most horrific circumstances and rendered aid to mutilated and dying men. These women served with little recognition for the work they did in helping men toward recovery or death.

Hannah Anderson Ropes (1809–1863)

Hannah Anderson Ropes was born in New Gloucester, Maine, in 1809 to a prominent attorney family. Her personal convictions were developed in childhood. She was strongly opposed to slavery. During the prewar era, she gained recognition as a reformer and abolitionist. It was only after the loss of her husband's support (he moved and left the family) and when she was left to raise two small children that she became increasingly active in the abolitionist movement and westward expansion. Ropes nursed sick family and friends, as many women did during that time. It was at this time in her life that she was deeply affected by a copy of Nightingale's *Notes on Nursing*, given to her by a family member. As a result, she volunteered to serve as a nurse when her son served in the Civil War. In 1862, Ropes worked in a Union hospital (Ropes, 1993). Conditions were appalling and extended beyond a lack of sanitation; they also included cruel treatment by those in charge of the care for the soldiers. She worked to provide good food and a clean environment and displayed a true sense of caring for the wounded. When Ropes witnessed soldier mistreatment by those in charge of providing their care (the steward and chief surgeon), she reported these behaviors directly to the secretary of war, which resulted in an official inspection of the conditions at the facility and the arrest of these two individuals, resulting in a change of administrators. Her efforts brought about remarkable changes for a woman in a male-dominated military environment. She was soon made head matron of the Union Hotel Hospital in Georgetown, a neighborhood outside Washington, D.C. With her prior contacts secured, in her roles of reformer and abolitionist, Ropes was able to secure supplies and care necessities for wounded soldiers. This allowed her to put sanitation components pioneered by Nightingale into place. She worked to put her beliefs related to healthy surroundings, good food, and humanitarian treatment into nursing practice. Her concerns over the brutally indifferent treatment of soldiers caused her to ruthlessly battle the system on their behalf. Like so many of the soldiers she cared for, she succumbed to typhoid pneumonia at age 54.

Dorothea Lynde Dix (1802–1887)

Dorothea Lynde Dix was a champion for the mentally ill and those in prisons. She initiated her work in Massachusetts after observing the ill treatment and extremely poor conditions of those in healthcare facilities and prisons. This was her life's work for more than 20 years. During this time, she campaigned from state to state, addressing state legislators to effect positive change. Dix went from institution to institution, systematically observing and documenting her findings. She was so successful in her ability to initiate change that she was appointed superintendent of the female nurses of the Army by the secretary of war. Although she had no formal nursing training, she was able to recruit more than 2,000 women to serve in the Union Army during the Civil War (American Nurses Association [ANA], 2011; Backus, 2021). In this position, Dix was in charge of all the female nurses working in army hospitals. She served in this position throughout the entire war period without compensation for any of her work. Her recruitment efforts of other women worked to verify that women could work effectively in these settings. She was the first to implement a dress code in order to give female nurses more credibility among the ranks of the military men. Dix labored to improve the welfare of nurses and patients alike, not only recruiting female nurses but also often soliciting resources from private sources when these were not supplied by the government. Following completion of her duty in the military, she returned to continue working with the mentally ill and promote a better lifestyle for these individuals (Norwood, 2017).

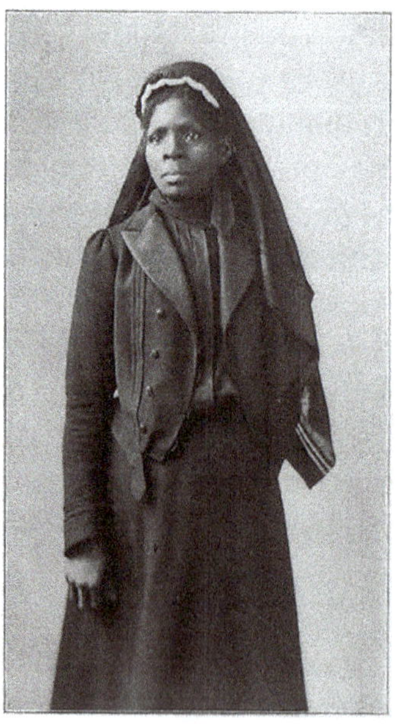

FIGURE 2.2 Susie Taylor King, First African American Army Nurse

Susie King Taylor (1848–1912)

Susie King Taylor was born a slave in the state of Georgia. She had a very different experience as a child and was a slave of the Grest family. Despite her slave status, she was treated affectionately by the plantation owner's wife, who set the standard for how King judged potential relationships between Blacks and Whites.

As a slave, she was not allowed to obtain an education. It was only after she visited her freed grandmother that her education began. During the war efforts, the family was moved in an attempt to secure safety. It was at this time that she met and married her husband. When she was living in Port Royal Island, off the South Carolina coast, her husband joined an all-Black unit, and she moved with him as the unit traveled about the area fighting. She served as nurse and caretaker, also teaching many men to read and write during this time. In 1863, King began to nurse the wounded as they returned, battle-weary and injured. She worked with Clara Barton when caring for Black soldiers in South Carolina. She volunteered for more than three years in this capacity, despite the fact that she had no formal medical training. After the war ended in 1865, she focused her teaching efforts on children. She worked in education until the 1870s, at which time she remarried and continued her nursing efforts by joining and later becoming president of the Women's Relief Corps. King worked for the organization until her death.

Mary Ann Bickerdyke (1817–1901)

Mary Ann Bickerdyke had a relatively uneventful lifestyle until age 43. After the loss of an infant daughter, she started reading books on medicine in an effort to learn about health. In a sermon, she heard how Union soldiers received poor medical care and became determined to work to improve this situation. She initiated a drive to collect medical supplies in her hometown and personally delivered these to the nearest Union base in Illinois. Upon seeing the terrible conditions of the camp's medical clinic, Bickerdyke stayed and started washing bedding and clothes, cooking, and cleaning soldiers' wounds. She enlisted a small group of volunteer women to help her continue this work. She later moved from the hospital to the front line, where she insisted on working alongside the medical staff. For her work, she was hired in an official capacity by the U.S. Sanitary Commission until it was disbanded at the war's conclusion. After that ended, Bickerdyke continued to work with recuperating soldiers. Her work extended to promoting services for Union veterans. She worked to get compensation that had been earned but never paid, along with pensions. For her work with the Union army, she is remembered as "Mother" by her grateful patients (Sartin, 2003).

Clara Barton (1821–1912)

Clarissa Harlowe Barton—or Clara, she wished to be called—did not start out working with the sick. This evolved as a result of an initiative she began in Massachusetts. While working in the U.S. Patent Office, she witnessed soldiers returning from war. As new recruits, these returning soldiers often had nothing more than the clothes on their backs. Their disheveled appearances and poor medical care on the battlefield meant that some were disfigured, and their appearance confused and frightened the townspeople. Barton recognized that something needed to be done and organized a relief effort for these men. Her independent campaign carried her into the battlefield, where she set up a makeshift hospital to care for sick and dying soldiers. From this work, she became known as the "Angel of the Battlefield" (Strickler, 2018). Due to the success of her soldier relief efforts, she was granted permission to travel with army ambulances to comfort the sick and wounded while nursing them. Barton continued this work for three years, becoming nationally known for her caring work with casualties from the Battle of the Wilderness and Bermuda Hundred. During this time, she wrote to families and informed them about their relatives in the field. Her work behind the lines prompted an appointment by President Abraham Lincoln to locate men listed as missing and, once she had obtained information, notify families of the disposition of their loved ones. She established the Office of Correspondence with Friends of the Missing Men of the U.S. Army, which she operated for four years. Barton was instrumental in answering more than 63,000 letters and identifying more than 22,000 missing men (American Red Cross, n.d.). In 1881, this work culminated in the establishment of the Red Cross. Today, locating missing loved ones and family reunifications or notifications has become a valuable service by the organization. The Red Cross was the fruit of all the efforts Barton made over her lifetime. She worked with the Red Cross until she resigned in 1904.

Other Women in U.S. Nursing

Linda Anne Judson Richards (1841–1930)

Linda Anne Judson Richards began her career as a schoolteacher, and after 10 years, she began working as a nurse at Boston Hospital in 1870. In 1872, she began training at the New England Hospital for Women and Children and was the program's first graduate. This program was run by female physicians who based their one-year program on Nightingale's principles. After graduation, she worked as night-shift supervisor at Bellevue Hospital in New York City. In 1874, she returned to Boston and was named superintendent of the Boston Training School. Due to her astute managerial skills, she was able to increase respect for the program, as it eventually became recognized as one of the best in the country. Richards traveled to England to work in an intensive nursing program of study. She studied at St. Thomas' Hospital in London. She was able to work with Nightingale, who recommended that she continue her studies at King's College Hospital and the Edinburgh Royal Infirmary in Scotland. Upon Richards' return to the states in 1878, she used her learned skills and expertise to assist in the organization of the Boston

City Hospital training program. She was subsequently named matron of the hospital and superintendent of the school. Richards worked in these positions until 1885. Later in this same year, she traveled to Japan to establish the first nurse training program there. She remained in Japan for five years to supervise the school at Doshisha Hospital Kyoto. She subsequently returned to the United States, where she worked in nursing for an additional 20 years. During this time, Richards established and directed nurse-training programs in Philadelphia, Massachusetts, and Michigan. Through her efforts, nursing programs progressed to an international level (American Association for the History of Nursing, n.d.b.; Holder, 2004).

Mary Eliza Mahoney (1845–1926)

Mary Eliza Mahoney was the first African American registered nurse (RN) in the United States (Kays, 2022). Her interest in nursing started in her teen years as a free individual (a person not born into slavery). She worked for 15 years performing domestic duties and serving as an unofficial nurse's assistant at the New England Hospital for Women and Children in Massachusetts. At age 33, she made a conscious decision to enroll in a very difficult nursing program of the time. Nursing classes were challenging, and the programs were rigorous. In her class of approximately 40 students, only four completed the program—Mahoney was the only African American (Prieto, 2022). Following graduation, she registered with the Nurses Directory in Boston and worked primarily as a private duty nurse. During her 30 professional years, she worked in states along the Eastern Seaboard of the United States and ended her maiden (never married) nursing career working for 10 years as director of the Howard Orphan Asylum for Black Children in New York City. In 1896, Mahoney was one of the original members of the predominantly White Nurses Associated Alumnae of the U.S. organization, which later became known as the ANA (ANA, 2018). She was co-founder of the National Association of Colored Graduate Nurses in 1908, which was later dissolved.

Isabel Adams Hampton Robb (1860–1910)

Isabel Adams Hampton Robb received her training at the Bellevue Hospital Training School. Upon her graduation in 1883, she moved to Rome and worked at St. Paul's House, a small hospital for English and American travelers. Following this time, she returned to the United States and was appointed superintendent of nurses at the Illinois Training School for Nurses at Chicago's Cook County Hospital. In this post, she was extremely instrumental in changing the training curricula for nurses. She abolished the practice of private-duty nursing as a clinical experience, affiliated with other hospitals to broaden nurses' experience, and developed the first grading policy in a school of nursing. In 1889, she became head of the newly established Johns Hopkins Hospital in Baltimore. Robb served in an administrator capacity and as an instructor for students and wrote a textbook. After a life change (she married), she moved to Cleveland and worked at Case Western Reserve University as a professor of gynecology. She continued to implement innovative ideas related to teaching and learning for nurses. She prompted the development of a hospital economics course, which served as a foundation for nursing. She was a founding member of the International Council of Nurses and a member of the founding committee for the American Journal of Nursing (American Association for the History of Nursing, n.d.a.; Sy, 2023).

Lavinia Lloyd Dock (1858–1956)

Lavinia Lloyd Dock was from a middle-class family and received a proper education in art, music, literature, and language. She saw her mother die at a young age and her father grow ill and no longer be able to support the family in keeping with its prior financial status. In the late 1870s, there was a strong belief that women of her life's station were to be wives and mothers. Throwing convention aside, she looked to nursing as a means of financial security after reading an article regarding a new profession for women in 1882. Dock decided to attend nursing school, even though this was not considered a job for proper young women. She graduated from Bellevue Training School for Nurses in 1886. Shortly after her graduation, she worked to begin a visiting nurse service in New York City. In 1887, Dock took a position as the first visiting nurse for a pioneer social organization called the United Workers of Norwich in Connecticut. After being asked to assist with the yellow fever outbreak in Florida by a classmate, she moved to Jacksonville, Florida, in 1888. She eagerly assumed responsibility for taking care of the sick and later returned home after two months. Upon her return, she was appointed as night superintendent at Bellevue. Even in this position, she continued volunteer relief efforts. During this time, Dock authored a textbook called *Materia Medica for Nurses* to promote an understanding of compounds used for medicines. She also authored a textbook on hygiene and morality, co-authored the first two volumes, and independently authored the remaining two volumes on the history of nursing. Dock also served as foreign editor of the *American Journal of Nursing*. In 1890, Dock worked with Lillian Wald at Henry Street Settlement in New York City. She realized that the settlement permitted her to use her abilities to their fullest. During the 1890s, she was a member of a group of women at the settlement who focused their efforts on improved education, promotion of nursing organizations, and the creation of a professional journal. This group included Isabel Robb, Adelaide Nutting, and Sophia Palmer. They used the *American Journal of Nursing* to provide education and information about women's health issues, such as venereal disease. She was a contributing editor between 1900 and 1923. This journal heightened awareness of women's issues to promote health and wellness. In 1896, Dock worked with Ethel Gordon Fenwick and founded the International Council of Nurses, serving as its secretary from 1900 to 1922. Dock was an advocate for women's rights.

Mary Adelaide Nutting (1858–1948)

Mary Adelaide Nutting was born in Canada but entered nursing school in 1889 after reading a newspaper article announcing the opening of the new Johns Hopkins Training School in Baltimore. Following her graduation in 1891, she remained at Johns Hopkins as head nurse and was later moved into the position of assistant superintendent of nurses. During that time in nursing's growth and evolution, education was financially supported by hospitals, which used student nurses as cheap labor. This type of educational arrangement did not promote learning as a priority. Students could spend in excess of 60 hours a week working, leaving little time for studying and other educational endeavors. Nutting promoted moving nursing education to universities (Govan, 2022). Using this philosophy, she limited the number of hours that students could perform bedside work in the hospital. In 1907, Nutting accepted employment at Teachers College, Columbia University, and was later appointed as chair of the new Department of Nursing Education. She was the first nurse in the country to be appointed to a university professorship. Her most significant contribution to nursing literature was the first two volumes of *The History of Nursing* that she co-authored with Lavinia Dock. Nutting was a strong supporter of university-based nursing education and contributed many written works, which served to bring focus to nursing education.

Annie Warburton Goodrich (1866–1954)

Annie Warburton Goodrich was born into a family of comfortable means. Due to her family's financial status, she was able to engage in foreign travel and have private tutors for her education (Daisy, 1991). Her first introduction to nursing was to see her sisters and then later her grandparents receiving care from a compassionate, knowledgeable nurse. The illness of her father saw the family financial situation take a turn downward. In an effort to become self-sufficient, she entered nursing school. She obtained her nursing education at New York Hospital. Goodrich completed her education and entered the profession as a registered nurse in 1892. Following this education, she obtained a position as head nurse at New York Hospital. She held nurse supervisory positions at Post-Graduate Hospital, St. Luke's Hospital,

Bellevue Hospital, Allied Hospital, and Visiting Nurse Service of Henry Street Settlement. She taught in the Department of Nursing and Health at Teachers College in Columbia University. She served for nine years (1914–1923) as a training school inspector for the New York State Department of Education. Goodrich started the United States Student Nurse Research, now known as the Army School of Nursing. In 1923, she became the first dean of the Yale University School of Nursing (Cedar Hill Foundation, n.d.; Schiff, 2011). In her lifetime, Goodrich received three honorary degrees. In 1921, she received an honorary degree from Mount Holyoke College (Doctor of Science); in 1923, she received an honorary degree from Yale University (Master of Arts); and in 1936, she received an honorary degree from Russell Sage College (Doctor of Laws). Goodrich also served in several professional organizations. She served a one-year term as president of the American Society of Superintendents of Training Schools for Nurses (1905–1906). She was president of both the International Council of Nurses (1912–1915) and the ANA (1916–1918). She served as the first president of the Association of Collegiate Schools of Nursing. Goodrich's achievements made a significant impact on the nursing profession.

Lillian Wald (1867–1940)

Lillian Wald was born at a time when city sanitation either was minimal or did not exist. As a result, infectious diseases were common. They affected all individuals, regardless of their social standing in the community. It was soon recognized that diseases did not just affect poor areas, but rather the plight of all citizens was linked, regardless of their financial standing. Communities attempted to address these conditions by hiring trained nurses for home care. Many organizations took up the charge to promote a healthier society. This was the society in which Wald lived and worked.

Wald's interest in nursing stemmed from a family crisis—the illness of her sister, who was tended by a private-duty nurse. Following her primary training at the New York Hospital Training School for Nurses, she went to work in a juvenile asylum. She left this position disheartened that nurses had so little influence on the institutional care of these children. This led her to working on the lower East Side of New York based on an identified need for immigrant education in home nursing. An 1893 life experience changed everything for Wald when she visited the home of one of her students in an effort to render care. Her walk "through 'evil' smelling streets, past open courtyard 'closets', up slimy steps of the rear tenement, and finally to the sick room" left her painfully aware of the significant need for reform (Buhler-Wilkerson, 1993, p. 1779). Following this incident, Wald and a fellow schoolmate moved to the neighborhood to work as nurses. Her continued work and solicitation of support allowed her to purchase a house on Henry Street. From this area, she worked to address societal needs that evidenced themselves in disease, poverty, and overcrowding. She pushed for reform from the perspective of health reform and an agenda that included industry, education, recreation, and housing. In 1895, Wald moved into a residence that was to become the Henry Street Nurses' Settlement (Fee & Bu, 2010). She started the settlement out of a community need for health care and educational, recreational, and family activities for children and families. By 1910, staff nurses of the settlement were working to address issues associated with public health, including but not limited to (a) a milk station; (b) a convalescent home; (c) country homes; (d) first-aid stations; (e) a maternity service and mother-baby health conferences; (f) home visits; (g) several social programs, one of which was a kindergarten; (h) skill classes, which included sewing, carpentry, art, music, and dance; (i) boys' and girls' clubs; and (j) a drama club. This demonstrated Wald's move toward social and health reform (Ruel, 2014).

Wald's nursing career is marked by two other innovative initiatives. The next included insurance coverage for home-based nursing care. She was convinced that home nursing was cost-effective and would improve the health of individuals and reduce deaths. This could be beneficial to insurance companies. Following a three-month pilot test by the Metropolitan Life insurance company, the program proved to verify this expectation. This relationship proved beneficial to the company and the visiting nurses' association, which received financial support as part of this endeavor. This was the first established national system of insurance coverage for home-based care. Another innovative initiative included the creation of a National Public Health Service. This was called the American Red Cross Public Health Nursing Service. Through this service, standardized public health nursing appeared in small townships across the country. This service kept communities engaged in care with nursing support.

Mary Breckinridge (1881–1965)

Mary Breckinridge came from a prominent family with international influence. Her immediate family included a grandfather who was vice president of the United States and her father, who was a U.S. ambassador to Russia. Her tutored education allowed her to travel with her family, which exposed her to various cultures and lifestyles. Following the abrupt death of her beloved husband, Breckinridge entered St. Luke's School of Nursing. She remarried and taught French and hygiene prior to becoming a mother to a son and daughter. She lost her second child, a daughter, who was born prematurely. A few years later, she lost her first son to appendicitis. Following the death of both children, she and her husband divorced. From these tragedies, her life in nursing began. She used nursing as a means of comfort and strength during this time of personal chaos. Breckinridge joined the American Committee for Devastated France after World War I. Following an introduction to nurse-midwives in France and Great Britain, she studied midwifery in an effort to bring this care to mothers and babies in America. During this time, women in U.S. rural areas had no access to health care and suffered a high maternal mortality rate. This is where Breckinridge decided to focus her efforts. She established the Frontier Nursing Service (FNS) in 1925 to provide health care to the poor residents of the Appalachian Mountains and eastern Kentucky (Fugate, 2023). These nurses traveled on foot and horseback to care for individuals who lived in these remote areas. She focused her efforts on mothers and on children up until age 1 year, but care was extended to anyone seeking it. Money or goods were accepted as payment for individual services. Through speaking engagements and personal connections, she was able to raise millions of dollars to fund the FNS. Through her efforts, both maternal and infant mortality rates dramatically decreased. The FNS staff started the American Association of Nurse-Midwives, which laid the groundwork for the American College of Nurse-Midwives (ACNM) (Castlenova, 2020). Breckinridge was a pioneer for midwifery and rural health care, and she changed the lives of thousands (Carter, 2018).

Margaret Sanger (1879–1966)

Margaret Sanger was one of 11 surviving children in a Catholic family. Her mother had numerous pregnancies, with some ending in miscarriages. Sanger believed that this was the reason her mother was in poor health and that these events were instrumental in her death. Seeking a reprieve from the life of poverty in which she grew up, Sanger attended school and moved on to study nursing during her educational endeavors. She married and moved to New York City, where she became involved in politics and union activities. She worked as a nurse on New York's Lower East Side, which was a predominantly poor immigrant neighborhood. While promoting help for the sick, she saw many women who had undergone abortions by individuals who were ill-educated or poorly equipped to perform these procedures as well as women who had tried to self-terminate their pregnancies. These situations resulted in significant suffering and disfigurement. In an effort to get health information to individuals who desperately needed it, Sanger started a monthly feminist publication called *The Women Rebel*, which was mailed to constituents. At that time, it was illegal to forward information of this nature through the mail, as it was considered constituting "obscene and immoral materials," according to the Comstock law. Sanger fled the country rather than face a five-year prison term for this action. She went to England, where she continued her work for women's birth control (a term she coined) rights. In England, she was able to research other forms of birth control, which she smuggled back into the United States in 1915 upon her return, following the dissolution of charges against her. She continued her work in the United States by touring to promote birth control and opened the country's first birth control clinic. Sanger was arrested nine days following the opening of the clinic, which resulted in her serving 30 days in jail. After appealing her conviction, the law was amended to permit doctors to prescribe contraception to their female patients for medical reasons. In 1921, Sanger established the American Birth Control League, the precursor to Planned Parenthood. She immersed herself in women's rights and worked to make it legal for doctors to freely distribute birth control by starting the National Committee on Federal Legislation for Birth Control. A significant victory occurred in 1936, when import permission was given by the U.S. Court of Appeals for birth control devices and related materials to be brought into the United States. Sanger was instrumental in establishing the International Planned Parenthood Federation in 1952 (Biography.com Editors, 2024). She was the impetus for research that resulted in the approval of the first oral contraceptive approved by the U.S. Food and Drug Administration (FDA) in 1960. During Sanger's lifetime, birth control was made legal by the Supreme Court for married couples in 1965, which stemmed from the legal case of *Griswold v. Connecticut*. These were huge milestones for women's rights.

A Move Toward Licensure

Nursing's evolution paralleled that of other professions. Prior to Nightingale's era, no credentials were available for individuals who called themselves nurses. Certificates of completion were the first credentials given to nurses early in nursing's professional development. Nursing programs varied in length, and some were as short as six weeks, while others extended to three years. Some programs had little true education classes, consisting mainly of apprenticeship-type work. This was an issue that nurse leaders addressed in 1893 in a meeting at the Columbian Exposition in Chicago. The ANA evolved in 1896 from this work. A formal directive to address this issue came from the ANA, when the association proposed permissive **licensure** for nurses. This concept did not require that all nurses be licensed but did regulate the use of the title *registered nurse*. Only nurses who met the standards for permissive license requirements determined by the state could use this title. It did not restrict the use of the word *nurse*. Anyone could and still can call themselves a nurse.

TABLE 2.1 Women in Nursing

Women in Nursing	Lifespan	Contributions
Florence Nightingale, "Lady with the Lamp"	1820–1910	She worked to improve the care of soldiers during the Crimean War and laid the foundation for mastering a body of knowledge specific to nursing through her publication *Notes on Nursing: What It Is and What It Is Not.*
Hannah Anderson Ropes	1809–1863	From her political activity and connections during the abolitionist movement, she was able to get changes made to improve sanitation and the appalling conditions in field hospitals for soldiers.
Dorothea Lynde Dix, 1976 ANA Hall of Fame Inductee	1802–1887	She was a champion for the mentally ill and those in prison. She traveled from state to state, working in jails and almshouses, making organized notes, and petitioning the state legislatures throughout the United States to improve conditions. She was able to successfully get laws and funding imposed to ameliorate living conditions. She also implemented the first nursing dress code.
Susie King Taylor	1848–1912	Born a slave, she traveled with her husband's all-Black army unit, caring for the wounded and teaching them to read and write. She became president of the Woman's Relief Corps.
Mary Ann Bickerdyke, "Mother to the Boys in Blue"	1817–1901	She enlisted volunteers to provide needed services, such as washing, cooking, and wound care, to soldiers. She provided care alongside the medical care in both the field hospitals and at the front line during a time when women were not allowed in all-male war camps.
Clara Barton, "Angel of the Battlefield"	1821–1912	Her organizational efforts locating and documenting the disposition of soldiers in battle became known as the American Red Cross.
Linda Anne Judson Richards, 1976 ANA Hall of Fame Inductee	1841–1930	She was the first graduate of the New England Hospital for Women and Children nursing program. She was instrumental in setting up a nurse training school at Boston City Hospital. She also set up the first patient record system.
Mary Eliza Mahoney, 1976 ANA Hall of Fame Inductee	1845–1926	She was the first Black woman to hold a nursing position in the United States. Her excellent work in providing nursing care paved the way for other Black nurses to obtain a nursing education. She was co-founder and a lifetime member of the NACGN.
Isabel Adams Hampton Robb, 1976 ANA Hall of Fame Inductee	1860–1910	She was an organizing member of the International Congress of Nurses in 1899 and a member of the founding committee for the *American Journal of Nursing.*

Women in Nursing	Lifespan	Contributions
Lavinia Lloyd Dock	1858–1956	She wrote one of the first nursing textbooks. She was a noted author and made significant contributions to nursing literature. She served as foreign editor of the *American Journal of Nursing*.
Mary Adelaide Nutting, 1976 ANA Hall of Fame Inductee	1858–1948	She made significant contributions to nursing through her advocacy of university-based nursing education. She was the first nurse to be appointed to a university professorship.
Annie Warburton Goodrich, 1976 ANA Hall of Fame Inductee	1866–1954	She developed Yale University's first nursing program, later becoming its dean. This program later became the Yale Graduate School of Nursing.
Lillian Wald, ANA Hall of Fame Inductee	1867–1940	She worked and solicited support to provide home nursing care and addressed societal needs. These public health efforts led to the establishment of the National Public Health Service. This was later called the American Red Cross Public Health Service.
Mary Breckinridge, 1982 ANA Hall of Fame Inductee	1881–1965	She was a pioneer for midwifery and rural health care. She established the Frontier Nursing Service (FNS) in 1925, which laid the groundwork for the American College of Nurse Midwives (ACNM).
Margaret Sanger, 1976 ANA Hall of Fame Inductee	1879–1966	She fought for women's right to birth control in the United States and abroad. She opened the first U.S. birth control clinic. She established the American Birth Control League, the precursor to Planned Parenthood. Instrumental in establishing the International Planned Parenthood Federation in 1952, she was the impetus for research that afforded approval for the first oral contraceptive by the Food and Drug Administration (FDA) in 1960.

Source: ANA, n.d.

During the early 1900s, nursing practice individual identification was merely a list of individuals who had been trained to carry out nursing activities. In 1903, North Carolina was the first state to enact permissive license legislation. This was on the heels of the 1900 initial release of the *American Journal of Nursing*, which merged the efforts of nurse leaders Lavinia Dock, Mary Davis, Mary Adelaide Nutting, Sophia Palmer, and Isabel Hampton Robb. This further served to identify credibility to nursing. By 1923, some 20 years later, all remaining states had permissive licensing for RNs. This was just a first step. Nurse leaders desired to take permissive licensing a step further by requiring mandatory licensure. This would further protect citizens by clearly identifying individuals who had successfully completed the strenuous program of study and met state requirements for licensure. The first mandatory licensure legislation was enacted in 1947 in the state of New

York. This landmark action legally protected use of the term *registered nurse*. The National League for Nursing assumed responsibility for administering the initial nationwide State Board Test Pool Examination in 1950 to validate individual proficiency and knowledge of RNs. Today, all states and territories require licensure for anyone who practices as an RN.

Summary

Throughout the course of wars—the Civil War, the Spanish-American War, and World War I—nurses played a major role in caring for the sick, injured, and dying. They cared for soldiers and the many afflicted by disease, such as the influenza epidemic in 1917. These women have been of White and African American heritage. Many of these women crossed historical paths. Their years of service have overlapped, demonstrating the many changes occurring in the evolution of nursing during these years. There were no men reportedly directly involved in the evolution of nursing, but they served to support many of these women through contributions and appointments to various offices. This acknowledgement allowed them to earn recognition, which further served to promote nursing. These nurses were but a few of the many who served to foster nursing and lay the groundwork for all levels of today's nurses. They worked in broad areas of nursing and rendered aid to those in need.

References

American Association for the History of Nursing. (n.d.a.). *Isabel Adams Hampton Robb 1860–1910*. https://www.aahn.org/robb

American Association for the History of Nursing. (n.d.b.). *Linda A. J. Richards 1841–1930*. https://www.aahn.org/richards

American Red Cross. (n.d.). *Founder Clara Barton*. http://www.redcross.org/about-us/who-we-are/history/clara-barton

American Nurses Association. (n.d.). *Hall of fame inductees 1976–1982*. https://www.nursingworld.org/ana/about-ana/history/hall-of-fame/1976-1982-inductees/

American Nurses Association. (2018). *The history of the American Nurses Association*. https://www.nursingworld.org/ana/about-ana/history/

Backus, P. G. (2021, June 1). *Female nurses during the civil war*. American Battlefield. https://www.battlefields.org/learn/articles/female-nurses-during-civil-war

Biography.com Editors. (2024, March 6). *Margaret Sanger*. Biography.com. http://www.biography.com/people/margaret-sanger-9471186

Buhler-Wilkerson, K. (1993). Bringing care to the people: Lillian Wald's legacy to public health nursing. *American Journal of Public Health, 83*(12), 1778–1786. https://doi.org/10.2105/ajph.83.12.1778

Carter, E. (2018, September 20). *The forgotten frontier: Nursing done in wild places.* National Library of Medicine. https://circulatingnow.nlm.nih.gov/2018/09/20/the-forgotten-frontier-nursing-done-in-wild-places/

Castlenova, G. (2020, April). *Mary Breckinridge (1881–1965).* The Truth About Nursing. http://www.truthaboutnursing.org/press/pioneers/breckinridge.html

Cedar Hill Foundation. (n.d.). *Annie Warburton Goodrich (1874–1954).* http://cedarhillfoundation.org/notable-residents/annie-warburton-goodrich/

Daisy, C. A. (1991). Searching for Annie Goodrich. *Western Journal of Nursing Research, 13*(3), 408–413. https://doi.org/10.1177/019394599101300310

Fee, E., & Bu, L. (2010). The origins of public health nursing: the Henry Street Visiting Nurse Service. *American Journal of Public Health, 100*(7), 1206–1207. https://doi.org/10.2105/AJPH.2009.186049

Fugate, A. (2023, July 21). *Mary Breckinridge's vision for Appalachian medical care turns 100 years old.* Mountain Association. https://mtassociation.org/energy/mary-breckinridges-appalachian-medical-care-turns-100-years/

Gandet, L. (1907). Brothers Hospitallers of St. John of God. In *The Catholic encyclopedia.* Robert Appleton Company. http://www.newadvent.org/cathen/02802b.htm

Garofalo, M. E., & Fee, E. (2010). Florence Nightingale (1820-1910): Feminism and hospital reform. 2010. *American Journal of Public Health, 100*(9), 1588. https://doi.org/10.2105/AJPH.2009.188722

Govan, J. (2022, October 3). *Today in history: Remembering Mary Adelaide Nutting.* Teachers College, Columbia University. https://library.tc.columbia.edu/blog/content/2022/october/today-in-history-remembering-mary-adelaide-.php

Holder, V. L. (2004). From handmaiden to right hand—The infancy of nursing. *AORN Journal, 79*(2), 374–390. https://doi.org/10.1016/s0001-2092(06)60614-5

Kays, H. (2022, April 4). *Breaking barriers: A history of Mary Eliza Mahoney.* American Association of Nurse Practitioners. https://www.aanp.org/news-feed/breaking-barriers-a-history-of-mary-eliza-mahoney

Norwood, A. R. (2017). *Dorothea Dix (1802–1887).* National Women's History Museum. https://www.womenshistory.org/education-resources/biographies/dorothea-dix

Prieto, L. (2022, February 24). *Activism in black and white: Mary Eliza Mahoney, pathbreaking nurse and voter.* City of Boston. https://www.boston.gov/news/activism-black-and-white-mary-eliza-mahoney-pathbreaking-nurse-and-voter

Ropes, H. (1993). *Civil war nurse: The diary and letters of Hannah Ropes.* University of Tennessee Press.

Ruel, S. R. (2014). Lillian Wald: A pioneer of home healthcare in the United States. *Home Healthcare Nurse, 32*(10), 597–600. https://doi.org/10.1097/NHH.0000000000000153

Sartin, J. S. (2003). "Commissioned by God": Mother Bickerdyke during the Civil War. *Military Medicine, 168*(10), 773–777.

Schiff, J. (2011). Yale's first female dean. *Yale Alumni Magazine*. https://yalealumnimagazine.org/articles/3090

Stanley, D. (2007). Lights in the shadows: Florence Nightingale and others who made their mark. *Contemporary Nurse, 24*(1), 45–51. https://doi.org/10.5172/conu.2007.24.1.45

Strickler J. (2018). Clara Barton: Angel of the battlefield. *Nursing, 48*(3), 43–45. https://doi.org/10.1097/01.NURSE.0000529805.60418.26

Sy, P. (2023). *Isabel Hampton Robb (1859–1910), founding president of the ANA*. Working Nurse. https://www.workingnurse.com/articles/isabel-hampton-robb-1859-1910-founding-president-of-the-ana/

Image Credits

Fig. 2.1: "Florence Nightingale," http://www.florence-nightingale.co.uk/cms/index.php/online-shop?page=shop.product_details&product_id=77.

Fig. 2.2: "Susie Taylor King: ," https://www.loc.gov/item/2003653538/, 1902.

CHAPTER 3

Nursing's Move Toward Professionalism

Objectives

Upon completion of this chapter, the learner will be able to do the following:

1. Describe the nursing educational shift from apprenticeship models to formalized education.
2. Validate characteristics and attributes that make nursing a profession.
3. Defend an occupation-profession model in nursing.
4. Identify challenges to nursing professionalism.
5. Integrate concepts of diversity, communication, and leadership into nursing professionalism.

Key Chapter Terms

- Professionalism
- Occupation
- Intellectual endeavor
- Evidence-based knowledge
- Theoretical framework
- Social values
- Code of ethics
- Miller Wheel of Professionalism in Nursing Model
- Social justice
- Advocacy
- Health equity
- Diversity

Nursing's Move Toward Professionalism

Nursing's professional status has been a point of inquiry, discussion, and debate for many years. Often, nurses hear the term *professional* in conversation but fail to truly understand the meaning of the word. Individuals also enter nursing and do not understand the attributes that constitute a professional identity. The term most often referred to when speaking of attributes is *profession*—a derivative of the term *professionalism*. Although many definitions have been offered for the term *profession*, many exhibit similarities and agree that it is an occupational group with a designated set of attributes and/or behaviors. Individuals who enter a profession often do so based on what they identify as their calling, or attitudes driven by commitment rather than profit. There is a service perspective adopted by those entering a profession that focuses on helping others. Upon entering a profession, individuals develop characteristic attributes and attitudes, inclusive of ways of thinking (e.g., the nursing process) and special attire (e.g., nurse's uniform) that allows others to recognize them as being a member of their specific profession.

Nursing ***professionalism*** is often defined by its attributes of providing care based on specific principles that include caring and altruism. The meaning of the word *professionalism* is difficult to define, quantify, or measure as it can vary across time, constraints, or cultures. The concept itself is multidimensional, and as a result, there is no clear definition of what constitutes a profession. This controversy extends to nursing, which continues its professional identify quest.

Occupations: Nursing's Beginning

An ***occupation*** usually begins with simple and basic survival tasks. From these tasks, individuals progress to skilled laborers. These skilled laborers learn their trade through repetitive task performance or under the tutelage of a master tradesman. Several professions evolved from these simple beginnings. The first identified professions were law, medicine, and the ministry. Individuals even today work in occupations in which they learn by doing and performing tasks that are assigned based on knowledge learned on the job. They do not consider this their life's work and seek employment to achieve a specific goal (e.g., a student who works in the fast-food industry while going to college). They work under the supervision of another person and accept the philosophical base of the occupation in which they work (e.g., the customer is always right; make the customer happy). Nursing has evolved from its early pre–Florence Nightingale days, during which simple tasks were performed by humans (e.g., manually taking blood pressures) to a technologically based entity in which machines have been introduced to promote care delivery (e.g., use of automatic electric blood pressure machines). There are distinct differences between an occupation and a profession in several categories (see Table 3.1).

TABLE 3.1 Occupation Versus Profession

Category	Occupation	Profession
Longevity	Temporary; frequently changing jobs	Lifelong
Educational preparation	May have minimal training; on-the-job training	University/professional degree program based on a foundation of core liberal arts
Decision-making	Guided by experience or trial and error	Based on evidence validated through research
Continuing education	Only what is required for a job or achieved for financial incentive	Lifelong learning with continuous efforts to improve knowledge base, skills, and abilities
Level of commitment	Varies; may be short-term, and the job may be related to attain personal needs	Long-term commitment to the profession and its organizations
Motivation	Self-interest; work is viewed as a means to an end	Service-oriented; work is viewed as a service to society
Accountability	Lies with a supervisor or an employer	Lies with the individual
Level of engagement	Work is supervised by others	Works autonomously
Expectations	Reasonable work for reasonable pay; work activities performed during specified hours	Activities related to work extend beyond the boundaries of work hours; will accept additional responsibilities that promote the good of society, which includes volunteering for organizational or community activities
Values and beliefs	Often adopts values and beliefs of the employing organization	Develops values and beliefs that transcend organizational boundaries and become part of the individual's personal life

Characteristics of a Profession

Abraham Flexner was a professional educator who identified specific characteristics to describe a profession in a 1915 paper about social work. This work became known as the *Flexner report*. It is a classic piece of literature regarding professional characteristics and was the impetus for medical education reform. This benchmark report is often used to form the educational foundation for professional status in disciplines. Flexner's 1915 criteria stipulate that the following must be present in order for a discipline to be considered a profession:

1. Professional activity is based on intellectual action accompanied by personal responsibility.
2. A profession is based on a body of research knowledge that is continuously expanded.
3. There is a practical application, and it is not just theoretically based.
4. Techniques are taught through specialized education.
5. There is an internal organizational structure with members who have a group consciousness.
6. Members are motivated by altruism (an unselfish desire to help others), working in some sense for the good of society.

Flexner (2015) identified ***intellectual endeavor*** as the first criterion. This relates to individuals who use critical and analytical reasoning in a professional capacity. A professional practice is based on a body of knowledge derived from experience and research. This knowledge base is founded on research evidence to validate and alter care activities. Nurses use the nursing process as a basis for critical thinking and decision-making. They progress in their knowledge base as they gain experience in their area of practice. Nurses use ***evidence-based knowledge*** or research to validate care activities and establish better patient outcomes (see Box 3.1). Evidence-based practice is a significant part of the profession of nursing.

Box 3.1

Use of a Comprehensive Program to Reduce the Incidence of Hospital-Acquired Pressure Ulcers (HAPUs) in an Intensive Care Unit (ICU)

Title:	Useofacomprehensiveprogramtoreducetheincidenceofhospital-acquired pressure ulcers in an intensive care unit (2016)
Authors:	Swafford, K. (clinical nurse specialist), Culpepper, R. (staff nurse and shift coordinator), & Dunn, C. (staff nurse and shift coordinator)
Journal and article info:	*American Journal of Critical Care, 25*(2), 152–155. https://doi.org/10.4037/ajcc2016963
Objective:	The objective of this quantitative assess the effectiveness of a formal, yearlong HAPU prevention program in an adult ICU. The goal was to achieve a minimum reduction of 50% in 2013 compared with 2011 results.
Setting:	This study was conducted in a 14-bed combined medical-surgical ICU.

Intervention: During the first quarter of 2013, the following were implemented:

- Braden scores were used to indicate specific steps for proper moisture, nutrition, mobility, friction, and shear management in hospitalized patients.
- A revised skin care protocol based on National Pressure Ulcer Advisory Panel guidelines for pressure staging were used to encourage proactive interventions prior to skin breakdown evidence.
- Fluidized repositioners behind the torso for all patients were used to help in repositioning and offloading pressure especially for obese patients for patients with a Braden score ≤14.
- Face-to-face staff education.

During the second quarter of 2013, the following was added:

- Requirement to use Allevyn Life silicone dressings on the sacrum of patients with a Braden score of ≤14

Outcome measures: Weekly skin audits were conducted, and real-time feedback was collected from staff.

Results: Prior to initiation of the interventions in 2011, there was a total of 45 hospital-acquired pressure ulcers (HAPUs) that occurred in 10% of patients. The financial cost of these patient HAPUs was approximately $1.7 million. Following intervention, the HAPU incidence was reduced by 69% (n = 17%, which equated to 3% of patients). The financial savings were approximately $1 million. This HAPU reduction occurred despite an increase in the patient load during this time frame.

Conclusion: Staff education and a focus on adherence can have a positive effect on patient outcomes. A proactive, comprehensive, collaborative approach for the prevention of HAPUs can be beneficial to reduce HAPUs in hospital ICUs.

In 1971, Ronald M. Pavalko offered eight dimensions to describe a profession. This scale allows professions to exhibit various degrees of these attributes and possess most, if not all, of these dimensions. An occupation would exhibit none of these dimensions. Professions would exhibit high quality in the work that results from engagement and demonstration of these traits. These can be correlated to nursing. Nursing as a profession has some degree of all dimensions, with some certainly at higher levels than others.

1. **Theoretical framework** as a basis for practice. Nursing is based on many theories that are borrowed from other disciplines, and some are adapted to fit the professional perspective. As a result, these theories have evidence-based knowledge that could not have been advanced by the profession alone. Through educational growth and preparation specialists, nursing theories have evolved, adding to the profession's theoretical framework for practice.

2. **A profession has relevance to social values.** From a historical perspective of nursing through today, nursing has exhibited altruism with a focus on service to others. Nursing focuses on the treatment of illness and the promotion of health as part of its goal. Nurses concentrate on patient education as part of these health promotion activities and serve as wellness coaches and managers to promote social values.
3. **A profession has a training (educational) period.** Nursing includes both a theoretical and a practice component, which was promoted by Nightingale. The educational process for the nurse focuses on establishing the knowledge base needed to practice evidence-based patient management. This process serves to progress scholarly endeavors that continue to advance the profession. The educational base for nurse preparation varies, and this has been the point of much debate. The diverse methods for entry into nursing practice will undoubtedly continue for many years to come.
4. **Elements of self-motivation address the way in which the profession serves the patient or family and larger social system.** Nurses work to service patients, families, and society at large. Through work in healthcare organizations, they directly serve these entities. Political activism is another way to translate social values into action. By working with government groups to develop social policies, they expand this objective beyond specific healthcare organizations.
5. **Members are autonomous and control their profession.** Nurses do not function completely autonomously. They work under both professional and legislative control in performing their work. Nurses' functions are based on the Nurse Practice Act, which identifies professional practice standards for their respective states. They are also governed by their State Board of Nursing.
6. **A profession has a commitment to lifelong work.** Many individuals who select nursing as a career see this as their life's work. This is not a means to an end or mechanism for moving into another profession outside of the nursing arena.
7. **Members have a common identity and distinctive subculture.** Professionalism is a social phenomenon in which members of the professional community assume some manifestation of a common identity and common destiny. The fates of the individual and the profession are intertwined.
8. **A profession has a code of ethics.** The first official code for professional nurses was adopted in 1950 by the American Nurses Association (ANA). As the profession has evolved, it has been revised to address issues that affect nursing.

This translates visually into a continuum model that demonstrates movement between an occupation and a profession for each dimension. This model is represented in Table 3.2.

TABLE 3.2 Occupation-Profession Model

Dimensions	Occupation		Profession
Theoretical framework as basis for practice	Absent	↔	Present
Relevance to social values	Not relevant	↔	Relevant
Training (education) period A	Short time frame	↔	Long time frame
B	Not specialized	↔	Specialized
C	Involves items of no symbolic value	↔	Involves items of symbolic value
D	Subculture not important	↔	Subculture important
Motivation	Self-interest	↔	Societal interest
Autonomy	Absent	↔	Present
Commitment	Short-term	↔	Long-term
Sense of community	Low	↔	High
Code of ethics	Low development	↔	High development

Source: Adapted from Pavalko, 1971.

Professionalism Concepts From a Nursing Perspective

Conceptual models and investigations of professionalism by nurse investigators have not been a prolific topic. Individuals who have contributed significant information include Lucie Kelly and Barbara Miller.

Miller developed a model in 1984 that has been used in nursing research studies that investigate professionalism (Miller et al., 1993; Miller et al., 1996). The **Miller Wheel of Professionalism in Nursing Model** was developed using sociologist Hall's five attitudinal attributes of a profession (Tanaka et al., 2015). This visual model can help nurses determine which behaviors Miller considered important to demonstrate professionalism in nursing. Behaviors include participation in professional organizations; being self-regulatory or autonomous; developing, using, and evaluating research; engaging in continuing education to maintain competence; performing community service; developing, using, and evaluating theory; adhering to a code of ethics for nurses; and having publications and communication. These behaviors are depicted as spokes on a wheel that center around nursing education (see Figure 3.1).

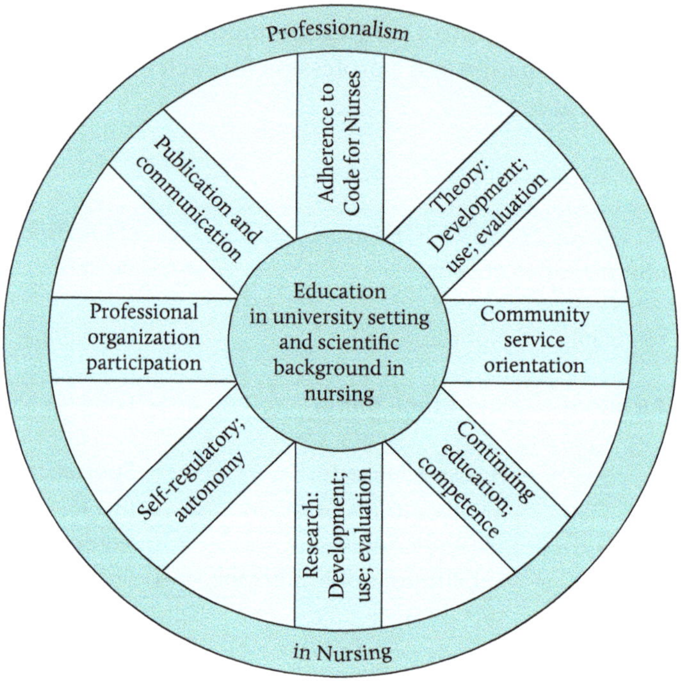

FIGURE 3.1 Miller Wheel of Professionalism in Nursing Model

Lucie Kelly compiled characteristics for nursing professionalism in 1981 that reflected themes from prior works. These foundational dimensions carry forward to nurses practicing from the time of identification into today's electronic age of care delivery. These characteristics consist of the following:

1. Services provided are vital to humanity and society's welfare.
2. There is a special body of knowledge that is continually grown through research.
3. Services offered involve intellectual activities and are accountable for these activities.
4. Practitioners are educated in institutions of higher education.
5. Practitioners are relatively independent and have control of their policies and activities.
6. Practitioners are altruistic (service-motivated) and consider this important in their lives.
7. A code of ethics guides practitioner decision-making and conduct.
8. There is an organization that encourages and supports high standards.

Components for professionalism that were presented individually by Flexner (1915), Pavalko (1971), Kelly and Joel (1995), and Miller (1988) are shown in Table 3.3 in an effort to provide a quick review and comparison.

There are many similarities among the presented professionalism models and concepts. It is difficult to grasp the likenesses and differences even when viewing these authors side by side. In an effort to add clarity to your understanding, these areas have been delineated based on their conceptual components or themes. Many themes carry through all professional characteristics identified. These include education, service, organization, and ethics. Four of the five authors address altruism and research. Autonomy and theory follow in order of frequency, with three out of five authors identifying this concept as a basis for professionalism which are in Table 3.4, which uses the numerical listings from Table 3.3 for each author.

BLE 3.3 Professionalism Characteristics by Author

lexner (1915)	Pavalko (1971)	Kelly & Joel (1995)	Miller (1988)
Professional activity is based on intellectual action accompanied by personal responsibility. A profession is based on a body of research knowledge that is continuously expanded. There is a practical application, and it is not just theoretically based. . Techniques are taught through specialized education. . There is an internal organizational structure with members who have a group consciousness. . Members are motivated by altruism (a desire to help others) working in some sense for the good of society.	1. There is a theoretical framework as a basis for practice. 2. A profession has relevance to social values. 3. A profession has a training (educational) period. 4. Elements of self-motivation address the way in which the profession serves the patient or family and larger social system. 5. Members are autonomous and control their profession. 6. A profession has a commitment to lifelong work. 7. Members have a common identity and distinctive subculture. 8. A profession has a code of ethics.	1. Services provided are vital to humanity and society's welfare. 2. There is a special body of knowledge that is continually grown through research. 3. Services offered involve intellectual activities and are accountable for these activities. 4. Practitioners are educated in institutions of higher education. 5. Practitioners are relatively independent and have control of their policies and activities. 6. Practitioners are altruistic (service-motivated) and consider this important in their lives. 7. A code of ethics guides practitioner decision-making and conduct. 8. There is an organization that encourages and supports high standards.	1. Participation in professional organizations 2. Being self-regulatory or autonomous 3. Developing, using, and evaluating research 4. Engaging in continuing education to maintain competence 5. Performing community service 6. Developing, using, and evaluating theory 7. Adhering to a code of ethics for nurses 8. Having publications and communication

TABLE 3.4 Comparison of Professionalism Components by Author

	Component							
Author	**Education**	**Service**	**Organization**	**Ethics**	**Altruism**	**Research**	**Autonomy**	**Theory**
Flexner (1915)	4	3	5	1	6	2	–	–
Pavalko (1971)	3	6	7	8	2, 4	–	5	1
Kelly & Joel (1995)	4	1	8	3, 7	6	2	5	–
Miller (1988)	4	5	1, 8	7	–	3	2	6

A concept analysis by Cao and several other authors in 2023 identified a theoretical definition and a conceptual model of professionalism in nursing. Their intent was to validate the concept as an essential step to providing quality patient care. Based on concept analysis, professionalism is three-dimensional and based on knowledge, attitudes, and behaviors. Knowledge in professionalism is a systematic body that has complex configurations. Attitudes represent a level of recognition and commitment. These are closely correlated with behaviors that the nurse exhibits in the Miller (1988) Wheel of Professionalism in Nursing Model. The concept analysis revealed that nursing professionalism is multidimensional (knowledge, attitude, behavior), dynamic (a socialization process, a process of interaction), and culture-oriented (affected by personal and employer culture) with three connotations, which are professionalism, caring, and altruism.

Challenges to Nursing Professionalism

Professionalism in nursing has not been without its challenges from inception to today. These challenges include varied educational preparation, nursing mental health and well-being, labor problems, social justice issues (Paquin, 2011), and diversity. It is only through identification and continued work to resolve these challenges that nursing will proceed to gain the full recognition and respect of a profession.

Varied Educational Preparation

In speaking with many individuals inside and outside of the nursing profession, the first challenge identified is the level of entry into the profession. There are a variety of educational backgrounds that mark individual entry into the profession. They are all linked to the term *nurse*, from licensed practical nurses to baccalaureate degree nurses. These individuals may be working side by side in a healthcare organization and identified by a patient as being at the same level on the professional continuum. Educational preparation is one common component of a profession identified by those who have worked to clarify the concept. It stands without argument that professional recognition, status, and power increase with educational preparation.

There is no other profession that allows entry into practice with less than a baccalaureate degree. Many now require master's-level preparation in order to be eligible for practice privileges. Nurses are currently prepared at three different entry levels, which include diploma (licensed practical nurse), associate degree (registered nurse [RN]), and baccalaureate degree (RN). Discussion of this topic brings about strong reaction from many nurses. This topic has been a divisive issue for the profession over many years and continues to evoke anger and defensive posturing among nurses. Only through a resolution of this issue will nursing evolve into the profession many desire.

Nurse Mental Health and Well-Being

Workplace Violence

Nurse mental health and well-being are challenged by workplace violence experienced in many settings. The U.S. Bureau of Labor Statistics (2021) identified that the rate of injuries resulting from assaults and violent acts by other persons for nursing and personal care facility workers was 21.8%. Based on these statistics, many healthcare workers will experience workplace violence at some point in their careers.

Workplace violence can be divided into two main groups: physical and psychological. This type of violence can increase job stress, decrease job satisfaction, increase absenteeism, increase nurse burnout, cause sleep disorders and fatigue, and result in post-traumatic stress disorder (Kafle et al., 2022; Labyak, 2002). Workplace violence can also affect the work environment, making it toxic and hostile. Some causes of violence include understaffing, increased nurse stress, and the demanding type and nature of nurse work.

Nurses must work to address the violence problem. It is important for nurses to educate themselves on how to recognize the potential for violence. There is online material and web-based information (e.g., webinars) that are free or have a minimal charge from organizations such as the American Association of Critical-Care Nurses (2016), American Hospital Association, ANA, and National Institute for Occupational Safety and Health, that address the issue of violence in nursing. It is important for the nurse to recognize violent situations and remove oneself, if possible. Know how to employ de-escalation techniques and how to seek assistance to prevent or respond to violent situations.

Type and Nature of Work

Nursing has many challenges on a professional level due to the type and nature of the work involved in patient care that challenge nurse mental health and well-being. Nurses may work long hours (12-hour shifts), have mandatory overtime requirements, face health care risks, have an increased emotional load due to dealing with individuals in various stages of grief, and deal with death and dying. The length of this work is extensive, and List 3.1 identifies just a small portion of the actual work of the nurse.

Nursing shift work varies, based on organizational structure. Some are structured in eight- or 12-hour increments, with 12 hours being a prevalent practice. Hours can range from early morning to late evening (7 a.m. to 7 p.m.), while others are structured in traditional eight-hour shifts (7 a.m. to 3 p.m., 3 p.m. to 11 p.m., and 11 p.m. to 7 a.m.). Shift work can have an impact on sleep, well-being, performance, and outcomes (nurse, patient and organizational) (Hernandez et al., 2022). Studies have identified that higher levels of night-shift stress were associated with increased sleep disturbance, which leads to poor quality-of-life outcomes (AL-hrinat et al., 2024).

Work required in the nursing field is fluid and changes based on setting (area of acute care setting), geographic location (rural or urban), state of practice (related to the Nursing Practice Act), and societal norms and expectations. The type of work that serves as a challenge to nurse well-being can be in a constant state of change due to these and other changes in the healthcare system, organizational structures, and emerging challenges, such as pandemics and other emergencies.

Labor Problems

A major labor problem that faces the profession of nursing is the shortage of nurses. This shortage results in reduced health service delivery and poorer patient outcomes. The nursing shortage was exacerbated by the pandemic. It has been identified that by 2035, the demand for nursing will reach 12.9 million (Adams et al., 2021), with 2023 showing a nursing shortage exceeding 500,000 (Valizadeh et al., 2016). The shortage is a global issue. Some of the research-based causes include “policy and planning barriers, barriers to training and enrollment, factors causing nursing staff turnover, and nurses’ stress and burnout” (Tamata & Mohammadnezhad, 2022, p. 1247). Policy and planning means addressing poor salaries and low job satisfaction and establishing incentives for nurses. Training and enrollment mean addressing training space and clinical sites as well as the large number of nurses turned away from academic programs due to low faculty numbers. Factors causing nursing staff turnover and nurses’ stress and burnout mean that addressing burnout and psychomotor disorders and mandatory and long work hours

List 3.1
Nurse Work That Can Challenge Mental Health and Well-Being

- Delivering care in various settings, including physical, mental, and emotional delivery
- Manipulating patients in the delivery of care activities, including movement (transfer and mobility challenges from full manipulation for patients confined to bed to assistance with patients requiring minimal ambulation assistance)
- Participating in interdisciplinary team management and decision-making conferences
- Developing individualized plans for nursing care
- Frequently assessing current patient health status to identify care needs
- Implementing appropriate nursing measures in the delivery of patient care
- Interpreting plans of care developed by other providers for initiation (e.g., physician orders)
- Delegating appropriate care activities to other care providers
- Supervising others in the delivery of patient care
- Observing and validating patient outcomes resulting from interventions for patient needs
- Providing counseling, guidance, and education to patients and families
- Initiating appropriate referrals and follow-up services for patients and families.
- Recording and reporting patient health status and other necessary information to healthcare providers
- Promoting patient self-care and understanding of current health status
- Interpreting organizational policies, objectives, and services for patients and families
- Assuming leadership roles

are crucial. The resolution to these issues is complex and multifaceted. It includes supportive leadership (American Nurses Association, 2023), nurse representation, and action at the local and national levels for policymaking. It will take intentional approaches by educators, state and federal legislators, and state boards of nursing to collaboratively address this significant labor problem in order to provide safe and effective care for the public.

Social Justice Issues

Social justice means providing equal and fair health care services to all individuals regardless of their characteristics or circumstances. The nurse is in a unique position to drive social justice for society at large. The issue of social justice is detailed in the ANA's (2025) code of ethics for nurses, which provides a framework for addressing nurse responsibilities for providing equal and fair care for all people from various backgrounds. It envelops nurses' responsibility to work for social change on behalf of vulnerable people.

Advocacy

Advocacy in nursing is a critical component of social justice, as it ensures that nurses champion the rights and well-being of their patients, particularly those from marginalized or vulnerable populations. Nurses often serve as the primary link between patients and the healthcare system. They promote culturally competent care. Nurses also address disparities that can arise due to socioeconomic status, race, gender, or other social determinants of health. This commitment to social justice means actively identifying and challenging inequalities in health care, which serves to create an inclusive and fair system.

Advocacy in nursing goes beyond individual patients and their rights to make informed decisions about their care and extends to policy reform and community engagement. Nurses can play a pivotal role in shaping healthcare policies that address systemic issues affecting marginalized populations. By being involved in legislative efforts or community outreach programs, they can influence changes that improve access to care, promote health equity, and reduce health disparities. Nurse advocacy is grounded in the profession's ethical responsibility to not only care for the individual but also work toward the betterment of society as a whole.

Health Equity

Health equity is defined as "the state in which everyone has the opportunity to attain full health potential and no one is disadvantaged from achieving this potential because of social position or any other socially defined circumstance" (National Academies of Sciences, Engineering, and Medicine et al., 2017, p. 32). Only when everyone has a fair and just opportunity to achieve their maximum level of heath, is health equity achieved. Nurses are in a unique position to address health equity as they conduct patient screenings, review these results and develop plans of care, and coordinate care with social workers and community health individuals for continuity of continued care from acute facilities to home or other intermediate care facilities. Nurses working in public health areas outside of acute care and clinic settings directly serve as community partners in addressing health equity. The pandemic identified the need for collaborative care in all nursing areas in managing infectious disease outbreaks and addressing the significant health issues that accompany them. This allows for nursing community engagement to address the variety of clinical and community-based needs that result from such events. It is important that nurses are knowledgeable regarding the community in which they live and work. This knowledge of organizational policies, legislations, public needs and resources, and community assistance organizations can improve health outcomes for individuals and populations.

Diversity in the Population

Diversity in the nursing population is minimal when it comes to gender. Nursing has historically been equated with the work of women, although there was a time in history where this was not the case. There is a significantly higher number of women in nursing than men. Many male nurses who are in the profession are not at the bedside, reducing the perception of their overall numbers. Many move through bedside nursing to specialties such as nurse anesthesia or nursing administration. Due to the high ratio of women to men in nursing, even with a gradual increase, there may never be an equitable distribution of men in the profession. Men serve as a force to change the mode of thinking from women's work to the work of professionals delivering nursing care (see Figure 3.2).

Men have been part of the nursing profession for hundreds of years—as far back as the 11th century in Europe, when they were members of religious orders. The number of men in nursing has increased considerably over the past 20 years. The perspective toward men early in the educational development of the school of nursing was to exclude them from entry. Only women were allowed to enroll and thus become nurses. This attitude perpetuated the typical female perspective of the nurse.

A report by the American Association of Colleges of Nursing (2023) reported that as of 2022, men comprised approximately 12% of the nursing workforce. The upward trend that existed over the past 20 years stalled at 12% to 13% between

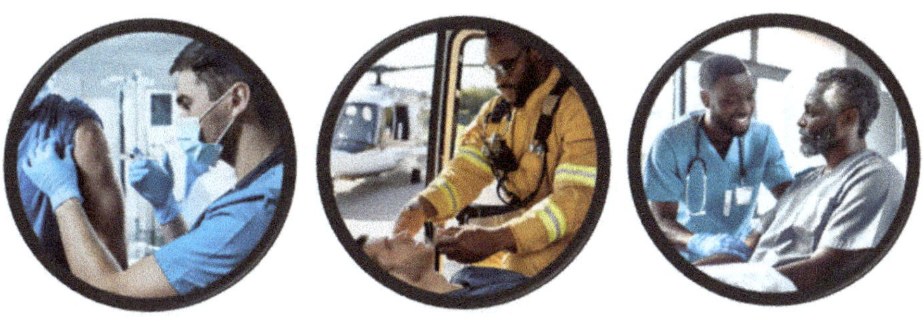

FIGURE 3.2 Men serve a vital function in the delivery of competent nursing care to clients, families, and communities.

2020 and 2022. Men in nursing were more likely to be older than their female counterparts (the median age for men was 35, compared with approximately age 31 for women) and work in hospitals. Men made up 12% of all employed RNs, yet they made up 41% of all certified RN anesthetists. The number of male licensed practical nurses and licensed vocational nurses increased by 4.2% from 1970 to 2021. The American Assembly for Men in Nursing (AAMN, n.d.) was established in 1974 to give men a voice in nursing. It is now unrestricted and open to all nurses, men and women, in order to address issues in the profession for all. The AAMN advocates for strengthening and humanizing health care; for men to grow professionally and increase the awareness of men's contribution to society; for continued research, education, and dissemination of information about men's health issues, men in nursing, and nursing knowledge; and for the support of member participation in the nursing profession.

Addressing Challenges

It is critical for nurses to address challenges that affect their quality of professional and personal life. No single intervention can address all challenges. Maintaining knowledge and skills to recognize one's limitations is a start. It is important to know what issues you can solve yourself and when to ask for help. Ensure that you have a sound support system for communicating your feelings and concerns. Take care of your physical health (e.g., eat well, rest, exercise) as well as your mental and emotional self (e.g., take breaks, establish activities that allow your brain to rest [such as art and music], and practice mindfulness [i.e., being present in the moment but using a technique such as slowly breathing in and out to prevent over reactions]). Contact a therapist before burnout or other challenges become too hard to manage.

Professionalism in a Digital World

Image of Nurses

Nurses took a front row seat during the pandemic, with the media focusing on their work and sacrifices. Media reports recognized the exceptional contributions and sacrifices made by nurses. They identified how nurses advocated for patients, connected patients with their families in order to facilitate their well-being, and functioned in the face of adversity during the pandemic; however, few members of the media focused on their working conditions. The media's reports during the pandemic identified not only challenges during this situation but also those faced by the nursing workforce on a daily basis. These reports went a long way to affect public perception of nursing as a profession. The image of nursing is closely linked to "the nurses' identity and role, the cultural context, the clinical practice, work satisfaction, and the quality of care" (Blau et al., 2023; Kumar, 2021). The image of nursing has been perceived more positively in the United States following the pandemic (Yavaş & Özerli, 2023), but there is still a long way to go for nursing to establish itself as an evidence-based profession with autonomy in managing patient care.

Increased Use of Technology for Care

Nursing professionalism is now manifested through digital media. The pandemic was the impetus for the increased use of mobile technology for communication inside and outside of organizations. It promoted the immediate implementation and use of remote healthcare technologies across the world. It moved nurses into identifying professional engagement and appropriate behaviors required to engage with technologies and adhere to confidentiality and security issues. It is important that nurses maintain an awareness of ethical use of technology and how it should be a tool for the promotion of safe care delivery (O'Connor et al., 2020).

A balance must be maintained between the digital needs of nurses with the perspectives of patients, families, health service managers, and others. In this digital environment, professionalism should be anchored in ethical principles and sound judgment. It is important that nurses use digital technology to demonstrate knowledge, skills, and moral orientation that are supported by colleagues and the larger organization. Engagement in the digital environment could serve to contribute to validating to society how nurses could professionally use technology to deliver high-quality care.

Summary

Attitudes and behaviors that characterize a profession cannot be learned through reading and studying alone. These must be actively acquired through the process of professional socialization, which starts at the beginning of the professional education process. Nursing recognized this early in its educational developmental process, and therefore, many programs offer professionalism courses at or near the beginning of their academic program of study. These concepts are then carried out through didactic and clinical courses. It is important to start attaining and demonstrating nurse professionalism during your educational process. Demonstration of professionalism includes being on time for class, clinical, and work; effectively communicating with patients and peers; showing compassion through sensitivity to others' suffering and demonstrating a willingness to help; being accountable and taking responsibility for your own actions; having a positive attitude; dressing the part in clinical and educational activities; demonstrating ethical behavior; putting patients first; showing respect and appreciation; and making sure that you take care of yourself in order to be the best possible you. These intertwine with the exemplary practice components (see Table 3.5) that reflect holistic patient management and grounding components for the profession as a whole (Riley et al., 2021). By being committed to these and adhering to standards of the profession, nurses can establish value and reward, which will be reflected in daily patient care activities.

In order to promote internal and external perceptions of nursing as a profession, nurses themselves must come to an agreement on how to define their profession. Nurses perform their care in some difficult work environments with a lack of autonomy. They are often required to take on tasks that are the responsibility of others in the healthcare organization when there is a need, regardless of the level of duty. They are called on to fill voids (e.g., the job of housekeeping on shifts when these individuals are reduced in staffing and patient beds must be cleaned for pending admissions). As a result, people do not see nurses as leaders with professional identity. The profession must acquire and demonstrate strong competencies and skills in order to achieve the level of respect attributed to other professions (e.g., physicians, lawyers, and clergy). This will only be achieved through leadership visibility and self-promotion to individuals who are at the helm of health care in the United States. This includes health insurance organizations, policymakers, media, and the public at large.

TABLE 3.5 Exemplary Practice Components

Pillar	Characteristics
Professionalism	Has the desire for lifelong learning, shared accountability, and a strong professional identity; is responsible and accountable
Scholarly practice	Synthesizes knowledge and caring; shares knowledge; develops, uses, and disseminates scholarship; collaborates
Leadership	Promotes vision, partners, empowers others, embraces leadership roles
Stewardship	Preserves and advances the profession, serves society, develops policies

Source: Riley et al., 2021.

References

Adams, D., & Miller, B. K. (2001). Professionalism in nursing behaviors of nurse practitioners. *Journal of Professional Nursing*, *17*(4), 203–210.

Adams, R., Ryan, T., & Wood, E. (2021). Understanding the factors that affect retention within the mental health nursing workforce: A systematic review and thematic synthesis. *International Journal of Mental Health Nursing, 30*(1), 1476–1497. https://doi.org/10.1111/inm.12904

AL-hrinat, J., Al-Ansi, A.M., Hendi, A., Adwan, G., & Hazaimeh, M. (2024). The impact of night shift stress and sleep disturbance on nurses quality of life: Case in Palestine Red Crescent and Al-Ahli Hospital. *BMC Nursing, 23*, 24. https://doi.org/10.1186/s12912-023-01673-3

American Association of Critical-Care Nurses. (2016). *AACN standards for establishing and sustaining healthy work environments: A journey to excellence.* https://www.aacn.org/~/media/aacn-website/nursing-excellence/healthy-work-environment/execsum.pdf?la=en

American Association of Men in Nursing. (n.d.). *The history of AAMN.* https://www.aamn.org/history

American Nurses Association. (2023, May 19). *Leadership in nursing: Qualities & why it matters.* https://www.nursingworld.org/content-hub/resources/nursing-leadership/leadership-in-nursing/

American Nurses Association. (2025). *Code of ethics.* https://codeofethics.ana.org/provisions

Blau, A., Sela, Y., & Grinberg, K. (2023). Public perceptions and attitudes on the image of nursing in the wake of COVID-19. *International Journal of Environmental Research and Public Health, 20*(6), 4717. https://doi.org/10.3390/ijerph20064717

Cao, H., Song, Y., Wu, Y., Du, Y., He, X., Chen, Y., Wang, Q., & Yang, H. (2023). What is nursing professionalism? A concept analysis. *BMC Nursing, 22*(1), 34. https://doi.org/10.1186/s12912-022-01161-0

Flexner, A. (1915). *Is social work a profession?* Social Welfare History Project. https://socialwelfare.library.vcu.edu/social-work/is-social-work-a-profession-1915/

Hernandez, A. F. J., Bautista, R. L. S., & Tan, C. C. (2022). Sleep disturbances during shift work. *Sleep Medicine Clinics, 17*(1), 1–10. https://doi.org/10.1016/j.jsmc.2021.10.001

Kafle, S., Paudel, S., Thapaliya, A., & Acharya, R. (2022). Workplace violence against nurses: A narrative review. *Journal of Clinical and Translational Research, 8*(5), 421–424.

Kelly, L., & Joel, L. A. (1995). *Dimensions of professional nursing* (7th ed.). McGraw Hill.

Kumar, M. (2021). Nursing as a profession beyond tropes of the image among public, media, and identify crisis: A discussion paper. *International Journal of Science and Healthcare Research, 6*(2), 53–57. https://doi.org/10.52403/ijshr.20210411

Labyak, S. (2002). Sleep and circadian schedule disorders. *Nursing Clinics of North America, 37*, 599–610.

Miller, B. K. (1988). A model for professionalism in nursing. *Today's OR Nurse, 10*(9), 18–23.

Miller, B. K., Adams, D., & Beck, L. (1993). A behavioral inventory for professionalism in nursing. *Journal of Professional Nursing, 9*(5), 290–295.

Miller, B. K., Adams, D., & Beck, L. (1996). Professionalism behaviors of hospital nurse executives and middle managers in 10 western states. *Western Journal of Nursing Research, 18*(1), 77–88.

National Academies of Sciences, Engineering, and Medicine, Health and Medicine Division, Board on Population Health and Public Health Practice, Committee on Community-Based Solutions to Promote Health Equity in the United States; Baciu, A., Negussie, Y., Geller, A., & Weinstein, J. N. (Eds.). (2017). *Communities in action: Pathways to health equity.* National Academies Press (U.S.).

O'Connor, S., Chu, C. H., Thilo, F., Lee, J. J., Mather, C., & Topaz, M. (2020). Professionalism in a digital and mobile world: A way forward for nursing. *Journal of Advanced Nursing, 76*(1), 4–6. https://doi.org/10.1111/jan.14224

Paquin, S. O. (2011). Social justice advocacy in nursing: What is it? How do we get there? *Creative Nursing, 17*(2), 63–67. https://doi.org/10.1891/1078-4535.17.2.63

Pavalko, R. M. (1971). *Sociology of occupations and professions.* F. E. Peacock Publishers.

Riley, J. M., Beal, J. A., & Ponte, P. R. (2021). The exemplary practice life of the nurse. *Journal of Professional Nursing: Official Journal of the American Association of Colleges of Nursing, 37*(5), 1018–1025. https://doi.org/10.1016/j.profnurs.2021.07.003

Swafford, K., Culpepper, R., & Dunn, C. (2016). Use of a comprehensive program to reduce the incidence of hospital-acquired pressure ulcers in an intensive care unit. *American Journal of Critical Care, 25*(2), 152–155. https://doi.org/10.4037/ajcc2016963

Tamata, A. T., & Mohammadnezhad, M. (2022). A systematic review study on the factors affecting shortage of nursing workforce in the hospitals. *Nursing Open, 10*(3), 1247–1257. https://doi.org/10.1002/nop2.1434

Tanaka, M., Taketomi, K., Yonemitsu, Y., & Kawamoto, R. (2015). An international comparison of professional behaviors among nurse leaders in the U.S.A. and Japan. *International Journal of Nursing and Clinical Practices, 2*, 113. http://dx.doi.org/10.15344/2394-4978/2015/113

U.S. Bureau of Labor Statistics. (2023). *Injuries, illnesses, and fatalities.* https://www.bls.gov/iif/home.htm

Valizadeh, L., Zamanzadeh, V., Habibzadeh, H., Alilu, L., Gillespie, M., & Shakibi, A. (2016). Experiences of Iranian nurses that intent to leave the clinical nursing: A content analysis. *Journal of Caring Sciences, 5*(2), 169–178. https://doi.org/10.15171/jcs.2016.018

Yavaş, G., & Özerli, A. N. (2023). The public image of nursing during the COVID-19 pandemic: A cross-sectional study. *International Nursing Review.* https://doi.org/10.1111/inr.12922

Image Credits

Fig. 3.1: Adapted from Barbara K. Miller, "A Model for Professionalism in Nursing," Today's OR Nurse, vol. 10, no. 9. Copyright © 1988 by Slack, Inc.

Fig. 3.2: Generated using Adobe Firefly..

CHAPTER 4

Core Values of Nursing

Sherin Tahmasbi, DNP, FNP-C

Objectives

Upon completion of this chapter, the learner will be able to do the following:

1. Articulate core professional values in nursing.
2. Explain the role of Caritas in nursing.
3. Demonstrate how core nursing values guide ethical decision-making.
4. Identify how respect for patient autonomy, dignity, and cultural differences is integral to providing holistic and individualized care.

Key Chapter Terms

- Core values
- Caring
- Integrity
- Diversity and inclusion
- Excellence
- Caritas
- Watson's Theory of Human Caring
- Ethical decision-making
- Autonomy
- Dignity
- Transcultural nursing
- Cultural competence
- Holistic care

Core Professional Values in Nursing

The field of nursing is guided by **core values** that shape actions, judgment, decision-making, and daily interactions in practice. These values are goals and beliefs that establish professional behavior and provide a foundation

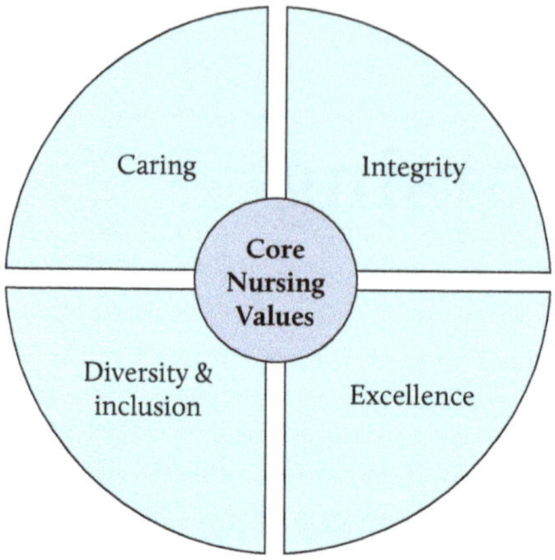

FIGURE 4.1 Core Nursing Values

for decision-making. They are rooted in ethics for the nursing profession (Epstein & Turner, 2015). According to the National League for Nursing (n.d.), these values include **caring, integrity, diversity and inclusion,** and **excellence** (see Figure 4.1).

The American Association of Colleges of Nursing (AACN; 2024a) emphasizes that the development of professional identity in nursing is built on these foundational core values.

Caring is integral and fundamental to the foundation of nursing and was demonstrated by Florence Nightingale in the early 1800s. Caring in nursing occurs through two domains: the act of caring (caring for another person who cannot care for themselves) and the context of concern (demonstration of compassion and kindness). This value uses empathy, which allows nurses to step into the shoes of another and view emotions and experiences from the patient's point of view. Nurses demonstrate the core value of caring toward patients and others (Arthur et al., 1999). The concept of caring involves actively listening, understanding a patient's unique situation, and providing support. Through a demonstration of compassion, empathy, and concern, the nurse fosters trust and promotes healing. Caring allows the creation of meaningful patient connections, which makes patients feel valued and respected and can therefore enhance care outcomes. Value and respect earned through caring allows the nurse to promote patient navigation through the complex healthcare system with dignity and confidence. Through the cultivation of caring, patients are empowered.

Integrity requires a commitment to ethical principles, honesty, and moral responsibility. Nurses demonstrate integrity by upholding high professional standards. They ensure that their actions align with professional values (Poorchangizi et al., 2019) and ethical guidelines. They prioritize patient safety and welfare and take accountability for their decisions and actions. This allows nurses to develop trust with patients, families, and colleagues. This trust is built through open communication, respect for confidentiality, and a commitment to fairness and justice. Integrity also drives accountability and self-reflection. Nurses who act with integrity continuously self-assess their practices, seek constructive feedback, and seek opportunities for growth and improvement. Nurses who demonstrate integrity strengthen the profession's reputation and ensure that patients receive high-quality care based on trust and respect.

Diversity and inclusion are essential values in nursing as they ensure equitable care for all patients regardless of their race, ethnicity, gender, socioeconomic status, religion, or other individual characteristics. Nurses embrace diversity by showing respect and value for an individual's unique background, experiences, and perspectives. They seek to understand and address the cultural, social, and linguistic needs of the population whom they serve. Inclusion involves creating a welcoming environment where patients feel safe, respected, and understood. Nurses who promote inclusion advocate for patients to ensure that their voices are heard and needs met. Diversity and inclusion enhance teamwork. This value promotes nurses embracing varied colleague perspectives, which allows for effective collaboration to generate creative solutions and promotes organizational equity. These values contribute to a fair healthcare system that responds to individual needs.

Excellence is the continued pursuit of high-quality patient care. This is achieved through continuous learning, professional development, and a commitment to using the best nursing practices. Excellence requires that nurses master clinical skills, stay up to date on evidence-based practices, and foster innovation. This allows nurses to achieve optimal results in the delivery of patient care delivery. Through a proactive approach, nurses are able to adapt to rapid changes in health care without compromising quality care delivery. Using high standards for themselves and others, they inspire a culture of improvement and accountability within their organization. Collaborative efforts in the delivery of excellence involve mentoring colleagues, sharing knowledge, and contributing to the collective expertise of the nursing profession. By embracing excellence, nurses elevate their practice, contribute to healthcare advancement, and ensure that patients continuously receive the best possible care.

Core values of nursing can help nurses make optimal decisions in situations in which ethical dilemmas may arise. Understanding how these values can help guide oneself in situations in which ethical dilemmas arise can reduce negative impacts or prevent them from arising. Values such as integrity and social justice can act as a moral compass when making decisions related to ethical dilemmas.

The professional values of caring, integrity, diversity and inclusion, and excellence form the structure in which nurses interact not only with patients but also with colleagues and the healthcare system in general (Fahrenwald et al., 2005). These values are not simply ideals—they are principles that guide nursing practice. Over time, these values have shifted and evolved due to societal changes, healthcare advances, and other factors. In modern times, it is crucial to uphold these core values in daily practice to maintain nursing's integrity and make sure patients receive high-quality care (Hemberg & Salmela, 2021).

The Role of Caritas in Nursing

Caritas is derived from the Latin word *carus*, meaning *dear* or *beloved*. The word *caritas* in Latin translates to the word *love*. The concept of Caritas has shaped the foundation of the nursing profession throughout the history of nursing. Between 1975 and 1979, Jean Watson, a professor of nursing, developed the **Theory of Human Caring** based on her personal perspective on nursing. This theory incorporates 10 Caritas processes, which emphasize holistic and compassionate care (see Table 4.1). An idea central to caring is

TABLE 4.1 10 Caritas Processes

Carita	Associated Terms	Meaning
1. Embrace	Loving-kindness	Sustaining humanistic-altruistic values through the practice of loving-kindness, compassion, and equanimity with self and others
2. Inspire	Faith, hope	Being authentically present; enabling faith/hope/belief system; honoring subjective inner, life-world of self/others
3. Trust	Transpersonal presence	Being sensitive to self and others by cultivating own spiritual practices; transcending ego-self to transpersonal presence
4. Nurture	Relationships	Developing and sustaining loving, trusting, and caring relationships
5. Forgive	Holding space	Allowing for expression of positive and negative feelings; authentically listening to another person's story
6. Deepen	Creative self	Creatively problem-solving/"solution-seeking" through caring process; full use of self and artistry of caring-healing practices via use of all ways of knowing/being/doing/becoming
7. Balance	Learning	Engaging in transpersonal teaching and learning within the context of caring relationship; staying within others' frame of reference; shift toward coaching model for expanded health/wellness
8. Co-create	Caritas field	Creating a healing environment at all levels; subtle environment for energetic authentic caring presence
9. Minister	Humanity	Reverentially assisting with basic needs as sacred acts; touching the mind, body, and spirit of others; sustaining human dignity
10. Open	Infinity	Opening to spiritual, mystery, unknowns—allowing for miracles

Source: Jean Watson, "10 Caritas Processes." Copyright © 1979 by Watson Caring Science Institute (WCSI). Reprinted with permission.

"human beings cannot be separated from themselves, others, nature, and the larger world" (Ghanbari-Afra et al., 2022). Watson's theory establishes a holistic, interpersonal connection between the caregiver and the care recipient (Akbari & Nasiri, 2022).

Watson's caring theory identifies these caritas processes as essential components of nursing practice as they guide nurses to integrate science and compassion into care delivery. These processes encourage nurses to use practices such as showing loving-kindness to patients by being "authentically present" (Carita 2: Inspire) and creating a healing environment (Carita 8: Co-create). In this way, nurses can connect with their patients on a deeper level, which will allow them to holistically address their emotional, spiritual, and psychological needs. These mindful and intentional interactions promote trust, as they demonstrate respect for patients' cultural and personal values. This serves to strengthen the therapeutic relationship, reduce patient anxiety, and promote positive patient health outcomes. The caritas approach promotes recognition of nurses as healers in their capacity to provide compassionate care.

Caritas in nursing emphasize the importance of intentionality and mindfulness in interactions with patients. Through practices such as actively listening, offering comfort, and respecting patients' cultural and personal values, nurses embody the essence of caritas. These actions support Watson's vision of a caring moment, where the nurse and patient engage in a meaningful exchange that benefits both parties. Such moments strengthen the therapeutic relationship, reduce patient anxiety, and contribute to positive health outcomes. Furthermore, the caritas approach recognizes the nurse as a healer (SadatHoseini et al., 2023), emphasizing self-care and personal growth to sustain their capacity to provide compassionate care.

Integrating caritas into nursing practice reinforces the profession's core values. It promotes the nurse-patient relationship and fosters a caring culture. By embracing Watson's caritas, nurses enhance their ability to address diverse needs and contribute to the profession's moral and ethical foundation. Caritas serve as a reminder in this technology-based healthcare environment that the patient is the most important component and that care should be patient-centered and grounded in love and compassion.

Core Values and Ethical Decision-Making

Ethical decision-making is a fundamental aspect of nursing practice. The core values of caring, integrity, diversity and inclusion, and excellence serve as guiding principles that shape how nurses' approach complex dilemmas while upholding high standards of care. These values are not only essential to fostering trust and respect in the nurse-patient relationship; they also ensure that decisions are compassionate, equitable, and evidence-based. By integrating these values into their practice, nurses approach ethical challenges from a holistic perspective. This promotes honoring individuality and dignity while still balancing professional obligations (Matiti et al., 2007).

Caring as a Guide to Ethical Decision-Making

Caring is a core nursing value that plays a central role in ethical decision-making by fostering empathy and compassion for patients. Caring motivates nurses to prioritize the well-being of individuals, ensuring that decisions are made with the patients' best interests in mind. For example, suppose that a nurse is faced with an ethical dilemma, such as whether to honor a patient's decision to refuse treatment. Using caring as a foundation for decision-making, the nurse would approach the situation with sensitivity and an understanding of the patient's emotional and psychological state. By engaging with the patient, the nurse can advocate for choices that represent the patient's wishes and values (Morris, 2025).

Integrity as a Foundation for Ethical Choices

Integrity provides the moral foundation for ethical decision-making by ensuring that nurses act with honesty, transparency, and accountability. It requires nurses to uphold professional standards and adhere to ethical principles, even when faced with complex or challenging situations. For example, when a nurse identifies a medication error, integrity drives them to report the mistake promptly, prioritize patient safety, and work collaboratively to resolve the issue. Integrity promotes a commitment to truthfulness and ethical conduct. This ensures that decisions are guided in a way that promotes trust between nurses and their patients, patient family members, and other healthcare providers.

Diversity and Inclusion in Ethical Decision-Making

Diversity and inclusion are crucial in guiding ethical decisions in order to show respect for the unique backgrounds and needs for each individual patient. Nurses must consider patients' cultural, religious, and personal values when making care decisions to ensure that they receive equitable and culturally competent care. For example, when developing a plan of care for a patient from a marginalized community, nurses guided by diversity and inclusion will address potential barriers to care, such as various socioeconomic issues of the patient. These issues might include poverty, unemployment, poor nutrition, low educational attainment, and housing insecurity. By addressing diversity and inclusion, nurses ensure that decisions are fair, nondiscriminatory, and responsive to the diverse needs of their specific patient population.

Excellence in Ethical Decision-Making

Excellence in nursing involves the nurse being committed to (a) using current evidence-based practice through research identification and critique, (b) lifelong learning through attending appropriate skill and education-based programs to improve knowledge or obtain further academic degrees or certifications, and (c) a continued pursuit of delivering the highest quality of patient care. Excellence ensures that ethical decisions are made using the best available evidence and addressing effective patient outcomes. For instance, when considering whether to adopt a new technology or treatment, excellence drives nurses to evaluate its ethical implications, weigh potential benefits and risks, and advocate for its appropriate use in best care delivery. By striving for excellence, nurses ensure that their decisions are not only ethical but also grounded in the most current knowledge and best practices. This will ultimately enhance patient care delivery.

Respecting Patient Autonomy, Dignity, and Cultural Differences

Respecting patient autonomy, dignity, and cultural differences is core to effective nursing care. These principles are essential for providing care that addresses the individual needs and values of each patient. They foster trust and help build meaningful patient relationships. Respect for patient autonomy empowers individuals to make informed decisions about their health, while upholding dignity ensures that patients are treated with compassion and respect, regardless of any circumstances being experienced. Embracing cultural differences enhances nursing practice by promoting inclusivity and improving the health care quality provided to diverse patients. It is important that nurses navigate patient scenarios with sensitivity, empathy, and cultural competence to ensure that care is both equitable and patient-centered. By respecting patient autonomy, dignity, and cultural differences, nurses can contribute to the physical, emotional, and spiritual well-being of their patients (Adib-Hajbaghery & Aghajani, 2015).

Respecting Patient Autonomy

Respect for patient **autonomy** is a foundational principle in nursing. It emphasizes the right for each patient to make decisions about their health care. Autonomy recognizes that patients are individuals with unique values, beliefs, and life experiences that influence their health care choices. Respect is given by nurses when they accurately and comprehensively provide information about diagnosis, treatment options, and potential outcomes, to patients in order to facilitate informed decisions. Nurse respect empowers patients to take ownership of their health. It fosters nurse-patient relationship trust and collaboration. Nurses actively listen and give respect when they accept patient choices, even when those choices differ from their professional opinion. It is important that nurses support patients without coercion or judgment. This can be difficult as nurses may feel strongly about the benefits of a specific treatment option. Upholding the ethical principle of respect for persons ensures that health care remains patient-centered. By demonstrating respect, nurses affirm patients' dignity and also build a foundation of trust that strengthens the nurse-patient relationship.

Upholding Patient Dignity

A nurse who provides patient ***dignity*** has "respect for human individuality and treating each individual as a unique human being" (Parandeh et al., 2016). It can be influenced by many things, including the level of independence, perceived control, symptom management, and healthcare provider attitude. Dignity reflects inherent worth, regardless of patients' health conditions or circumstances. Factors that influence dignity and reflect its inherent worth make the word *dignity* multidimensional. In order to uphold patient dignity, it is important for nurses to know their patients. Dignity can be promoted by treating patients with kindness, humanity, respect, and compassion; seeing patients as people beyond their illness; getting to know the whole person; and including patients in all conversations and decisions. These practices promote physical comfort and affirm patients' emotional and psychological well-being.

By demonstrating patient dignity, nurses represent a commitment to ethical and compassionate care and reaffirm their role as patient advocates. This focus on preserving dignity fosters an environment of respect and safety, encouraging patients to engage more actively in their care and overall recovery.

Embracing Cultural Differences

The **Transcultural Nursing** theory was introduced by Madeleine Leininger in 1991. Leininger's transcultural nursing is also called *Culture Care Theory* in the literature. Leininger (1995) defined *transcultural nursing* as:

> a substantive area of study and practice focused on comparative cultural care (caring) values, beliefs, and practices of individuals or groups of similar or different cultures with the goal of providing

> culture-specific and universal nursing care practices in promoting health or well-being or to help people to face unfavorable human conditions, illness, or death in culturally meaningful ways. (Nursing Theory, n.d.)

Based on Leininger's work, cultural knowledge for nurses is important to understanding variations necessary to support patient compliance with care requirements, promote healing, and assist patients in achieving overall wellness (Busher Betancourt, 2015).

Transcultural nursing is an essential aspect of nursing today as the ever-increasing U.S. population becomes multicultural. Nursing has not significantly increased in diversity and falls far behind the multicultural population whom nurses serve. Nursing is mostly a homogenous group. According to the American Association of Colleges of Nursing (2024b), 80% of nurses are White/Caucasian. Other races fall far behind, with 7.4% being Asian, 6.3% Black/African American, 0.4% Native American or Alaskan Native, and 0.4% Native Hawaiian or Pacific Islander. This poses a significant challenge for nurses to provide individualized care that is holistic in nature.

The ever-changing population landscape requires nurses to be competent in the cultural care they provide. ***Cultural competence*** is defined by Paric and colleagues (2021) as "a set of beliefs, attitudes, knowledge, and skills that can be adapted to manage cultural differences in work settings" (p. 2). It is essential in order for nurses to provide care that is respectful of and responsive to the diverse backgrounds of their patients. Cultural competence is the ability to effectively work with and care for a variety of patients regardless of their heritage or background (Tosun et al., 2021). It is a process that requires "self-awareness, cultural humility, and the commitment to understanding and embracing culture" (National Association of Social Workers, 2015, p. 4).

Embracing cultural differences involves understanding that every patient's values, beliefs, and practices are shaped by their unique cultural identity. Nurses demonstrate awareness of cultural differences by seeking to learn about the cultural norms and expectations of their patients. They then incorporate this knowledge into their daily patient care activities. They work to accommodate cultural identities regardless of their personal opinions or beliefs. For example, they refrain from calling patients by their first name and instead respectfully address them as *Mr.*, *Mrs.*, or *Ms.* They strive to work with

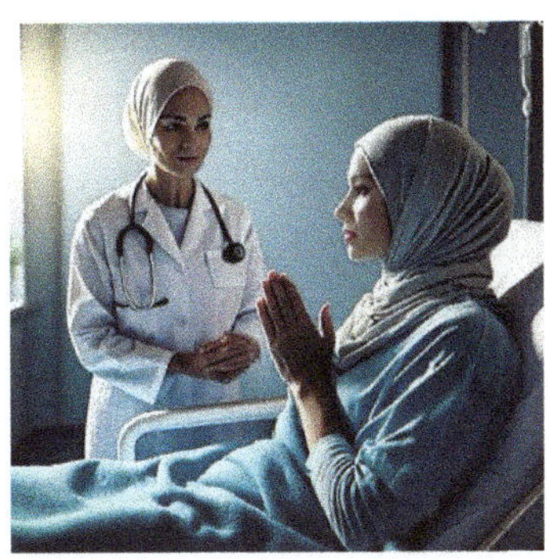

FIGURE 4.2 Patient Praying Before a Procedure

dietary resources in order to ensure that patients' meals align with cultural dietary requirements. Nurses respect their patients' desire to say a prayer as they are prepared for a procedure to be performed by the physician at the bedside (see Figure 4.2). These actions demonstrate cultural respect.

Embracing diversity for nurses also extends beyond accommodating cultural practices and respect for patients. It means that nurses must address structural barriers that may hinder equitable care for patients. Nurses must advocate for patients who face language barriers by requesting interpreters or using communication aids. They must address practices that are discriminatory and that reduce the ability of patients to receive equitable care. They must be knowledgeable of resources to assist patients in facing socioeconomic challenges. Embracing diversity activities fosters an inclusive patient care environment, helps build a positive nurse-patient relationship, and promotes trust.

Integrating Respect Into Holistic Care

Nursing is grounded in holistic principles. These principles provide an in-depth understanding of patients and their needs from a total healthcare perspective. This care is comprehensive and goes beyond treating illness. The whole-person perspective involves addressing physical, emotional, social, and spiritual needs. All play a part in patients' recovery and return to wellness as well as maintaining that state of wellness. Nightingale (1859) said it best, as she emphasized the importance of nature in the healing process along with nursing's role:

> It is often thought that medicine is the curative process. It is no such thing. ... Surgery removes the bullet out of the limb, which is an obstruction to cure, but nature heals the wound. So it is with medicine; medicine so far as we know, assists nature to remove the obstruction, but does nothing more. And what nursing has to do in either case, is to put the patient in the best condition for nature to act upon him. (pp. 74–75)

Holistic care is key to addressing all parts of patients' health. Respecting autonomy, dignity, and cultural differences is integral to the practice of holistic nursing care. It promotes nurse recognition that a patient's well-being extends beyond their physical condition and treatment, encompassing their total individual experiences, values, and goals. By integrating respect for autonomy, dignity, and culture into care, nurses create a personalized approach that honors the uniqueness of each patient. The importance of holistic care can be demonstrated by incorporating items that address areas other than treatment activities on patients' care plan, such as spirituality.

This would demonstrate nurse recognition that spirituality plays a key role in the patients' healing process. Such activities could be identified through collaboration with patients to identify items of importance from their culture or heritage. This collaboration empowers patients and creates a supportive healthcare environment in which they feel seen, heard, and valued.

Summary

The core nursing values of caring, integrity, diversity and inclusion, and excellence emphasize that the profession extends beyond merely providing hands-on care to patients. It requires an ability to enhance patients' psychological and emotional self as related to their illness and recovery to health. Caritas are fundamental elements of the nursing profession. They play a vital role in shaping how nurses care for diverse patient populations. Nurses adopt a multifaceted approach that includes respecting patient autonomy, dignity, and cultural differences. These are important to promote advocacy, respect for patients and families, and an understanding of patients from various cultural backgrounds. They can serve as foundations for addressing ethical dilemmas that may arise. While the field of nursing is complex, embracing core nursing values can help alleviate the sense of being overwhelmed that nurses may feel as they strive to deliver high-quality care.

References

Adib-Hajbaghery, M., & Aghajani, M. (2015). Patients dignity in nursing. Nursing *and Midwifery Studies*, *4*(1), e22809. https://pmc.ncbi.nlm.nih.gov/articles/PMC4377527/

Akbari, A., & Nasiri, A. (2022). A concept analysis of Watson's nursing Caritas process. *Nursing Forum*, *57*(6), 1465–1471. https://doi.org/10.1111/nuf.12771

American Association of Colleges of Nursing. (2024a). *Enhancing diversity in the nursing workforce*. https://www.aacnnursing.org/Portals/0/PDFs/Fact-Sheets/Enhancing-Diversity-Factsheet.pdf

American Association of Colleges of Nursing. (2024b). *Nursing* workforce *fact sheet*. https://www.aacnnursing.org/news-data/fact-sheets/nursing-workforce-fact-sheet

Arthur, D., Pang, S., Wong, T., Alexander, M. F., Drury, J., Eastwood, Johansson, I., Jooste, K., Naude, M., Noh, C. H., O'Brien, A., Sohng, K. Y., Stevenson, G. R., Sy-Sinda, M. T., Thorne, S., van der Wal, D., & Xiao, S. (1999). Caring attributes, professional self concept and technological influences in a sample of Registered

Nurses in eleven countries. *International Journal of Nursing Studies*, *36*(5), 387–396. https://doi.org/10.1016/s0020-7489(99)00035-8

Busher Betancourt, D. A. (2015). Madeleine Leininger and the Transcultural Theory of Nursing. *The Downtown Review*, *2*(1). https://engagedscholarship.csuohio.edu/tdr/vol2/iss1/1

Epstein, B., & Turner, M. (2015). The nursing code of ethics: Its value, its history. *OJIN: The Online Journal of Issues in Nursing*, *20*(2). https://doi.org/10.3912/ojin.vol20no02man04

Fahrenwald, N. L., Bassett, S. D., Tschetter, L., Carson, P. P., White, L., & Winterboer, V. J. (2005). Teaching core nursing values. *Journal of Professional Nursing: Official Journal of the American Association of Colleges of Nursing*, *21*(1), 46–51. https://doi.org/10.1016/j.profnurs.2004.11.001

Ghanbari-Afra, L., Adib-Hajbaghery, M., & Dianati, M. (2022). Human caring: A concept analysis. *Journal of Caring Sciences*, *11*(4), 246–254. https://doi.org/10.34172/jcs.2022.21

Hemberg, J., & Salmela, S. (2021). Integrity and efficiency in nursing leadership: An integrative review. *International Journal of Caring Sciences*, *14*(2), 1496–1513.

Leininger, M. (1995) *Culture Care Diversity & Universality: A theory of nursing.* National League for Nursing Press.

Matiti, M., Cotrel-Gibbons, E., & Teasdale, K. (2007). Promoting patient dignity in healthcare settings. *Nursing Standard*, *21*(45), 46–52.

Morris, G. (2025, October 27). *How nurses can advocate for patients.* NurseJournal.org. https://nursejournal.org/articles/how-to-advocate-for-patients/

National Association of Social Workers. (2015). *Standards and* indicators *for cultural competence.* https://www.socialworkers.org/LinkClick.aspx?fileticket=PonPTDEBrn4%3D

National League for Nursing. (n.d.). *Core values.* https://www.nln.org/about/about/core-values

Nightingale, F. (1859) *Notes on nursing: What it is and what it is not.* Harrison and Sons, London.

Nursing Theory. (n.d.). *Culture care theory.* https://nursing-theory.org/theories-and-models/leininger-culture-care-theory.php

Parandeh, A., Khaghanizade, M., Mohammadi, E., & Mokhtari-Nouri, J. (2016). Nurses' human dignity in education and practice: An integrated literature review. *Iranian Journal of Nursing and Midwifery Research*, *21*(1). https://doi.org/10.4103/1735-9066.174750

Paric, M., Kaihlanen, A. M., Heponiemi, T., & Czabanowska, K. (2021). Nurse teacher's perceptions on teaching cultural competence to students in Finland: A descriptive qualitative study. *Nurse Education Today*, *99*, 104787. https://doi.org/10.1016/j.nedt.2021.104787

Poorchangizi, B., Borhani, F., Abbaszadeh, A., Mirzaee, M., & Farokhzadian, J. (2019). The importance of professional values from nursing students' perspective. *BMC Nursing, 18*, 26. https://doi.org/10.1186/s12912-019-0351-1

SadatHoseini, A., Shareinia, H., Pashaeypoor, S., & Mohammadi, M. (2023). A cross-cultural concept analysis of healing in nursing: A hybrid model. *BMC Nursing, 22*(1), 252. https://doi.org/10.1186/s12912-023-01404-8

Tosun, B., Yava, A., Dirgar, E., Şahin, E. B., Yılmaz, E. B., Papp, K., Tóthova, V., Hellerova, V., Prosen, M., Licen, S., Karnjus, I., Tamayo, M. D. B., Leyva-Moral, J. M., Claeys, A., & Tricas-Sauras, S. (2021). Addressing the effects of transcultural nursing education on nursing students' cultural competence: A systematic review. *Nurse Education in Practice, 55*, 103171. https://doi.org/10.1016/j.nepr.2021.103171

Watson Caring Science Institute. (n.d.). *10 Caritas processes*. Watson Caring Science Institute. https://www.watsoncaringscience.org/about-wcsi/jean-bio/caring-science-theory/10-caritas-processes/

Image Credits

Fig. 4.2: Generated using Adobe Firefly.

CHAPTER 5

The Healthcare Delivery Setting

Objectives

Upon completion of this chapter, the learner will be able to do the following:

1. Describe various settings for patient management and care delivery.
2. Explain the unique features, services provided, and patient populations typically served in various healthcare delivery settings.
3. Analyze how the roles and responsibilities of nurses vary depending on the healthcare setting.
4. Assess challenges faced by nurses in various healthcare settings.

Key Chapter Terms

- Nursing workforce
- Acute care hospital
- Primary care clinic
- Specialty care clinic
- Urgent care center
- Home health care
- Long-term care
- Nursing home
- Assisted living facility
- Hospice care
- Rehabilitation center
- Mental health facility
- Telehealth

The Healthcare Delivery Setting

Nurses deliver health care in a variety of settings. These range from organizational delivery within the confines of a designated area, such as **acute care hospitals**, rehabilitation centers, community health centers, and clinics, to areas outside organizations, such as home care. Technology has now been integrated into the setting with telehealth and computer-based delivery settings lacking brick-and-mortar components. For optimum care delivery, organizations offer a variety of services or include access to these services. Nurses interact with individuals and other healthcare providers in these settings to promote continuity of care delivery. Patients can move through the system with nurse assistance and guidance. This interdisciplinary approach to the delivery of care works to promote the best outcomes for patients and families.

The Nursing Workforce

In 2022, there was an estimated 4,349,377 licensed registered nurses (RNs) in the United States, with 3,459,209, or 80%, employed in various healthcare settings (see Figure 5.1).

General or specialty inpatient settings employed the greatest number of the RN workforce (N = 795,682; 23%). Ambulatory care settings employed the next highest number (N = 452,013; 13%) of nurses. Overall hospitals employed 57.5% of RNs. Trends for employment settings have changed for nurses (see Table 5.1 and Figure 5.2). Between 2017 and 2022, there was an increase in the number of nurses working in hospitals, ambulatory care, and public health. There was no significant change in other areas of nursing employment settings (Health Resources and Services Administration, 2024).

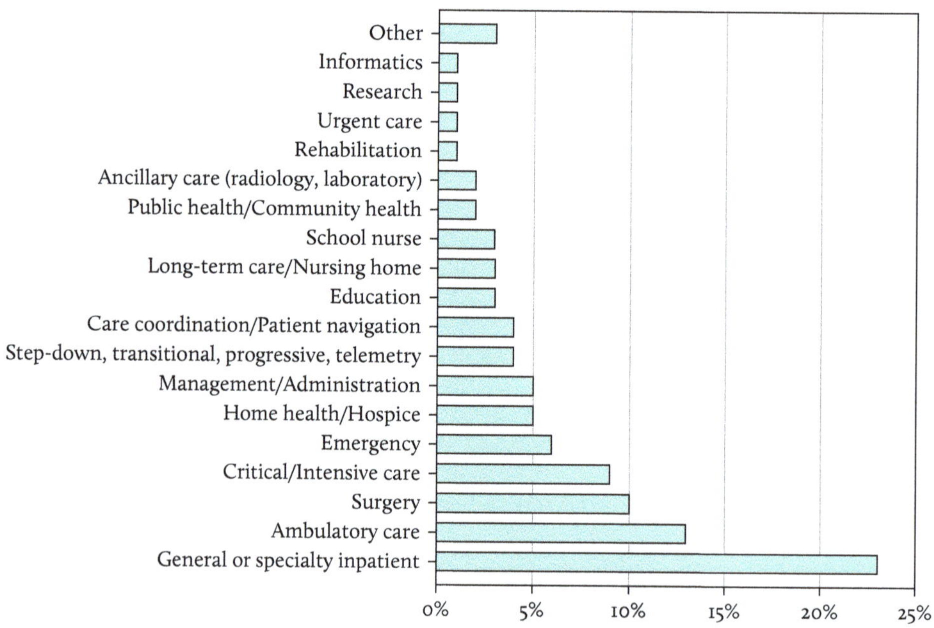

FIGURE 5.1 Employment Settings of Registered Nurses by Percentages

TABLE 5.1 Employment Settings of Registered Nurses, 2017–2022, by Number (Rounded)

Type	2017	2020	2022
Hospital	21,647	18,442	133,912
Ambulatory care	296,030	326,843	387,190
Home health care	136,765	150,025	124,744
Hospice	61,471	67,365	66,623
Education	83,466	95,318	78,324
Long-term care/nursing home	150,865	148,526	143,994
School health services	83,178	105,678	86,826
Public health/community health	539	408	3,832.20
Correctional facility	23,918	27,743	24,338
Other	310,178	327,483	358,155

Source: Developed by the author from data retrieved from Smiley et al., 2023.

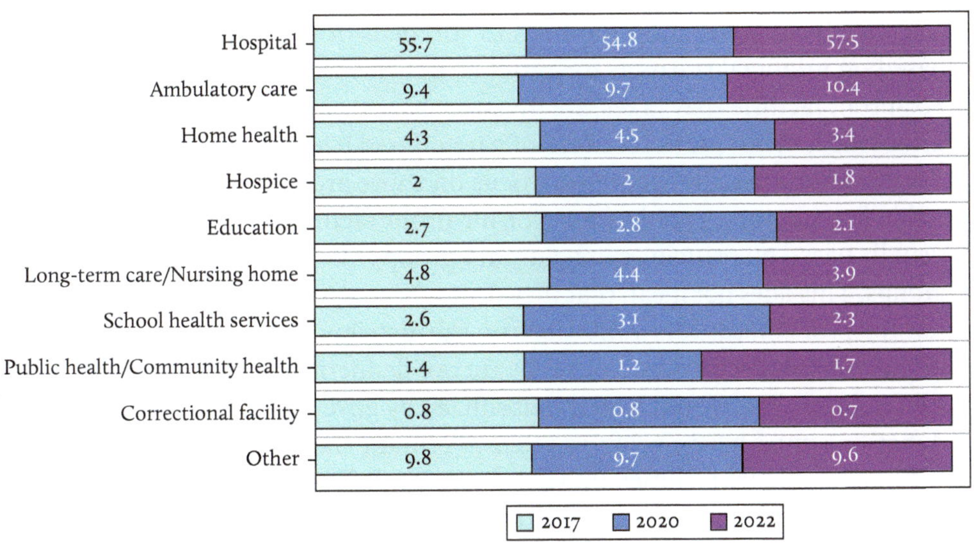

FIGURE 5.2 Employment Settings of Registered Nurses, 2017–2022, by Percentage

Types of Healthcare Delivery Settings

Acute Care Hospital Settings

Hospitals are large medical centers that offer care for a wide range of situations (Liu & Kelz, 2018). Some situations may require overview and

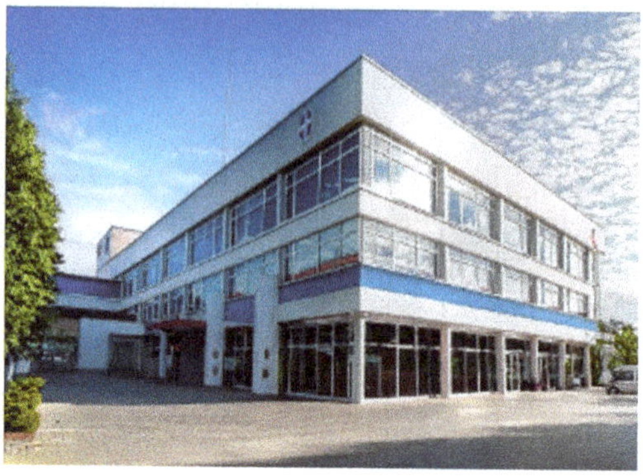
IMAGE 5.1 Hospital

intermittent interventions that would be difficult to obtain in another setting (e.g., trauma care). They are designed to provide 24-hour emergency care. They handle emergencies, perform surgeries, and provide intensive care for critically ill patients. Hospitals are typically divided into departments that focus on specific care areas, such as cardiology, oncology, surgery, maternity, and pediatrics. This division allows specialized care for patients, ensuring that they receive the appropriate treatments based on specific health needs. Hospitals are equipped to handle life-threatening conditions, such as heart attacks, strokes, severe injuries, and other urgent medical crises. They have intensive care and trauma units for patients who require constant monitoring and advanced life support.

Hospitals are generally classified based on their size and specialty. Hospitals can vary from fewer than 100 beds to 500 beds or more. Facilities are also based on financial status as for-profit or not-for-profit (Bazzoli et al., 2010). For-profit facilities pay taxes, are investor-owned, and provide care based on achieving a mean profit for areas of care offered (Cronin et al., 2021). These organizations usually attempt to focus on those areas of care that are profitable for their geographic area. Not-for-profit facilities are tax-exempt and usually based on principles or voluntary groups like religious or community groups. This does not mean that they do not have a positive profit margin. The not-for-profit status sets limitations on the distribution of profits, the ability or inability to receive donations that are tax-deductible, and tax exemptions. All facilities that are not heavily subsidized by government funds or private donations must have a profit in order to remain viable in health care.

Many acute care facilities are accredited in an effort to be eligible for federal grants and work with educational programs. This accreditation is offered by The Joint Commission, which has a vision of safe, high-quality, best-value care. Additional information may be retrieved from http://www.jointcommission.org/. Joint Commission accreditation is voluntary but considered to be an indication of status and verification of quality. Nurses working in these organizations during accreditation site visits work within the organizational goals and objectives to achieve a successful outcome.

Some organizations have also achieved Magnet Recognition Program® status. This program recognizes healthcare organizations that have achieved a high level of quality care, excellence in nursing, and nursing practice innovations (Abuzied et al., 2022). Consumers identify Magnet designation as validation of high-quality nursing care. Magnet Recognition was developed by the American Nurses Credentialing Center (ANCC). The mission of the Magnet Recognition Program is to "continually elevate patient care around the world in an environment where nurses, in collaboration with the interprofessional team flourish by setting the standard for excellence through leadership, scientific discovery and dissemination and implementation of new knowledge" (ANCC, n.d.). Characteristics of Magnet organizations include low RN turnover (12.47%), nurse longevity (average 12.26 years), a high percentage of RN decision-makers certified by a nationally recognized organization (68.10%), many nurses certified by a nationally recognized organization (48.44%), and a high number of RNs with bachelor/university degrees or higher (72.39%; ANCC, 2022). Many nurses desire to work in these nurse-focused organizations.

Nurses work shifts that cover services 24 hours a day, seven days a week. They offer orientation or internship periods that may range from a few weeks for general care areas to several months for specialty care areas. Working in this type of facility, whether for-profit or nonprofit, allows the nurse to identify an area that appeals to their personal interest and move within the same organization, which can be beneficial for continuity of benefits and longevity. Benefits for the nurse to remain within the same healthcare organization include eligibility for educational benefits and the ability to transition up a clinical ladder (a multistep program that begins with entry staff positions and progresses in identified steps based on experience, education, and certification). Salary and position eligibility increase as one progresses up the ladder. Nursing responsibility also increases with subsequent steps in the hospital care arena.

Primary and Specialty Care Clinics

Primary Care Clinics

Primary care clinics are healthcare facilities that serve as the first point of contact for individuals seeking medical attention. These clinics can be staffed or owned by family practice physicians or family nurse practitioners who are educated to manage a wide range of health

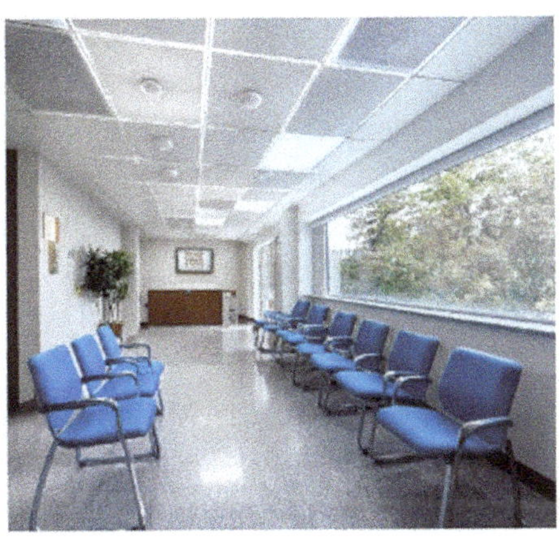

IMAGE 5.2 Clinic

conditions. Nurses in private practice are nurse practitioners or clinical specialists. They may be the only healthcare provider in a designated area. They usually work under protocols and may be in contact with a physician for additional healthcare information. These nurses may diagnose illnesses, admit patients to healthcare facilities, refer patients for further diagnostic treatment or immediate care intervention to a hospital, and/or prescribe medications as needed by patients. Nurses in these situations function within their scope of practice based on their state of residency and/or practice. These nurses own or manage their clinic as a business venture and must continue to balance care and financial obligations. Nurses who own their own businesses must manage employees and all situations that accompany this responsibility (e.g., payroll, contracts, employee tax requirements); appropriate business taxes; advertising for services; fees for services offered; and patient records maintained in a confidential manner. This responsibility list may be increased by activities that involve collaboration with state or federal organizations or academic institutions. Nurse-owned clinic settings are usually owned by nurses with graduate degrees. Nurse employees who work in these settings may work variable hours. These offices may offer eight or 10 daytime work hours with no or minimal weekend work hours. These offices are often closed on major holidays.

One of the key roles of primary care is early identification and management of chronic diseases such as diabetes, hypertension, heart disease, asthma, and arthritis. Patients with chronic diseases often require regular checkups in primary care clinics in order to monitor their health and make needed adjustments to treatment plans, including medications. They can refer patients to specialists if more advanced care is needed. Many primary care providers have long standing relationships with their patients and help them with health management and well-being.

Primary care clinics offer a wide range of preventive services, including immunizations, cancer screenings (e.g., mammograms), blood pressure monitoring, cholesterol checks, and advice on lifestyle components, such as diet and exercise. Health education offered serves as a guide to weight loss, smoking cessation, and other health-related patient concerns. Healthcare providers in these clinics collaborate with patients to ensure continuous, comprehensive care.

Specialty Care Clinics

Specialty care clinics are facilities focused on specific areas of health care. They offer advanced diagnosis and treatment for particular medical conditions. These clinics are often staffed by specialists—doctors with advanced training in areas such as cardiology, dermatology, orthopedics, neurology, and oncology. Patients are usually referred to these clinics by a primary care provider when they require treatments or interventions that are beyond the scope of general medicine. Specialty care clinics provide outpatient consultations and perform diagnostic or therapeutic procedures that do not require hospitalization.

Services offered in specialty care clinics can include cardiology-specific tests for diagnosis and management (e.g., stress tests, echocardiograms) and heart disease management (e.g., arrhythmias, heart failure, and coronary artery disease). Orthopedic clinics may provide services such as physical therapy, joint injections, and treatments for musculoskeletal disease and injuries. Oncology clinics focus on diagnosing and treating cancer and offering chemotherapy, radiation therapy, and access to clinical trials for the latest treatments. Specialty care clinics may have advanced diagnostic equipment, such as magnetic resonance imaging scanners, computed tomography scanners, and specialized lab services in order to identify and manage complex conditions.

Specialty care clinics allow patients to receive patient-focused care. These clinics often work in conjunction with hospitals and other healthcare providers to ensure comprehensive, coordinated care for patients. Specialists in these settings may also work closely with researchers to offer patients access to cutting-edge treatments and clinical trials.

Nurses play a vital role in these organizations. Roles for the nurse can include patient assessment, monitoring, education, and coordination of care in specialty care clinics. They perform complete admission assessments for patients reporting for care and interventions. They reassess patient conditions as needed to evaluate responses to treatments. They provide disease management education that is specific and at the patient level of understanding. Nurses function in a consultative and collaborative role to healthcare providers in managing patients. They provide follow-through and support to assist patients with managing their conditions. In the specialty care clinic, they promote integration of holistic care management, moving the patient toward desired healthcare outcomes.

Urgent Care Centers

Urgent care centers provide immediate medical care for conditions that are not life- threatening but still require prompt attention. These centers are designed to fill the gap between primary care and emergency care, offering services outside of typical office hours. They require no appointment. Patients visit urgent care centers for minor injuries, such as sprains, cuts, and fractures, as well as common illnesses, such as the flu, ear infections, and strep throat. Urgent care centers are typically staffed by physicians, nurse practitioners,

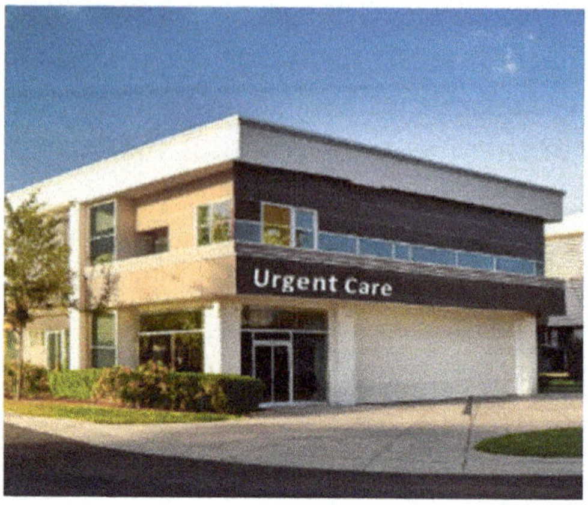

IMAGE 5.3 Urgent Care

and physician assistants who can diagnose and treat a wide range of conditions.

Urgent care centers offer a variety of diagnostic and treatment services. Many have on-site laboratories to quickly diagnose infections and imaging equipment, such as X-rays, to diagnose fractures. They also provide services such as wound care, splinting, and stitches for lacerations, making them a convenient option for patients who need immediate care but do not require hospitalization. For common illnesses, urgent care providers can prescribe medications, offer vaccinations, and provide treatments such as intravenous (IV) fluids or breathing treatments for asthma attacks.

Nurses working in these areas triage patients while gathering information. Following examination by a physician, nurse practitioner, or physician assistant, the nurse will perform any tasks needed for additional diagnosis (e.g., drawing blood or starting an IV line for fluid or medication administration). Nurses may also process blood for on-site test results. This area can be fast-paced, requiring the nurse to continuously employ critical thinking skills and multitask, reprioritizing tasks based on the changing patient situation.

Urgent care centers serve as intermediaries and promote streamlining healthcare systems. Nurses in these environments work to ensure that patients receive an appropriate level of care based on their needs. Urgent care centers are often part of larger health systems, allowing for better coordination of care if a patient needs to be referred for follow-up treatment or interventions beyond the scope of the center (e.g., surgical intervention). These centers serve to promote timely intervention for non–life-threatening situations.

Home Health Care

Home health care refers to a range of medical and support services provided in a patient's home for those who are recovering from an illness or surgery or managing chronic conditions (Home Care Association of America, 2016). Services are often prescribed by a physician and may include skilled nursing care, physical therapy, and assistance with activities of daily living (ADLs). Home care services may be given by physicians, home care aides, nurses, and therapists who collaboratively work to promote out-of-facility care and keep the patient in their home, promoting independence and improving quality of life. Home care is a cost-effective and convenient type of care. An individual plan of patient care is developed based on needs. This type of plan involves (a) addressing needed services; (b) identifying healthcare professionals to provide the identified services; (c) determining the frequency of needed services; (d) determining the medical equipment needed for effective care or personal activities (e.g., walking [e.g., tripod, walker or crutches], toileting needs [e.g., high-rise lift on toilet seat or bathroom railing supports]); and (e) addressing expected results from treatment regimens.

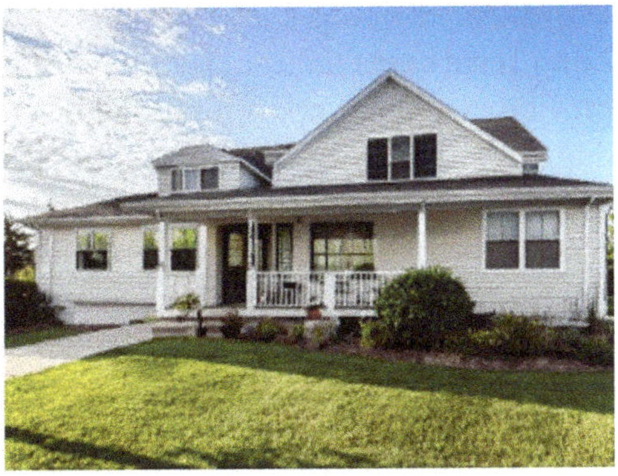

IMAGE 5.4 Home Health Care

Nurses provide specialized care such as changing wound dressings, administering medications, and monitoring vital signs. They also educate patients and caregivers on disease management, helping patients adhere to their plan of care. Physical, occupational, and speech therapy may also be provided at home, allowing patients to regain strength, mobility, and communication skills without the need to travel for care. Therapists work with patients to improve their ability to perform daily tasks, enhancing their independence. Nurses assess patients to identify results from therapies and work to prevent complications such as wound infections. They also teach the patient, family members, and friends included in the care circle to effectively implement care activities, recognize complications, and know whom to contact for healthcare problems.

Nurses usually work for a specific agency and implement specific physician-approved plans of care. Hours of work may vary from agency to agency and state to state. This type of nursing may require traveling to various counties based on area of coverage by the agency and caseload (i.e., the number of patients to be seen and type of nursing care to be administered). Confidence in patient management abilities and astute assessment skills are important components of this type of care. Validation of care is essential to reimbursement, so nurses may keep electronic or paper information. Nurses have access to physicians and other healthcare providers when referral care or specific orders are needed based on patient assessment. As society ages, home healthcare opportunities are increasing. This type of care is a flexible, patient-centered option that meets the evolving needs of individuals in their own homes.

Long-Term Care Facilities

Long-term care facilities, such as nursing homes and assisted living centers, provide care and support for individuals who are unable to live independently due to age, disability, or chronic illness. Long-term care is comprised of a variety of services that provide care to individuals who have chronic diseases or conditions that do not allow for self-care. These facilities offer 24-hour supervision and medical care, along with assistance with activities of daily living (ADLs), such as eating, bathing, dressing, and mobility. Long-term care facilities are designed for residents who require constant monitoring and support, whether due to physical limitations (e.g., 32-year-old male quadriplegic following an automobile accident), cognitive impairments such as dementia (e.g., 76-year-old woman who wanders), or complex medical needs (e.g., 80-year-old man who suffered a stroke and has right-sided paralysis, facial weakness, and difficulty swallowing). They serve a variety of age ranges and have a homelike environment where individuals can receive care. Individuals in these facilities often retain control of their care and are given opportunities to retain as much independence as they desire. Long-term care communities are designed to offer variety in care based on personal need.

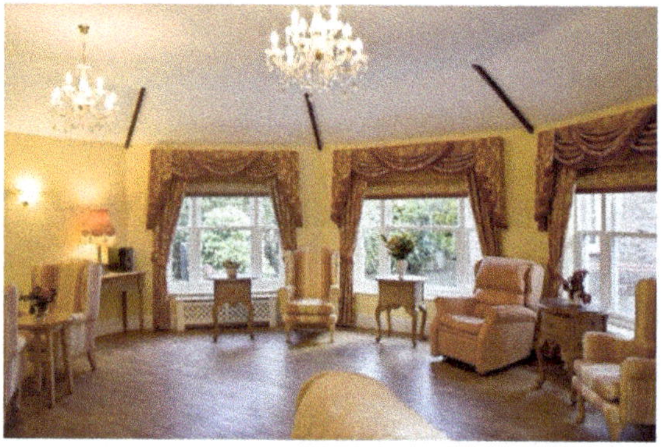

IMAGE 5.5 Assisted Living

Nursing homes, a common type of long-term care facility, offer skilled nursing services to individuals who need regular medical attention (Moilanen et al., 2022). RNs, licensed practical nurses (LPNs), and certified nursing assistants provide around-the-clock care. RNs and LPNs administer medications, perform wound care, and monitor chronic conditions such as heart disease and diabetes. In addition to medical care, nursing homes also offer rehabilitation services, such as physical therapy and occupational therapy, to help residents maintain or regain functional abilities (Gutenbrunner et al., 2021). Many facilities also offer specialized units for individuals with memory care needs, providing tailored support for those with Alzheimer's disease or other forms of dementia.

Nursing homes are not just for older individuals who can no longer manage their own care due to illness or debilitation. These places may offer an alternative to individuals with injuries or acute illnesses or those needing additional postoperative care with the need to recover outside a hospital. Many nursing homes are set up organizationally like acute care hospitals with limited diagnostic and therapeutic departments. They can offer both long-term and short-term care based on residents' need. They may also be affiliated with an acute care facility or a hospital with transfer capabilities when a higher level of care is required for residents. The level of skill and expertise offered by nursing homes can vary widely. Some provide a continuum of care for individuals ranging from home care to skilled nursing care. They may have the ability to implement sustainable interventions, such as IV fluids for dehydration and enteral feedings (administration of nutrition through a feeding tube placed through the nose or mouth into the stomach) to maintain nutritional status. Oxygen administration may be implemented to increase circulating oxygen levels in the blood to accelerate activity tolerance. Some nursing homes have subacute or specialty units. A subacute unit offers a continuum of care that may be initiated in an acute care hospital but at a lower level of intensity while providing needed support, such as rehabilitation. This intermittent care may be provided until the person can return to a prior living arrangement. Specialty units may exist for individuals with (a) Alzheimer's disease or other forms of dementia, (b) respiratory care needs beyond oxygen administration or for patients who have tracheostomies or are on ventilators (breathing machines) to assist with breathing, or (c) kidney failure needing renal dialysis (the use of a machine to perform the normal functions of the kidneys, such as removal of waste and fluid). Some of these units have residents who require sophisticated, labor-intensive, 24-hour care. Nurses working in subacute units perform care much like that administered in an acute care hospital but for individuals who need to be maintained instead of having interventional, episodic care. Nurses who work in long-term care facilities enjoy working with geriatric individuals, as many of the residents of these facilities are older. They like the interaction and assistance they can provide individuals as they age. They can work with individuals and their families in managing health situations, administering care, and offering referrals for the health care of older individuals (Zimmerman et al., 2022).

Assisted living facilities cater to individuals who may not need intensive medical care but still require some degree of help with personal care and daily activities. These facilities offer a more independent living environment, where residents have private or semiprivate rooms and access to communal dining, social activities, and transportation services. Residents may be assisted with ADLs, given reminders regarding medication administration, or given support activity services through enrichment classes such as jewelry-making or dance classes. Assisted living can be offered in facilities that are standalone buildings or as floors in a continuing-care retirement community building.

The physical environment is designed to influence psychological health through a more homelike appearance. Buildings may also be set up in an apartment style with various rooms and layout alternatives, from private rooms to suites. Many assisted living facilities have common areas that are designed for relaxation and comfort and promote meaningful activities and resident interactions. They may have garden areas and atriums with fireplaces. Some offer central dining areas with pleasant surroundings and entertainment. Nurses in these facilities assess and monitor resident health conditions and assist with medication management. These state-regulated facilities use nurses based on the degree of care provided. Hours of work can vary, and some with in-resident care are set up with shift work like that in acute care facilities. They may offer eight- to 12-hour shifts. Nurses assess and manage situations related to the residents' health care. Other on-site staff are available to perform housekeeping tasks and meal preparation, which allows residents to maintain a higher level of autonomy while receiving the support they need. Nurses create individualized care plans that are adjusted over time based on assessment results.

Long-term care facilities provide a social and community-based environment, which promotes resident well-being. Recreational activities, social events, and group programs are offered to encourage collective engagement and prevent isolation. Many facilities provide spiritual care, various therapies, and mental health support to help residents cope with the emotional aspects of aging or chronic illness. Long-term care facilities offer personalized care in a secure, structured setting to meet residents' physical, emotional, and social needs to improve quality of life.

Hospice Care

Hospice care is applicable to hospitals, home health care, and long-term care facilities. Hospice care is focused on end-of-life care (Wajid et al., 2021). This means that it promotes improving the quality of a patient's last weeks or months of life. Hospice care reflects a holistic philosophy, meaning that it works to address issues related to the whole person. This type of care provides evidence-based physical, emotional, psychological,

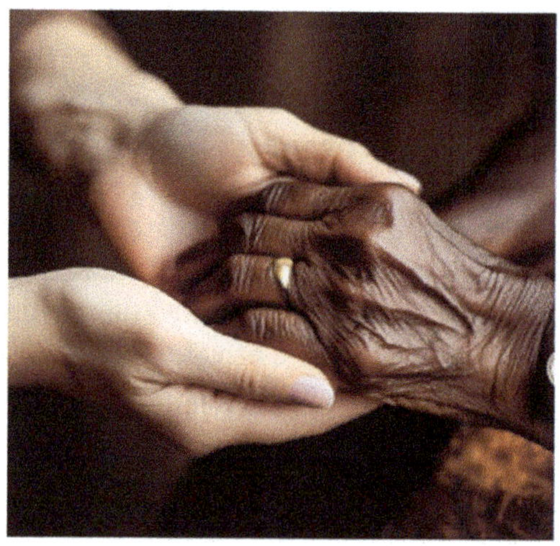

IMAGE 5.6 Hospice Care

and spiritual care to individuals and their families during times of an imminent life-limiting illness. According to the National Hospice and Palliative Care Organization's (2022) standards of practice hospice care is a set of services "coordinated by an interdisciplinary group to provide to provide for the physical, psychosocial, spiritual, and emotional needs of a terminally ill patient and/or family members, as delineated in a specific patient plan of care" (p. 179). Hospice nurses work with patients and their families from identification of the imminent end of life through death and the family bereavement period (American Nurses Association, 2024; Kwon & Byun, 2024).

Hospice care is divided into four levels of care: routine home care, general inpatient care, continuous home care, and respite care. Routine home care can include pain management, symptom management, emotional support, and spiritual counseling for the patient and family. It can also include assistance with daily tasks and services such as nutritional and therapeutic requirements. Home care is provided at whatever site is considered home for the patient, whether a facility or a personal residence. Continuous hospice care is also referred to as *crisis care*. It is initiated when a patient experiences a medical crisis or when disease symptoms require intensive management. This care is offered around the clock or for extended periods of time. Inpatient hospice care occurs when a patient's symptoms can no longer be managed at home. Goals for this type of care include severe pain control and symptom stabilization. This may allow the patient to return home. Respite care allows for occasional, short-term stays in an inpatient center for home hospice patients to give family care providers a break from providing continuous home care activities to a loved one with an advanced illness.

Hospice care incorporates a mixture of care, including home care and care within a facility (Lysaght & Ersek, 2013). Hospice care involves collaborative care between healthcare professionals (e.g., physicians, nurses, social workers, pharmacists, occupational therapists, nutritionists, speech therapists, bereavement coordinators, and pastoral services), family members, and volunteers. Members work within a circle of collaborative care to provide services. Healthcare individuals may enter and leave the circle based on patient needs. Some work techniques by specified healthcare members and volunteers can be seen in Figure 5.3. This list is not all-inclusive, because the number and type of individuals involved in the hospice plan of care will differ based on patient need. The goal of hospice care is to give the dying individual comfort, peace, and dignity in the last days, weeks, or months they have remaining to live. It involves a philosophy that includes interdisciplinary healthcare providers, community members, the patient, and their family. Family members are assisted in coping with the death and loss of the individual they once knew, as the patient's type of life changes from one of independence to dependence. Family will also ultimately deal with the loss of their loved one. Nurses are an integral part of hospice care. They interact with healthcare providers, the patient, and the family. They often become an integral part of their patients' lives and serve to coordinate care between various types of hospice options (e.g., routine home care to respite care). Nurses make home or facility visits and serve to notify other members of the collaborative team of situations that may require further intervention. Although hours may not be continuous, working in this type of healthcare option may require varied hours, from daytime to evening and night.

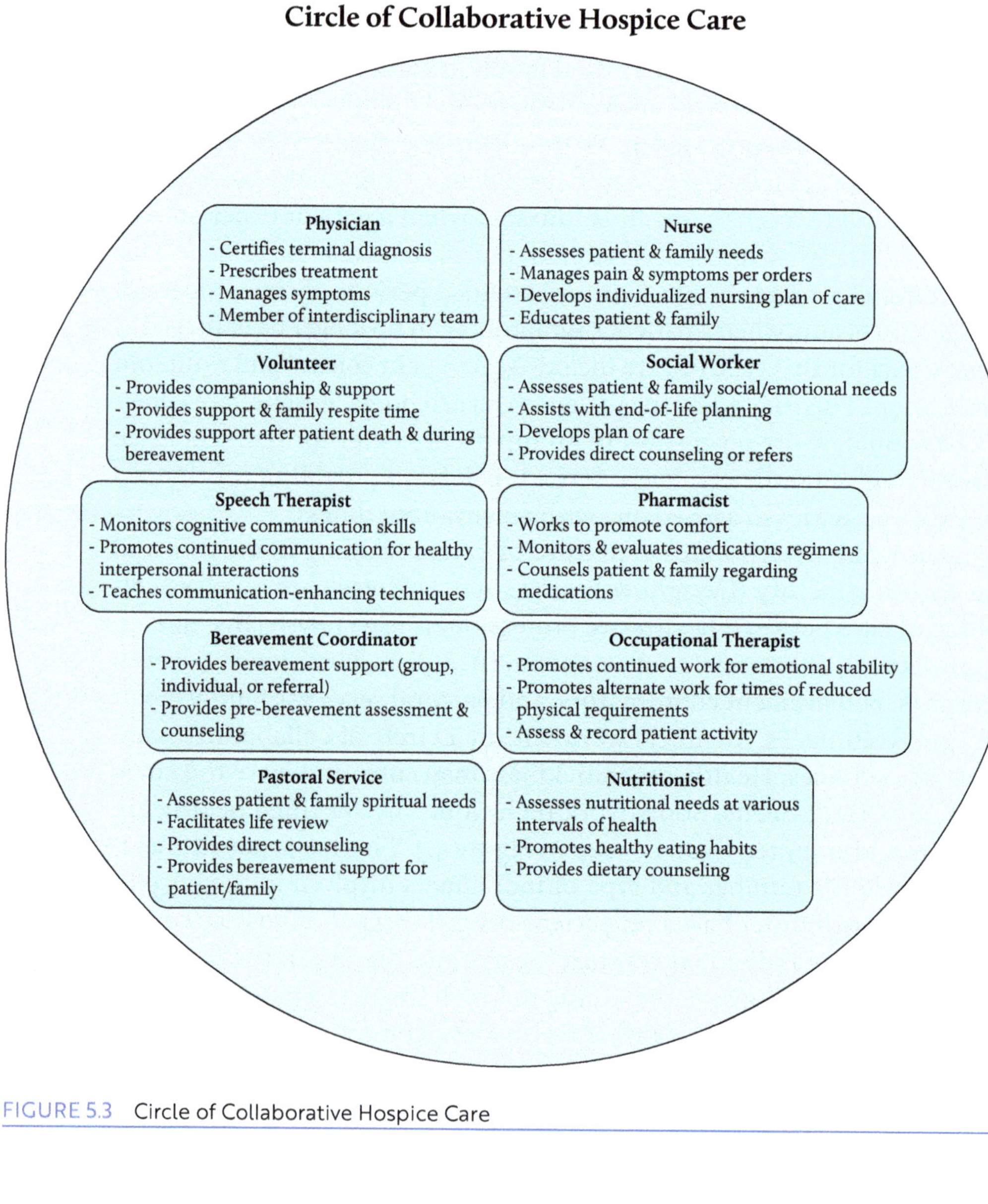

FIGURE 5.3 Circle of Collaborative Hospice Care

Rehabilitation Centers

Rehabilitation centers provide specialized care and therapy to help individuals remain as independent as possible and participate in meaningful life roles. These facilities offer both inpatient and outpatient services designed to restore physical, mental, or cognitive function after a debilitating event. Rehabilitation centers are staffed by a multidisciplinary team of healthcare professionals, including physical therapists, occupational therapists, speech therapists, rehabilitation nurses, and physicians. These centers help patients regain independence, improve mobility, and achieve the highest possible quality of life following a serious health event.

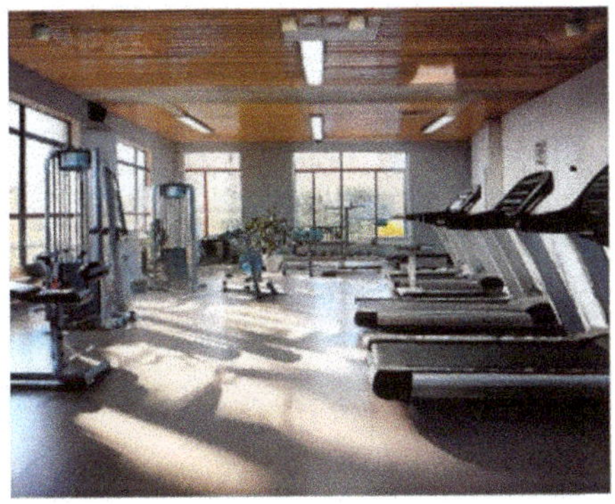

IMAGE 5.7 Rehabilitation Center

In physical rehabilitation centers, patients recovering from orthopedic surgeries, strokes, or traumatic injuries receive individualized treatment plans to improve their strength, balance, and coordination. Physical therapists work with patients to regain movement, manage pain, and improve functional abilities through exercises, manual therapy, and the use of assistive devices such as walkers or braces. Occupational therapists focus on helping patients relearn the skills necessary for daily living, such as dressing, cooking, and bathing, as well as recommend modifications to patients' homes to ensure safety and accessibility. For patients recovering from neurological events such as strokes or brain injuries, speech therapy and cognitive rehabilitation is available. Speech therapists help individuals who have difficulty speaking, swallowing, or communicating due to injury or illness. Cognitive rehabilitation therapists assist patients in regaining memory, attention, and problem-solving skills. The role of the rehabilitation nurse is multifaceted in the rehabilitation setting. They work as a member of the multidisciplinary team to promote the restoration and maintenance of functioning and prevention of complications.

Mental Health Facilities

Mental health facilities offer specialized care and treatment for individuals with emotional difficulties, psychiatric disorders, and substance use disorders (SUDs). They include inpatient psychiatric hospitals, outpatient counseling centers, residential treatment programs, and crisis intervention centers. These facilities are designed to offer a safe and supportive environment

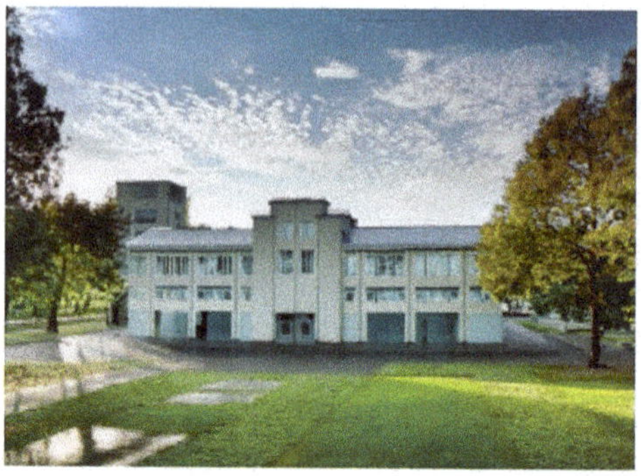

IMAGE 5.8 Rehabilitation

where individuals can receive professional care to manage and overcome their mental health condition, which can include anxiety, depression, schizophrenia, bipolar disorder, and addiction. Services are often delivered by an interdisciplinary team of mental health professionals such as psychiatrists, psychologists, therapists, social workers, and nurses specialized in psychiatric patient management.

Inpatient psychiatric hospitals or facilities offer intensive individualized care for persons experiencing severe mental health crises such as suicidal thoughts, psychosis, or acute emotional distress. These facilities offer 24-hour medical intervention and supervision. Services include medication management, psychotherapy, and crisis stabilization. Inpatient care delivery is usually short-term and focused on patient condition stabilization prior to transition to outpatient care or to an environment that is less restrictive. Inpatient hospitals and facilities may support patients during recovery by offering group therapy, recreational therapy, and family counseling.

Outpatient mental health facilities offer ongoing treatment for individuals who do not require hospitalization. Facilities such as counseling and therapy centers provide a range of services that include individual therapy, group therapy, cognitive behavioral therapy, and medication management. Outpatient care is designed to help individuals manage their symptoms, cope with life stressors, and develop strategies for sustaining long-term mental wellness. Patients often attend regular sessions with a counselor or therapist, which allows them continuous support while maintaining daily routines at work and home.

Residential treatment programs offer long-term care for individuals with chronic mental health conditions or SUDs. These facilities provide a structured environment where patients receive intensive therapy, life skills training, and rehabilitation services over an extended period of time. Residents usually participate in a combination of individual and group therapy sessions, educational programs, and recreational activities. These programs focus on assisting individuals in developing coping mechanisms, improving social skills, and preparing for a successful transition back into their community.

Telehealth

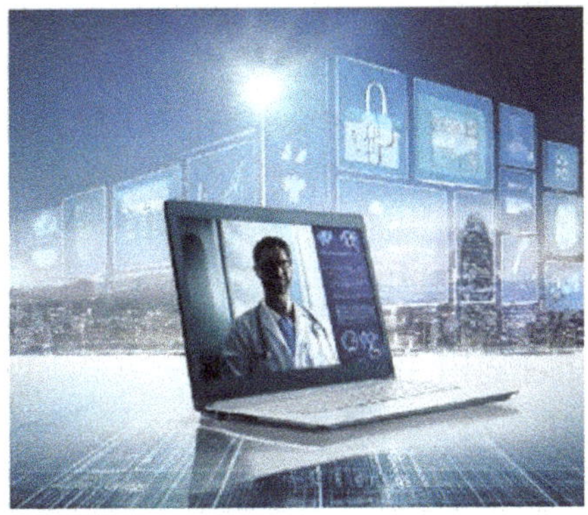

IMAGE 5.9 Telehealth

Telehealth is the delivery of health care services through digital platforms. This enables care to be delivered remotely for consultations, diagnoses, and treatment options. It uses technology-based platforms such as video conferencing, mobile apps, and secure messaging services to connect care providers with patients for care delivery. It is particularly valuable for individuals who reside in rural or underserved areas who may not have easy access to healthcare facilities or providers. It provides options for persons who prefer not to travel to a healthcare destination or are unable to travel due to their medical condition, time constraints, or lack of suitable transportation. Telehealth existed prior to the pandemic; however, during and after this time, it significantly expanded. It provided options for individuals who suffered from pandemic effects or other illnesses and needed the services of a healthcare provider but were unable to go to an office due to distancing measures, which limited face-to-face care delivery.

Telehealth services encompass a wide variety of healthcare delivery, from routine care and follow-ups to specialist appointments for chronic condition management. Patients can schedule virtual appointments with their primary care or other provider for discussions regarding concerns about symptoms, medications, and health monitoring results. Remote monitoring and wearable devices can relay information about an individual's heart rate, blood pressure, blood glucose, oxygen level, and electrocardiogram, to name several. These devices can allow for continuous or intermittent assessment and transmission of data for conditions such as hypertension, diabetes, and heart disease. This helps healthcare providers make informed decisions about treatment plans without requiring a patient clinic visit for data retrieval.

Telehealth also supports mental health services, which allow individuals to privately and remotely receive therapy and counseling. Telepsychiatry and teletherapy allows patients to obtain mental health services from the comfort of their homes, which can reduce barriers such as the stigma of entering an office or transportation required to visit a facility. Telehealth for mental health services offers a safe and confidential space for patients to discuss their concerns in therapy sessions, manage medications, and engage fully in their care. These services have been particularly helpful to promote access to individuals in rural areas or with limited mobility or transportation.

Telehealth supports preventive care educational resources, virtual wellness programs, and access to lifestyle coaches. Health information and guidance available through telehealth services include such topics as nutrition, exercise, stress management, and smoking cessation. This can serve to empower individuals and encourage them to take an active role in their health. Many telehealth services integrate into the patient's electronic health record, which ensures continuity of care. This allows tracking of progress over time. Telehealth has been identified to offer a flexible, accessible, and patient-centered approach to care promoting critical access to many individuals.

Summary

Healthcare delivery offers a variety of settings for all levels of prepared nurses to enjoy throughout their professional careers. Many nurses work in various settings until they identify the setting of their choice and preference. This allows them to experience areas that correlate to their preference, related to their work environment (acute to long-term care) and their life situation (full-time work with a family or part-time work while attending a program of higher education). This allows the nurse to experience satisfaction with their career choice.

References

American Nurses Association. (2024). *Nurses' roles and responsibilities in providing end-of-life care and support at the end of life.* ANA Position Statement. https://www.nursingworld.org/~4932e6/globalassets/docs/ana/practice/official-position-statements/nursesrolesandresponsibilitiesinprovidingcareandsupportattheendoflife_revised_bod-approved_final.pdf

American Nurses Credentialing Center. (n.d.). *About Magnet: The new 2020 Magnet mission and vision statement.* https://www.nursingworld.org/organizational-programs/magnet/about-magnet

American Nurses Credentialing Center. (2022, May). *Characteristics of Magnet organizations.* https://www.nursingworld.org/organizational-programs/magnet/about-magnet/why-become-magnet/characteristics-of-magnet/

Abuzied, Y., Al-Amer, R., Abuzaid, M., & Somduth, S. (2022). The Magnet Recognition Program and quality improvement in nursing. *Global Journal on Quality and Safety in Healthcare*, 5(4), 106–108. https://doi.org/10.36401/JQSH-22-12

Bazzoli, G. J., Clement, J. P., & Hsieh, H. M. (2010). Community benefit activities of private, nonprofit hospitals. *Journal of Health Politics, Policy and Law, 35*(6), 999–1026. https://doi.org/10.1215/03616878-2010-036

Cronin, C. E., Franz, B., Choyke, K., Rodriguez, V., & Gran, B. K. (2021). For-profit hospitals have a unique opportunity to serve as anchor institutions in the U.S. Preventive *Medicine Reports, 22*, 101372. https://doi.org/10.1016/j.pmedr.2021.101372

Gutenbrunner, C., Stievano, A., Stewart, D., Catton, H., & Nugraha, B. (2021). Role of nursing in rehabilitation. *Journal of Rehabilitation Medicine—Clinical Communications, 4*, 1000061. https://doi.org/10.2340/20030711-1000061

Health Resources and Services Administration. (2024, March). *National sample survey of registered nurses (NSSRN)*. https://bhw.hrsa.gov/data-research/access-data-tools/national-sample-survey-registered-nurses

Home Care Association of America. (2016). *Caring for America's seniors: The value of home care*. https://www.hcaoa.org/uploads/1/3/3/0/133041104/value_of_home_care___secured.pdf

Kwon, S., & Byun, J. (2024). Clinical experience of nurses in a consultative hospice palliative care service. *Journal of Hospice and Palliative Care, 27*(1), 31–44. https://doi.org/10.14475/jhpc.2024.27.1.31

Liu, J. B., & Kelz, R. R. (2018, September 11). Types of hospitals in the United States. *Journal of the American Medical Association, 320*(10), 1074.

Lysaght, S., & Ersek, M. (2013). Settings of care within hospice: New options and questions about dying "at home." *Journal of Hospice and Palliative Nursing, 15*(3), 171–176. https://doi.org/10.1097/NJH.0b013e3182765a17

Moilanen, T., Suhonen, R., & Kangasniemi, M. (2022). Nursing support for older people's autonomy in residential care: An integrative review. *International Journal of Older People Nursing, 17*(2), e12428. https://doi.org/10.1111/opn.12428

National Hospice and Palliative Care Organization. (2022). *NHPCO's standards of practice*. https://www.nhpco.org/wp-content/uploads/Standards_of_Practice.pdf

Smiley, R. A., Allgeyer, R. L., Shobo, Y., Lyons, K. C., Letourneau, R., Zhong, E., Kaminski-Ozturk, N., & Alexander, M. (2023). The 2022 National Nursing Workforce Survey. *Journal of Nursing Regulation, 14*(1), S1–S90.

Wajid, M., Rajkumar, E., Romate, J., George, A. J., Lakshmi, R., & Simha, S. (2021). Why is hospice care important? An exploration of its benefits for patients with terminal cancer. *BMC Palliative Care, 20*(1), 70. https://doi.org/10.1186/s12904-021-00757-8

Zimmerman, S., Carder, P., Schwartz, L., Silbersack, J., Temkin-Greener, H., Thomas, K. S., Ward, K., Jenkens, R., Jensen, L., Johnson, A. C., Johnson, J., Johnston, T., Kaes, L., Katz, P., Klinger, J. H., Lieblich, C., Mace, B., O'Neil, K., Pace, D. D., ... & Williams, K. B. (2022). The imperative to reimagine assisted living. *Journal of the American Medical Directors Association, 23*(2), 225–234. https://doi.org/10.1016/j.jamda.2021.12.004

Image Credits

Fig. 5.1: U.S. Department of Health and Human Services, "Employment Settings of Registered Nurses by Percentages," https://data.hrsa.gov/topics/health-workforce/nursing-workforce-dashboards, 2002.

Fig. 5.2: Richard A. Smiley, Richard L. Allgeyerm Yettu Shobo, Elizabeth Zhong, Nicole Kaminski-Ozturk, and Maryann Alexander, "Employment Settings of Registered Nurses, 2017 – 2022 by Percent from The 2022 National Nursing Workforce Survey," Journal of Nursing Regulation, vol. 14, no. 1. Copyright © 2023 by Elsevier B.V.

IMG 5.1: Generated using Adobe Firefly.

IMG 5.2: Generated using Adobe Firefly.

IMG 5.3: Generated using Adobe Firefly.

IMG 5.4: Generated using Adobe Firefly.

IMG 5.5: Generated using Adobe Firefly.

IMG 5.6: Generated using Adobe Firefly.

IMG 5.7: Generated using Adobe Firefly.

IMG 5.8: Generated using Adobe Firefly.

IMG 5.9: Generated using Adobe Firefly.

CHAPTER 6

Acute and Chronic Care

Objectives

Upon completion of this chapter, the learner will be able to do the following:

1. Distinguish between acute care, which addresses immediate and short-term health needs, and chronic care, which addresses long-term management of persistent health problems.
2. Analyze how the nursing role differs in managing acute versus chronic health conditions.
3. Identify the importance of interdisciplinary management for acute and chronic health conditions.
4. Articulate the need for effective care coordination, communication, and continuity of care for patients.

Key Chapter Terms

- Acute care
- Chronic care
- Urgent health care
- Acute care services
- New-graduate internship
- Clinical ladder
- Teach-back method
- Healthcare literacy
- Interdisciplinary management

Acute and Chronic Care

Nurses function in care settings that can descriptively be divided into two components based on illness: acute and chronic care. ***Acute care*** is care given for an illness that starts abruptly and is usually short-lived. ***Chronic care*** is care for an illness that develops gradually and persists for an extended period of time. These concepts will be presented in this chapter in an effort to help delineate the care required for management of individuals in both settings.

Acute Care

Most nurses in health care work in acute care settings. These settings provide outpatient and inpatient care. Some individuals who come for care in these settings have conditions or situations that cannot be addressed in an office or a clinic. Some individuals require care that cannot be provided in these settings that offer limited medical care. Acute care facilities offer services at higher levels than that given in offices or clinic settings.

What Is Acute Care?

Acute care is **urgent healthcare** attention given to individuals experiencing situations that require short-term treatment or intervention. This care is often administered in an acute care facility, which services individuals with a point of entry such as an emergency room or emergency department. Health care interventions for situations that bring an individual to these doors may be brief or extended, based on severity.

Acute care facilities are usually hospitals that have various settings, with services that extend from immediate treatment and discharge to treatment and admission for further care. Acute care institutions offer services that go beyond home treatment and office care. Many acute care facilities offer these services in an effort to allow recovery from an illness or accident. The philosophy of most acute care facilities is treatment to promote recovery and discharge as soon as possible in an effort to reduce costs of care and promote return to society.

Acute care services include but are not limited to the following:

- Medical units (e.g., medical-surgical, pediatric, maternity, labor and delivery)
- Surgical services (e.g., cardiovascular surgery, orthopedic surgery, plastic surgery)
- Laboratories (e.g., blood chemistry and microbiology, pathology, management of blood products for distribution to other areas of the acute care facility)
- Radiology (e.g., X-rays of various body parts, ultrasound, computed tomography, magnetic resonance imaging)

- Cardiac services (e.g., electrocardiogram, echocardiogram, stress testing)
- Emergency department
- Pharmaceutical services
- Respiratory services
- Dietary services

Acute care services are generally delivered by individuals specially trained in a specific area. Many services are available 24 hours a day. For services with limited access during night and weekend hours, many can be initiated instantly in the event of an emergency situation that requires intervention services. These services may have reduced staff in the facility during nonpeak hours but have access to other personnel who are capable of responding to an immediate call for specific services. Personnel features include licensed nursing personnel, physicians, dietitians, social workers, rehabilitation specialists, recreation therapists, and pharmacists, to name several.

Acute care organizations employ the majority of nurses in health care and offer a variety of opportunities for nurses. Although many positions are bedside- and nursing-based, there are other positions, including the supervision of nurses and other healthcare professionals, the education of nurses and the public, or research to improve patient outcomes. Nursing is the largest healthcare profession, according to the 2022 National Sample Survey of Registered Nurses, conducted by the Health Resources and Services Administration (2024). In 2022, there were more than 4 million registered nurses (RNs) nationwide with 3.5 million (80%) of all licensed RNs employed in nursing. Of this number, more than half (51%) worked in acute care organizations.

Acute Care Opportunities

RNs working in acute care facilities include those educated at the associate degree, baccalaureate degree, master's degree, and/or doctoral degree level. Licensed practical nurses who graduate from vocational programs of study also work in acute care organizations. Many new graduates enter the workforce through the acute care– or hospital-based route. Many organizations offer **new-graduate internship** opportunities. These extend orientation timelines to afford graduate nurses an opportunity to develop skill proficiency and improve critical thinking. This timeline gives new nurses a safe environment in which to develop coping skills in adjusting to a new profession. These provide nurses with resources to successfully transition from school to the work environment.

Nurses can also extend their educational bases to promote specialization in the management of individuals requiring acute intervention in hospitals.

Nurses working in areas such as surgical intensive care units, coronary care units, burn units, trauma units, and postoperative open-heart surgical units require specialized knowledge to care for patients in these settings. These patients have a higher acuity level and require an intensive level of care. Critical care and trauma units house individuals with serious conditions that require intense nursing management. Nurses working in these specialized areas can increase their knowledge bases through continuing education, higher academic levels of education, and certification. Many generalist or specialist certification opportunities exist for nurses working in acute care– or hospital-based care organizations. These opportunities extend to medical surgical nursing, critical care nursing, emergency room nursing, and neonatal nursing. Acute care organizations offer numerous opportunities for nurses in various areas of patient care in general or specialty positions.

These organizations may offer programs for progressing upward in mobility from entry levels for nurses called a ***clinical ladder***. These programs provide professional enrichment and growth for nurses. As nurses gain experience, they are able to move beyond the entry level. These often require more

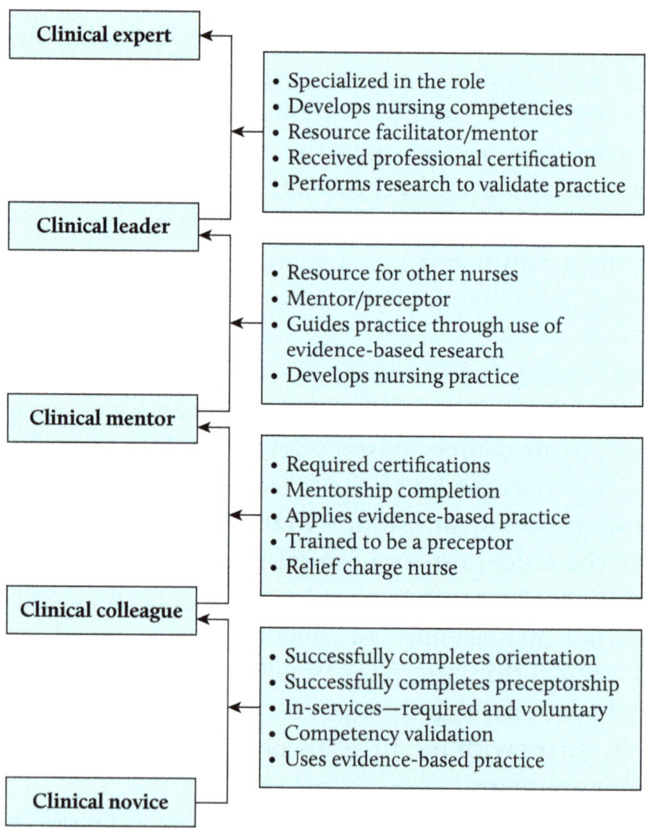

FIGURE 6.1 Example of Nursing Clinical Ladder With Required Competencies/Activities

eligibility components in addition to experience such as full-time employment, direct patient care, and completion of a probationary period. These components may also include continuing education, demonstration of clinical competence in a specific area, obtaining certification in a designated area, or pursuing formal education to achieve a specific degree level (e.g., baccalaureate degree in nursing or master's degree in nursing). As these levels are achieved, nurses are able to move up the rungs or steps of the ladder (see Figure 6.1).

Responsibility, specialization, and salary increase as nurses progress up the clinical ladder. There are dual benefits to the clinical ladder concept. These include increased nursing status while continuing to work at the bedside and retention of nurses proficient in care and use of evidence-based research. See Box 6.1 for an example of how evidence-based research can be used in acute care management.

Box 6.1

Use of Evidence-Based Research in Acute Care Management

Title: A nurse-driven oral care protocol to reduce hospital-acquired pneumonia (2019)

Authors: Warren, C., Medei, M. K., Wood, B., & Schutte, D.

Journal and article info: *American Journal of Nursing, 119*(2), 44–51. https://doi.org/10.1097/01.NAJ.0000553204.21342.01

Background: Hospital-acquired infections have a significantly negative impact on health and cost of patient treatment. One factor that contributes to these infections is the connection between oral care and pneumonia (Imai et al., 2021). Potentially, the mouth harbors more than 600 varieties of microorganisms that colonize in the oral mucosa and the tooth surface (Dewhirst et al., 2010). Some are potentially harmful and can colonize the oral cavity (Gluch, 2009). The lack of oral care may lead to the development of pneumonia.

Aim: This study was developed to implement an oral care protocol and evaluate its impact on the incidence of hospital-acquired pneumonia.

Methods: Specialized suction toothbrush kits were introduced specifically for long-term and short-term patient stays that included a baking soda toothpaste and an alcohol-free antiseptic mouthwash. Medical records were examined retrospectively over two seven-month periods to identify the presence or absence of patient hospital-acquired pneumonia.

Participants: The study employed a total of 417 patients. The intervention group consisted of 202 patients, and the baseline group consisted of 215 patients.

Ethical considerations: Retrospective chart reviews did not require patient consent.

Procedures: Study participants were randomized into one of two groups: intervention group or baseline group.

Data analyses: Chart audit information was placed in an Excel spreadsheet for analysis. The Statistical Package for Social Sciences was used to determine significance. Summary statistics and chi square analyses were done.

Results: This nurse-initiated and nurse-driven oral care protocol that included a "hospital-wide implementation of a multicomponent oral care bundle, including a decision-making algorithm, tailored oral care product kits, and embedded patient education, resulted in" a 50% reduction of hospital acquired pneumonia with $1.04 million in avoided costs through prevention (Warren et al., 2019).

Conclusion: Results demonstrate the positive results of a high-priority, high-impact, daily intervention tailored by nurses in providing oral care. Findings highlight the significance of nurse involvement in patient care management. It is imperative for nurses to address issues by initiating implementations, tracking outcomes, and validating protocols that improve patient outcomes.

References used for synopsis:

- Dewhirst, F. E., Chen, T., Izard, J., Paster, B. J., Tanner, A. C., Yu, W. H., Lakshmanan, A., & Wade, W. G. (2010). The human oral microbiome. *Journal of Bacteriology, 192*(19), 5002–5017. https://doi.org/10.1128/JB.00542-10.
- Gluch, J. I. (2009). Exploring the connection: The relationship between respiratory diseases and oral health. *Dimensions in Dental Hygiene, 7*(10), 54–57.
- Imai, K., Iinuma, T., & Sato, S. (2021). Relationship between the oral cavity and respiratory diseases: Aspiration of oral bacteria possibly contributes to the progression of lower airway inflammation. *Japanese Dental Science Review, 57*, 224–230. https://doi.org/10.1016/j.jdsr.2021.10.003
- Warren, C., Medei, M. K., Wood, B., & Schutte, D. (2019). A nurse-driven oral care protocol to reduce hospital-acquired pneumonia. *American Journal of Nursing, 119*(2), 44–51. https://doi.org/10.1097/01.NAJ.0000553204.21342.01

Use of evidence-based nursing practice leads to better patient outcomes and reduced health care costs. Work hours may also vary based on the clinical ladder position of the RN. While many acute care organizations typically maintain 12-hour shifts with variable holiday and weekend schedules, some higher-level nursing positions reduce these hours to be more consistent with eight-hour days, five days a week. Variable shifts may also be available for the nurse at higher ladder positions (e.g., four 10-hour shifts per week; variable eight-, 10-, or 12-hour shifts). Nurses at all levels in acute care organizations work with patients and families to promote the best outcomes possible and improve the quality of care for patients upon discharge (see Figure 6.2).

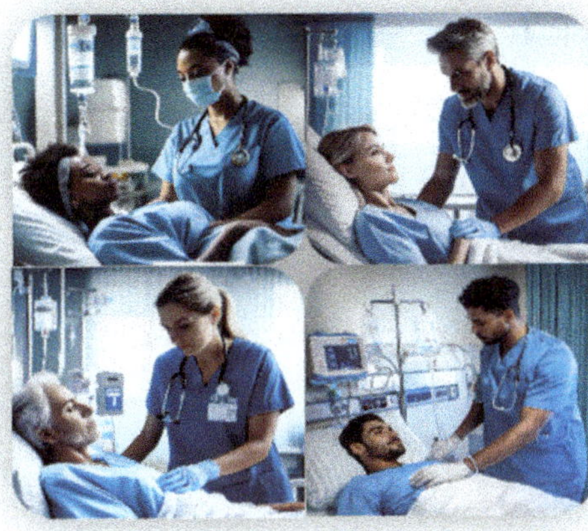

FIGURE 6.2 Acute Care–/Hospital-Based Nursing Care

Chronic Care

Unlike acute care, chronic care involves multiple interactions with the healthcare system. This type of care occurs when an individual has a condition that requires intermittent evaluation and/or adjustments to care activities or pharmaceutical interventions. More than 133 million people, or more than half the U.S. population, live with some form of chronic illness. At least 45% of the population have at least one chronic disease (World Health Organization, 2024). There is projected to be more than a 1% increase in this number by the year 2030. This will increase the estimated number of individuals with chronic illnesses to 171 million. Patients with chronic conditions may be managed in a home setting or an extended care setting based on disease and level of disability.

Nurses play a crucial part in management of the chronic care patient population (Anderson, 2010). Nurses need to have the skills to work within a collaborative system to manage these individuals, as many will have multiple illnesses. These illnesses will include but not be limited to diabetes, heart disease, high blood pressure, chronic obstructive pulmonary disease, depression, asthma, and renal failure. It will take skill and interactions within health systems that involve health organizations, community centers, and individual care providers to assist in maintaining the health of these individuals to a state of wellness that will allow them to contribute to their family social system and society. Nurses will need to use evidence-based care initiatives to promote the highest quality of care. Evidence-based care will allow delivery of care that is validated through the research process. See Box 6.2 for an example of how evidence-based research can be used in chronic care management.

Use of Evidence-Based Research in Chronic Care Management

Title: Self-care management of patients with diabetes: Nurses' perspectives (2020)

Authors: Ahmad, N. A. A., Sallehuddin, M. A. A., Teo, Y. C., & Rahman, H. A.

Journal and article info: *Journal of Diabetes and Metabolic Disorders, 19*(2), 1537–1542. https://doi.org/10.1007/s40200-020-00688-w

Background: Education is critical for proper self-care management of diabetes. It is important for these individuals to execute day-to-day knowledge on proper nutrition, proper exercise, self-monitoring, and medication management to accomplish identified goals (Shrivastava et al., 2013). Exploring health education perception and experiences of diabetic nurse educators had not been explored in order to identify its impact on self-care management.

Aim: The study was designed to explore nurses' experiences providing patient self-care management education to individuals diagnosed with diabetes.

Methods: A qualitative phenomenological study using semistructured focus group interviews.

Participants: Nine nurses certified as diabetes nurse educators.

Ethical considerations: The study protocol was approved by the designated research and ethics committees. Participants signed a written consent form. No participant-identifying information was obtained, and each participant had a specific code assigned by the researcher.

Data analyses: Audio recordings were transcribed verbatim and analyzed through thematic analysis.

Results: Three themes were identified in this research study. These were:

> 1) Factors of effective teaching strategies that emphasizes on assessing patients' knowledge and education level to provide individualised instructional plan, which need to follow latest ministerial guidelines and effective pedagogy; 2) Barriers to provide effective education including psychological, financial, and lack of familial support; 3) Overcoming barriers through parallel health education and counselling, referring to medical social worker and non-governmental organizations, and inclusion of family members and carers in plan of care. (p. 1537)

Conclusion: "Diabetic nurse educator plays a crucial role to ensure patient with diabetes achieved competency and compliance with long term self-care management. Nurses' need to ensure psychological preparedness and patient literacy assessment when designing individualised health education session" (p. 1541). Although this study focused on a specific type of nurse, it shows that foundationally nurses of all educational preparations should focus on diabetes education, as this is critical to patient self-management.

Methods used such as teach-back and focusing on the seven principles of self-care management (i.e., healthy diet, exercise, adherence to medication, glucose level monitoring, problem-solving, reducing risks, and healthy coping) can be implemented by all nurses.

References used for synopsis:

- Ahmad, N. A. A., Sallehuddin, M. A. A., Teo, Y. C., & Rahman, H. A. (2020). Self-care management of patients with diabetes: Nurses' perspectives. *Journal of Diabetes and Metabolic Disorders, 19*(2), 1537–1542. https://doi.org/10.1007/s40200-020-00688-w
- Shrivastava, S. R., Shrivastava, P. S., & Ramasamy, J. (2013). Role of self-care in management of diabetes mellitus. *Journal of Diabetes and Metabolic Disorders, 12*(1), 14. https://doi.org/10.1186/2251-6581-12-14

Nurses managing patients in chronic care settings need to be skilled in various patient education techniques, such as the **teach-back method**, in which patients are asked to repeat information taught to them in their own words to validate understanding. They need communication techniques that encourage patients to adhere to healthcare initiatives, such as listening, repetition, and demonstrations of concern and empathy. It is important for nurses to work with patients to establish goals and objectives that are attainable and focused. Patients need to learn about care activities that promote self-management.

Nurses need to facilitate coordination of care activities in individuals with chronic diseases (Griffin, 2017). This patient-centered approach promotes individualized care. Individualized care activities are necessary, since patients present with various combinations of chronic diseases. This allows specialized care to use interventions that promote the best patient outcomes.

Individuals with chronic diseases may be managed in the home setting or, based on disease severity, may be required to stay in a facility with varying degrees of assistance. Chronic care facilities are often referred to as *long-term care facilities* since patients there are housed in these facilities for extended lengths of time. Chronic care or long-term care facilities offer several levels of care. These levels include custodial care for active individuals who require minimal assistance; long-term personal assistance for individuals who need more than custodial but less than intensive care; or skilled care, which is the level of assistance required for individuals who need intensive 24-hour care. Persons with debilitating conditions may require assistance but not intensive care and may use facilities called *nursing homes, board and care homes, sheltered care homes*, or other names that imply care on an extended basis without intensive interventions.

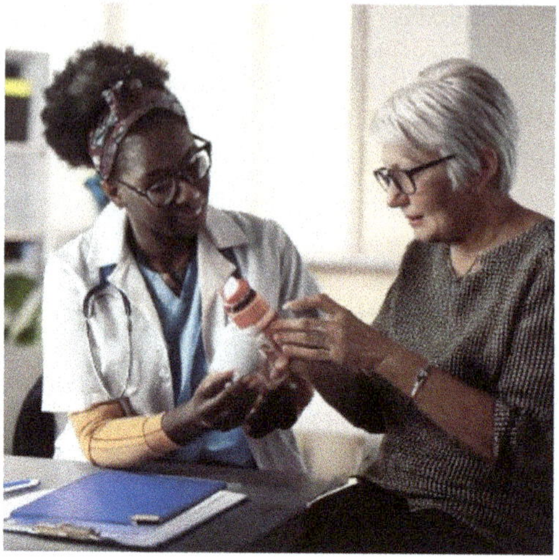

FIGURE 6.3 Healthcare Literacy in Chronic Care

Nurses need to promote the use of evidence-based interventions to promote quality care outcomes for individuals with chronic diseases (Duda-Sikuła & Kurpas, 2024). Evidence-based care supports improvements for care at all levels of the chronic care organization (Afenigus & Sinshaw, 2025; American Association of Colleges of Nursing, 2019).

Nurses are important in promoting **healthcare literacy** for patients with chronic diseases. Since many individuals with chronic illnesses present to healthcare areas with combinations of diseases, their care can be complex. They are likely to have multiple prescriptions and to require interactions with care providers on a more frequent basis. In addition to promoting compliance with visits to healthcare providers, it is important to promote literacy in facilitating medication adherence (see Figure 6.3).

Healthcare literacy is the ability of patients to interpret health information in order to make informed choices for care and manage current health situations. Individuals with chronic conditions can have frequent healthcare encounters that relate to current and new diseases. If patients do not understand their care activities and diseases, they cannot make informed decisions regarding activities that may affect their health. As a result, conditions deteriorate, and individuals lose the ability to contribute to society and family goals.

Chronic care management by promoting the understanding of care activities, inclusive of medications, is an important component of patient safety. Information should be tailored to the educational level of the individual's healthcare vocabulary. Explanations that use plain language or enlist the assistance of an interpreter allow accurate understanding. This fundamental information is important to promote accurate self-monitoring and disease management. Making sure that patients have a level of health literacy that allows them to make healthy and informed choices about health care is important. Only through the promotion of patient education and confirmation of a patient's healthcare literacy level will nurses work to improve the quality of life for individuals with chronic health conditions.

Interdisciplinary Management in Care Delivery

Interdisciplinary management in both acute and chronic care situations for management of specific health conditions that require immediate and long-term intervention is critical. In acute care settings, patients can come to these areas with life-threatening issues that must be addressed swiftly and efficiently. Communication between healthcare providers is essential for distribution of critical information that requires diagnostic tests that are the foundation for immediate treatment plan development and interventions to prevent complications. All care providers must be aligned in their approach to care, risk minimization, and promote accurate communication to prevent jeopardizing patient recovery.

Interdisciplinary management is even more important in chronic care. This is because patients with chronic conditions often require long-term management and multiple healthcare visits. Chronic diseases such as diabetes, hypertension, and heart disease require ongoing monitoring and changes to medications and treatment plans over time. Effective care coordination ensures that patient receive consistent care by various providers over multiple healthcare settings. This prevents gaps in care received that could result in worsening of the patient's condition and unnecessary hospitalizations. Communication among healthcare providers ensures synchronized care.

Patients with chronic conditions need to also be part of the collaborative team for management. This shared decision-making enhances adherence to medications and treatment regimens. This promotes better engagement and self-care management of their chronic condition. This partnership between healthcare providers and patients promotes better long-term self-care outcomes for chronic diseases.

Both acute and chronic care environments benefit from interdisciplinary collaboration, in which each member of the healthcare team contributes their expertise. This continuity of care promotes better patient outcomes and enhances efficiency of the healthcare system by reducing service duplication, preventing complications, and ensuring efficient use of all resources for the best patient outcomes.

Summary

Nursing management of acute and chronic diseases varies. These must be individualized and nursing-focused, directed toward immediate intervention or promotion of self-care. Patients continue to move between these areas of care, and as society ages, this will continue to be a challenge for nurses as care providers. Interdisciplinary management enhances efficiency for the best patient outcomes through the collaborative use of multiple healthcare providers' areas of expertise. Nurses as members of the interdisciplinary team for the provision of patient care are a must.

References

Afenigus, A. D., & Sinshaw, M. A. (2025). Developing nursing approaches across the chronic illness trajectory: a grounded theory study of care from diagnosis to end-of-life in Western Amhara, Ethiopia. *Frontiers in Health Services*, *5*, 1502763. https://doi.org/10.3389/frhs.2025.1502763

American Association of Colleges of Nursing. (2019, April). *Creating a more highly qualified nursing workforce*. https://www.aacnnursing.org/Portals/42/News/Factsheets/Nursing-Workforce-Fact-Sheet.pdf

Anderson, G. (2010). *Chronic care: Making the case for ongoing care*. Robert Wood Johnson Foundation. https://publichealth.jhu.edu/sites/default/files/2023-04/jhdaai-chartbook-2010.pdf

Ahmad, N. A. A., Sallehuddin, M. A. A., Teo, Y. C., & Rahman, H. A. (2020). Self-care management of patients with diabetes: Nurses' perspectives. *Journal of Diabetes and Metabolic Disorders*, *19*(2), 1537–1542. https://doi.org/10.1007/s40200-020-00688-w

Duda-Sikuła, M., & Kurpas, D. (2024). Enhancing chronic disease management: personalized medicine insights from rural and urban general practitioner practices. *Journal of Personalized Medicine*, *14*(7), 706. https://doi.org/10.3390/jpm14070706

Griffin, C. D., CPHQ, & CCM (2017). A primary care nursing perspective on chronic disease prevention and management. *Delaware Journal of Public Health*, *3*(1), 78–83. https://doi.org/10.32481/djph.2017.03.011

Health Resources and Services Administration. (2024, March). *National sample survey of registered nurses (NSSRN)*. https://bhw.hrsa.gov/data-research/access-data-tools/national-sample-survey-registered-nurses.

Warren, C., Medei, M. K., Wood, B., & Schutte, D. (2019). A nurse-driven oral care protocol to reduce hospital-acquired pneumonia. *American Journal of Nursing*, *119*(2), 44–51. https://doi.org/10.1097/01.NAJ.0000553204.21342.01

World Health Organization. (2024, May 21). *World health statistics 2024: Monitoring health for the SDGs, sustainable development goals*. https://www.who.int/publications/i/item/9789240094703

Image Credits

Fig. 6.2: Generated using Adobe Firefly.
Fig. 6.3: Generated using Adobe Firefly.

CHAPTER 7

Patient Rights

Objectives

Upon completion of this chapter, the learner will be able to:

1. Identify key patient rights, which include informed consent and privacy.
2. Analyze the legal principles of autonomy, confidentiality, and non-discrimination that underpin patient rights.
3. Justify the responsibilities of nurses in ensuring that patient rights are respected and protected throughout the patient care process.
4. Analyze how the protection and promotion of patient rights contribute to improved healthcare outcomes, patient satisfaction, and trust in the healthcare system.
5. Recognize potential barriers and challenges to upholding patient rights.

Key Chapter Terms

- Patient rights
- Emancipated minor
- Mature minor
- Mature Minor Doctrine Clarification Act
- Parental rights
- Patient Care Partnership Rights
- Advocacy
- Confidentiality
- Privacy
- Notice of Privacy Practices
- Consent
- Confidentiality
- Right to refuse treatment
- Patient awareness
- Time constraints
- System pressures
- Biases (cultural and societal)
- Constraints (legal and institutional)
- Policy reform

Patient Rights

As health care has changed, so have patient rights. These have been the center of attention in the new electronic age. Nurses serve to support and enhance patient rights while administering quality care. They do this through advocacy activities and adherence to privacy and confidentiality. Nursing care is part of this partnership and included in expectations that are to be fulfilled. Nurses must work to address rights from all perspectives of the organization, those initiated by other healthcare organizations, and those promoted by nursing as a profession. This chapter will review patient rights and nurses' role in promoting care and advocating for patient rights.

Patient Rights and Health Care

Patient rights are those items related to health care to which an individual is entitled in the process of having their healthcare needs fulfilled. These fundamental rights must be addressed and respected by nurses as their patients navigate through the healthcare system. Awareness and understanding are imperative to promoting compliance. These patient rights are based on guidelines that include the Health Insurance Portability and Accountability Act of 1996 (HIPAA) and organizations such as the American Hospital Association (AHA).

Fundamentally, patient rights include the right to make choices in their treatment. As long as the patient is considered intellectually sound, it is important to give factual information in order to promote decisions that are right for them. This goes back to the ethical right to informed consent. Patient options may include medicinal treatment, surgical treatment, radiological intervention, or a combination of any or all of these. Patients also have the right to refuse any or all treatment options. This right can be exercised regardless of the opinions of the healthcare provider. Patients have the right to make decisions about their own end-of-life care options. This can be done prior to being admitted to any type of organization through an advanced directive. The advanced directive is a legal document regarding end-of-life care. It often includes who can make decisions for the individual when they are no longer able to make such decisions due to illness or taking medication that may interfere with decision-making capacity (e.g., pain medication). Each state has its own criteria regarding this type of document and how legally binding it is regarding health care. It is important for patients to not only have an advanced directive but also to speak with family members and make their wishes known. This will allow family discussion and identification of important care activities that the patient may or may not desire in end-of-life decision-making.

It is also important for nurses to have an awareness of **parental rights** related to health care for a child (an individual younger than age 18 years of age). These rights have continued to change and expand as society has evolved through recognition of minors as individuals (Bosch et al., 2024; Ciranka & vanden Bos, 2019). These can vary considerably from state to state (SchoolHouse Connection, 2023). One state may allow minors to be treated for a sexually transmitted disease (STD) without parental knowledge, while another may not (English, 2007). There may be times when the wishes of the parents are overturned by the court system. This can occur if the child is believed to be in imminent danger and their life depends on receiving a designated treatment (e.g., a child whose parents refuse to allow the administration of blood due to religious convictions after a trauma has resulted in considerable blood loss, and it is believed that their survival depends on blood administration). Some states recognize teenagers ages 15 and older as "**mature minors**" and will occasionally adhere to the wishes of these individuals. This variability is the result of debates and various ways of thinking over parental responsibilities, the potential immaturity and vulnerability of children, and emancipation rights of children from parental decisions. Generally, parents are considered legal guardians of their children, and therefore they have the right to make health care decisions. In some cases, parental rights have legally been granted to others, and this right passes to them. Many states recognize parental rights up to age 12 years for a child. It is the teenage years where this thought differs among states. An ***emancipated minor*** is an individual who has terminated parental rights, which means that parental consent is not necessary for health care decisions, regardless of severity. The *mature minor* is an individual who is usually older than age 13 years of age and can provide informed consent through demonstration of understanding of the designated procedure (and the procedure is usually not serious in nature). The mature-minor status may be implemented when minors request contraception or, in some states, STD treatment, as these services are identified as right-to-privacy situations (Fiscus, 2021). A state that has a mature-minor doctrine allows minors to give consent for some medical procedures. This has been seen in most cases with individuals 16 years or older who demonstrate understanding of the designated procedure and the procedure is not serious. The concept has been in use since 2002, and some states have enacted the doctrine as a statute, which means it is law. An example of a state mature minor doctrine is in Box 7.1. As a result of the coronavirus disease 2019 pandemic, the Tennessee General Assembly, Senate Bill No. 1111 and House Bill No. 1380, enacted the **Mature Minor Doctrine Clarification Act**. This act limited the powers of adolescents to consent to immunizations (Arshagouni, 2006). The "parental rights" bill overrides the mature Minor Mature Doctrine by stipulating that clinicians may not administer immunizations to a minor without obtaining informed consent from the parent or legal guardian. "The new law also prohibits employees or agents of the state, such as the Tennessee Department of Children's Services, from mandating that minors in state custody receive immunizations. Biological parents of children in foster care must give consent to their children to receive immunizations while in state custody" (Hijano & Yaun, 2024, p. 155).

Mature Minor Doctrine Example

Mature Minor Doctrine, Tennessee

An emancipated minor is someone under the age of 18 who is independent of parental control and support. Legally, an emancipated minor is treated the same as an adult and can make his own health care decisions. He can also appoint a health care agent or surrogate.

For a minor who is not emancipated, the underlying rule is that a physician must get parental (or guardian) consent before rendering medical treatment, except in cases of emergency. However, the legislature and the courts have carved out exceptions to this rule that allow a minor to consent to medical treatment under certain conditions.

By statute in Tennessee, a physician can treat a minor without parental consent for certain health issues, such as drug abuse, venereal disease (STD/STI), contraception, and prenatal care. Also, by statute, a physician may render emergency care to a minor without parental consent. After a reasonable effort has been made to contact a minor's parent or guardian, a physician may render emergency medical treatment to a minor without parental consent if the physician has a good faith belief that the emergency treatment is necessary to save the life of the minor or prevent further deterioration of the minor's condition. In Tennessee, an un-emancipated minor cannot obtain an abortion without parental consent or judicial bypass.

The courts in Tennessee have also adopted the "mature minor" doctrine that allows a physician to treat a mature minor without parental consent. In determining who is a "mature minor," Tennessee follows the "Rule of Sevens."

- Under the age of 7 there is no capacity, and the physician must have parental consent to treat (unless a statutory exception applies).
- Between the ages of 7 and 14, there is a rebuttable presumption that there is no capacity, and a physician generally should get parental consent before treating (unless a statutory exception applies).
- Between the ages of 14 and 18, there is a rebuttable presumption of capacity, and the physician may treat without parental consent unless the physician believes that the minor is not sufficiently mature to make his or her own health care decisions.

Source: Tennessee Department of Health, "Mature Minor Doctrine, Tennessee," HIV/STD Program.

Nurses also work to promote patient rights identified by the American Hospital Association. This organization has identified six patient care partnership expectations, rights, and responsibilities, which are (a) high-quality hospital care; (b) a clean and safe environment; (c) involvement in one's care; (d) protection of privacy; (e) help when leaving the hospital; and (f) help with billing claims. Specifics related to **Patient Care Partnership Rights** are identified in Table 7.1.

TABLE 7.1 Patient Care Partnership Rights

Right	Explanation
High-quality hospital care	Care delivered with compassion, skill, and respect to the patient when needed, which includes management of pain and the identity of individuals administering care (e.g., students, residents, nursing assistants, physicians, nurses).
Clean and safe environment	Policies and procedures to prevent healthcare errors, abuse, or neglect. All incidents and any resulting changes that may be necessary as a result (e.g., additional tests or procedures required to address problems) will be reported to the patient.
Involvement in one's care	Decisions will be joint between patients and providers and include discussion of medically appropriate choices, treatment plan discussions, identification of health and coverage to promote appropriate decisions, an explanation of personal health care goals and values, and an explanation of who should make decisions about care when patients are unable to do so.
Protection of privacy	Confidentiality of the relationship between patients and caregivers is respected, and a notice of privacy is made available that describes the way private information is used, disclosed, and safeguarded as well as how a copy of the patient record can be obtained.
Help when leaving the hospital	Community resources will be identified for follow-up care, and any relationship between entities (hospitals and organizations) will be disclosed. Patient education, which includes information and training, will be given (e.g., dressing changes needed for wound care, information regarding when to contact a care provider or when emergency care is needed).
Help with billing claims	Care organizations will file health insurance forms, including those for private and federal programs (e.g., Medicare and Medicaid). For individuals who do not have insurance, the facility will provide assistance in locating financial help or making arrangements for payment. Billing questions will be addressed by the organization.

Source: AHA, 2003.

Rights are universal and relate to other patient rights components such as HIPAA, which has been discussed under the legal aspects of nursing. Fundamentally, patient rights are affected by legal and ethical decisions, which can intertwine to make this a complex situation for the nurse.

Advocacy as a Right

The role of patient advocate has been in the functional role of nurses since the days of Florence Nightingale. Nurses act as liaisons between patients and healthcare providers. The American Nurses Association (ANA) includes the word ***advocacy*** in its definition of nursing.

Serving as a patient advocate is a means of supporting and promoting patient safety, the right of every patient (Abbasinia et al., 2020). Nurses serve to defend the rights of patients when they are at their most vulnerable. They assist patients and their families to navigate the sometimes-complex healthcare system, not making decisions but promoting understanding in order to assist in an informed decision regarding treatment. Advocacy is not necessarily an innate skill. Nurses may have an introduction to it in their early educational nursing experience but often learn through identifying and mimicking the behaviors of expert nurses. Advocacy is important in demonstrating that the fundamental nursing concepts of caring underlie the moral value system of the nursing profession (Morris, 2023). The process of patient advocacy starts with establishing a trusting relationship and works through various steps terminating with upholding patient/family decisions (see Figure 7.1).

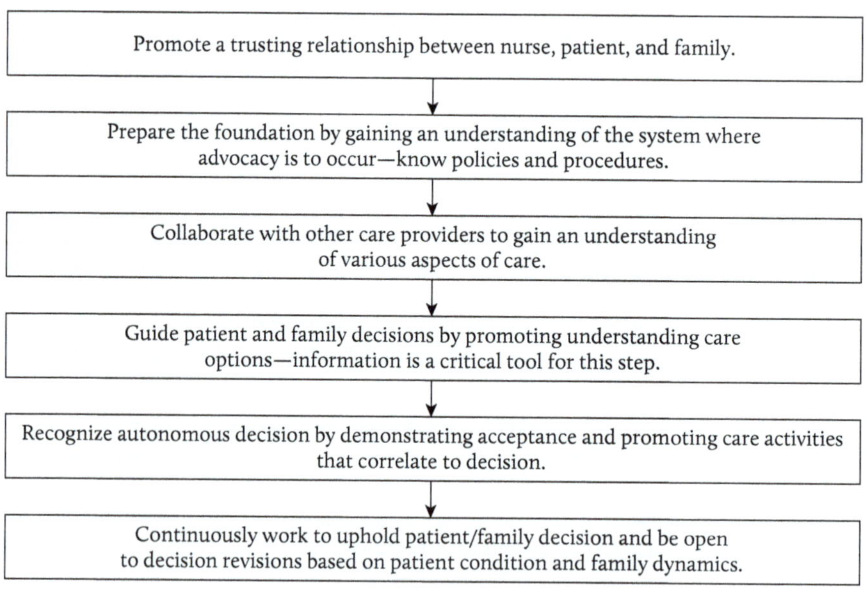

FIGURE 7.1 Steps in the Advocacy Process for Nurses

Advocacy in nursing has its theoretical basis in nursing ethics. The ANA's Code of Ethics for Nurses includes the following language in Provision 3, which relates to this function of the nurse: "The nurse promotes, advocates for, and strives to protect the health, safety, and rights of the patient" (ANA, 2025). Nurses promote the patient's right to privacy. When administering care, nurses are responsible for maintaining reasonable privacy of the physical space. This includes visual and auditory privacy. Patients are often exposed during assessments and other care activities or procedures. During assessments and physical examinations, curtains should be drawn, patient room doors should be closed, and all possible provisions should be made to keep patients from being viewed by others. Procedures that may physically expose patients should be done at a time when visitors are reduced in numbers, or visitors should be requested to step out of the room during these situations. During transport, patients should be covered, whether they are in wheelchairs or on stretchers. Family members should only remain upon patients' request and/or approval. It is important during the exchange of information to ensure that nurses lower their voice to prevent accidental information transmission to other care providers, patients, and family members who do not have a need to know. It is imperative that patient information not be accidentally transferred to others. These activities are nurses' responsibility.

Some nurses are uncomfortable with the advocacy role as part of their responsibility. Nurses must work through barriers that may occur to promoting this patient right in order to promote patient safety. Barriers may be personal or interpersonal. Personal barriers include discomfort due to inexperience. Working with a mentor who is experienced in promoting advocacy can assist with this obstacle. Interpersonal barriers can be nurse-to-patient or nurse-to–care provider (Ramsay et al., 2022). Establishing a trusting relationship begins with the first nurse-patient encounter. Introductions can present an open perspective of nurses by encouraging patients to ask questions and responding to patient needs as soon as possible. Nurses should listen actively and communicate clearly, giving factual information regarding care to promote understanding by the patient and family. Nurse-to-care provider relationships can be promoted through presenting one's self as a knowledgeable, competent professional. Working to complement care of other care providers while performing those tasks identified as nursing responsibilities can assist in promoting a cohesive approach to advocacy for a specific patient and eliminate this interpersonal barrier.

Right to Confidentiality and Privacy

Confidentiality is closely linked to ***privacy***. All patient information is treated in this manner. Only individuals who have a "need to know" are given patient information. Violations of confidentiality and privacy can jeopardize trust and have a negative impact on the nurse-patient relationship. This could result in patients not disclosing information that could affect safety and progression toward wellness. Transmission of information should be guarded in all methods, verbal, written, or electronic. Some organizations have patient codes for relaying information to family members over the phone. If in doubt, it is better to err on the side of caution when giving phone updates.

It is important to know organizational policy and procedures regarding disclosure of information. Disclosure of information may be required in certain situations. These may specifically relate to situations that address safety. Situations that may require disclosure could include:

- Patient protection from harm or injury—abuse situations
- Safety of others—threats to others
- Public health threat (e.g., anthrax, *Chlamydia trachomatis* infections, diphtheria, gonorrhea, hepatitis, human immunodeficiency virus [HIV] diagnosis, Lyme disease, malaria, measles, mumps, syphilis, tetanus, tuberculosis)

Healthcare organizations and entities collect protected and personal health information. A privacy rule exists that identifies how this information is used by the patient's specific healthcare provider. These rights must be addressed and individuals must be notified of these rights. These are disclosed in the **Notice of Privacy Practices**. These rights include the patient's right to (a) know how personal health information is used in the organization or practice, (b) know who has accessed their information, (c) access their own information, (d) request an amendment to or correct their individual health information, and (e) file a complaint about the use of their health information. An amendment was made to the rule in 2024 to support reproductive healthcare privacy (U.S. Department of Health and Human Services [DHHS], 2024).

Nurses should know policies and procedures related to confidentiality and privacy of information. One place to start is the organization's Notice of Privacy Policy (U.S. Department of Health and Human Services, 2025, 45 *Code of Federal Regulations* §164.520–§164.528). Each healthcare organization is required to describe how information is used for care and statement(s) about individual rights regarding use of the information. The Notice of Privacy Policy must include the items in Table 7.2.

TABLE 7.2 Notice of Privacy Policy

Required Inclusions
1. Information about whom and for what purpose health information is kept, which includes types of uses for treatment, payment, and healthcare operations
2. Descriptions of other uses of information with disclosures that may be made without individual consent or authorization
3. Other uses of information that is collected, such as appointment reminders, fundraising purposes, release of information to healthcare sponsors, and marketing
4. How patients can access, inspect, amend, or correct their information
5. Guidelines for filing a complaint about a privacy violation by the specific provider and a notification that the patient can file a complaint with the Department of Health and Human Services
6. Penalties that may occur for individuals who may violate privacy laws and violations as well as patient confidentiality

Often patients ask nurses how to engage components of the privacy notice. Nurses should be familiar with notice components. Not adhering to compliance is not only an ethical violation but a legal one as well.

It is important to protect all information regardless of the source or form. Sources of patient information can include obvious and not-so-obvious items. These can include but are not limited to the following:

- Copies of paperwork with patient-identifying information
- Laboratory or radiological patient data
- Pharmacy records of medications dispensed to be administered (medications can give a clue to a patient's diagnosis, such as medication used specifically for the treatment of HIV, Acquired Immune Deficiency Syndrome [AIDS], or a sexually transmitted disease)
- Packages used to dispense medications, such as intravenous medications hung via secondary infusion sets (these medications come with full patient identification for proper identification prior to administration)
- Computer screens accessed for data entry at the bedside, unit station, or office or in more public areas on mobile wireless computerized entry components (e.g., medical carts, workstations on wheels; see Figure 7.2)

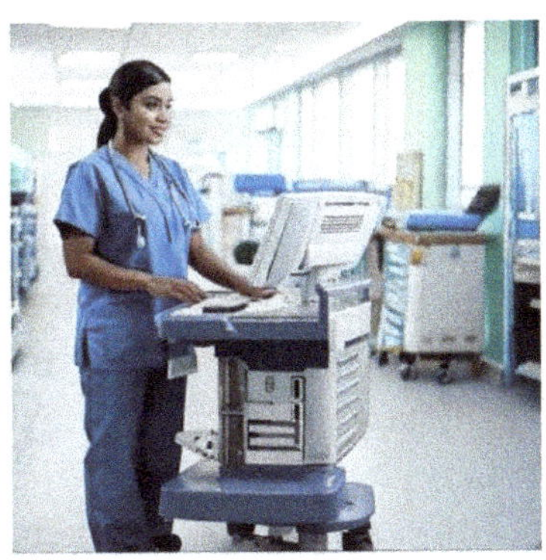

FIGURE 7.2 Wireless Workstation

- Personal devices for data access or entry (some healthcare providers have access to patient information via personal computerized handheld devices)
- Surveillance information that may be held in data sets

Items with patient-identifying information should be managed based on the organization's policy. Some require obliteration of identifying information on the object with special markers. There may be disposal in special places for internal or external shredding for security. This can include collection and disposal by special companies who specialize in the disposal of sensitive information.

Legal Principles That Underpin Patient Rights

Legal principles underpin patient rights. These include informed **consent**, **confidentiality**, and the **right to refuse treatment**. *Informed consent* is the right for patients to understand their treatment options and make autonomous decisions about their care. This stems from the ethical principle of autonomy which emphasizes the right for patients to control what happens to their body. Legally, healthcare providers are obligated to explain risks, benefits, and alternative treatments, ensuring that patients are fully informed in order to make a care decision. A failure to obtain informed consent can lead to claims of medical malpractice.

Confidentiality is another key legal principle and critical to maintaining trust between patients and healthcare providers. This ensures that patient information is kept private and shared only with individuals who have a need to know or have been approved by patients to receive such information. This right is protected under HIPAA (Alder, 2023). Violating patient confidentiality can result in legal penalties for healthcare providers and organizations. It can even lead to dismissal from employment.

Patients have the legal *right to refuse treatment*, even if a recommended treatment could potentially save the patient's life. This directly stems from the right for patient autonomy and ensures that individuals are not subjected to medical interventions against their will. If a patient is unable to make a decision for themselves, tools such as advanced directives or a legally appointed healthcare proxy can guide providers in addressing the patient's desires.

Laws have been enacted to ensure that there is non-discrimination in health care based on race, gender, religion, or socioeconomic status. Laws such as the Americans with Disabilities Act and Civil Rights Act protect patients from discrimination and guarantee that they receive fair and equitable care.

Healthcare institutions are legally required to accommodate the unique needs of diverse patient populations. This involves providing interpreters for non-English-speaking patients and facilitating access to individuals with disabilities. This reinforces the idea that every person is entitled to quality health care, without prejudice or bias.

Barriers and Challenges to Upholding Patient Rights

Upholding patient rights is essential to ethical healthcare, but various barriers and challenges can hinder its consistent implementation. One significant challenge is lack of **patient awareness**. Many patients may not fully understand their rights. This can be due to low healthcare literacy, language barriers, and/or unfamiliarity with medical terminology. Patients are less likely to exercise their rights if they are unaware of them. Some patients may feel overwhelmed or intimidated, which further compromises their ability to exercise their rights. Education and communication are key strategies healthcare providers can use to improve patient awareness. This can be accomplished through signage, brochures, or electronic resources. It is important for healthcare providers to be open to addressing questions and demonstrate compassion and caring when explaining medical procedures and options. Interpreters can also bridge communication gaps and assist patients to make informed decisions.

Time constraints and **system pressures** are other healthcare challenges. Healthcare providers often face heavy workloads and time limitation requirements, which can make it difficult to dedicate enough time to address patient concerns and respond to questions. Time constraints can result in patient rights being overlooked or treated as secondary to urgent care delivery. In fast-paced environments, due to system pressures, staff may prioritize efficiency over communication.

To address these issues, workflow adjustments and team collaboration are essential. Healthcare institutions can implement systems that allow for more time for provider-patient interactions, such as scheduling longer appointment times for complex patient visits or using patient advocates to assist with education and procedure consent processes. Fostering an environment where interdisciplinary teamwork is not just encouraged but expected can help more evenly distribute the workload, allowing for more patient engagement time.

Cultural and societal biases can affect how patient rights are upheld. Discrimination based on race, gender, or socioeconomic status can lead to unequal treatment and access to care. This can lead to a reduction in communication and explanation of procedures, which can make the patient feel dismissed by the provider. The result of this can be a failure to ensure patients' right to informed consent and equitable treatment. These biases can be addressed through an organization's commitment to employee cultural competence and bias training. Creating a more inclusive healthcare environment allows for the protection of patient rights regardless of background.

Legal and institutional constraints can pose barriers to upholding patient rights. Healthcare providers can feel restricted by institutional policies, insurance regulations, or legal fears that influence their ability to respect patient autonomy. Bureaucratic hurdles can delay access to care, which can undermine a patient's right to timely treatment.

Policy reform and advocacy are crucial to addressing barriers and challenges to upholding patient rights. It is important for healthcare institutions to evaluate and update policies to ensure that barriers to patient rights are addressed. Legal protections, such as advanced directives, can help uphold patient autonomy and reduce provider liability concerns. By working together, healthcare leaders and policymakers can streamline regulations and ensure that legal constraints do not compromise patient rights or care.

Summary

Nurses are on the front line in providing patient care. As patient advocates and protectors of information, they must be involved in compliance. They must strive to create a work environment where communication complies with laws. The patient care environment must also be structured to reduce the accidental communication of patient information to other individuals who do not have a right to know. Nursing communication habits in the work environment must drastically differ from social interactions. Communication of patient information must occur in a private setting and not a public forum, such as in a busy office setting or an elevator. Nurses should seek private areas for the exchange of private patient information, such as an empty care room or a place out of earshot of other individuals. This mindset is imperative to maintain confidentiality of private information and prevention of financial fines and personal sanctions for violations.

Nurses must be aware of the legal requirements for patient care and ensure that care is delivered in a nondiscriminatory manner. This allows for care to be given to all persons regardless of their race, gender, religion, or socioeconomic status. Legal ramifications can be severe for violations of legal principles that underpin patient rights. Knowledge of laws, barriers, and challenges allows nurses to remain confident in their ability to deliver quality care.

References

Abbasinia, M., Ahmadi, F., & Kazemnejad, A. (2020). Patient advocacy in nursing: A concept analysis. *Nursing Ethics, 27*(1), 141–151. https://doi.org/10.1177/0969733019832950

Alder, S. (2023, November 10). *HIPAA notice of privacy practices*. HIPAA Journal. https://www.hipaajournal.com/hipaa-notice-of-privacy-practices/

American Hospital Association. (2003). *Patient care partnership: Understanding expectations, rights, and responsibilities*. https://www.aha.org/system/files/2018-01/aha-patient-care-partnership.pdf

American Nurses Association. (2025). *Code of ethics for nurses with interpretive statements*. https://www.nursingworld.org/practice-policy/nursing-excellence/ethics/code-of-ethics-for-nurses/

Arshagouni, P. (2006). "But I'm an adult now ... sort of": Adolescent consent in health care decision-making and the adolescent brain. *Journal of Health Care Law and Policy, 9*(2), 315–364. http://digitalcommons.law.umaryland.edu/jhclp/vol9/iss2/8

Bosch, I., Siebel, H., Heiser, M., & Inhestern, L. (2024). Decision-making for children and adolescents: A scoping review of interventions increasing participation in decision-making. *Pediatric Research*. https://doi.org/10.1038/s41390-024-03509-5

Ciranka, S., & vanden Bos, W. (2019). Corrigendum: Social influence in adolescent decision-making: A formal framework. *Frontiers in Psychology, 11*. https://doi.org/10.3389/fpsyg.2020.598347

English, A. (2007). Sexual and reproductive health care for adolescents: Legal rights and policy challenges. *Adolescent Medicine: State of the Art Reviews, 18*(3), 571–581.

Fiscus, M. (2021, May 12). *Tennessee "Mature Minor" doctrine and co-administration of COVID-19 and routine immunizations*. Tennessee Department of Health. https://wpln.org/wp-content/uploads/sites/7/2021/06/MatureMinor_COVID19Coadministration_May122021.pdf

Hijano, D. R., & Yaun, J. A. (2024). Mature Minor Doctrine Clarification Act: A setback in pediatric immunizations. *Journal of the Pediatric Infectious Diseases Society, 13*(2), 155–158. https://doi.org/10.1093/jpids/piae006

Morris, G. (2023, June 20). *How nurses can advocate for patients*. Nurse Journal. https://nursejournal.org/articles/how-to-advocate-for-patients/

Ramsay, A., Birks, P. M., & Hartin, D. P. (2022). Advocacy in nursing: Speaking truth to power? *Collegian (Royal College of Nursing, Australia), 29*(5), 549–550. https://doi.org/10.1016/j.colegn.2022.09.001

SchoolHouse Connection. (2023, June). *State laws on minor consent for routine medical care*. https://schoolhouseconnection.org/article/state-laws-on-minor-consent-for-routine-medical-care

Tennessee Department of Health, HIV/STD Program. (n.d.). *Mature minor doctrine, Tennessee.* http://www.pediatricspecialistsofmarioncounty.com/pdf/mature_minor_doctrine-form.pdf

U.S. Department of Health and Human Services. (2024, April 26). HIPAA privacy rule to support reproductive health care privacy. *Federal Register.* Office of Civil Rights, Office of the Secretary. https://www.federalregister.gov/documents/2024/04/26/2024-08503/hipaa-privacy-rule-to-support-reproductive-health-care-privacy

U.S. Department of Health and Human Services. (2025, September 11). *Subpart E-privacy of individually identifiable health information- 45 CFR §164.520 through §164.528.* https://www.ecfr.gov/current/title-45/subtitle-A/subchapter-C/part-164/subpart-E

Image Credits

Fig. 7.2: Generated using Adobe Firefly.

CHAPTER 8

Problem-Solving in Nursing Practice

Objectives

Upon completion of this chapter, the learner will be able to do the following:

1. Apply critical thinking techniques to analyze and resolve patient care issues.
2. Use the steps of the problem-solving process in addressing nursing issues.
3. Recognize typical challenges that nurses face when using clinical reasoning and critical inquiry to solve clinical problems.
4. Justify the importance of interdisciplinary collaboration in problem-solving for patient management.

Key Chapter Terms

- Critical thinking
- Level of expertise
- Cognitive skills
- Nursing process
- Subjective data
- Objective data
- Nursing diagnosis
- Medical diagnosis
- NANDA International (NANDA-I)
- Maslow's hierarchy of needs
- Clinical reasoning
- Critical inquiry
- Interdisciplinary collaboration

Problem-Solving in Nursing

Nursing is fast-paced, and nurses are continually faced with complex patient situations that require thoughtful analysis and quick resolution.

Problem-solving by nurses is an important foundation to identification of essential physiological changes that can affect patient safety in the healthcare environment. Nurses are the contact liaison between patients and physicians or advanced practice nurses. There are key components that facilitate this foundational element for nurses. They are integrated components in the educational process—both in the classroom and clinical.

Critical Thinking

Critical thinking is the foundation of effective nursing practice. It is an essential element in nursing practice and a point of focus in nursing education. It involves actively questioning, analyzing, and evaluating information. *Critical thinking* is defined by the Foundation for Critical Thinking (2019) as "the intellectually disciplined process of actively and skillfully conceptualizing, applying, analyzing, synthesizing, and/or evaluating information gathered from, or generated by, observation, experience, reflection, reasoning, or communication, as a guide to belief and action." The American Nurses Association (2024) identifies *critical thinking* as involving problem identification, best solution determination, and implementation of the most effective resolution. The American Association of Colleges of Nursing (2021) has defined *critical thinking* as "the skill of using logic and reasoning to identify the strengths and weaknesses of alternative healthcare solutions, conclusions, or approaches to clinical or practice problems" (p. 57). The combination of these definitions is used to identify the scope and key elements for critical thinking in many nursing programs. This allows programs to validate critical thinking in applying learned knowledge and skills to the identification of patient problems and performing appropriate nursing actions for promotion of positive patient outcomes. Critical-thinking skills are cultivated in all aspects of nursing education using foundational liberal arts and science courses taken outside the nursing curriculum.

Critical Thinking: An Essential Component of Nursing Practice

Critical thinking is potentially the single most important factor that determines success or failure in nursing practice (Elder & Paul, 2010). Activities used by nurses in the workplace incorporate independent and collaborative problem-solving, resource allocation, integration of data and information using technology, and the acquisition and evaluation of numerous amounts of information. Success in using these activities requires that nurses possess basic educational skills such as reading and writing; personality attributes that promote personal interaction and trust, such as self-esteem, self-confidence, and self-awareness of limitations; and thinking skills that include the ability to reason, generate ideas, and problem-solve.

Critical thinking allows nurses to examine current scenarios, analyze all relevant information, and make decisions based on the best course of action. This promotes competent care delivery. Nursing experience enhances the ability to think critically. This ability is described by Patricia Benner (1984) in her research and work, describing five **levels of expertise**, from novice to expert (see Table 8.1).

TABLE 8.1 Benner's Five Levels of Nursing Expertise

Level of Experience	Descriptors
Novice	• Beginner with no experience • Taught general rules to assist with performing tasks • Rules are context-free and applied universally • Rule-governed behavior is limited and inflexible
Advanced beginner	• Demonstrates acceptable (marginal) performance of tasks • Has difficulty generating priorities and may view situations as having the same level of importance • Has gained prior experience in real situations to recognize recurring meaningful components • Principles are based on experiences and form a foundation to guide actions
Competent	• Demonstrates competence in task performance with usually two to three years of experience • Gains perspective from planning own actions based on conscious, abstract, and analytical thinking • Thinks abstractly and efficiently organizes activities for simultaneous implementation
Proficient	• Perceives and understands situations as part of a whole • Uses holistic understanding to improve decision-making • Learns from prior experience what to expect in certain situations • Uses prior experience to modify plans for situational management
Expert	• Does not rely on principles, rules, or guidelines to determine actions • Has an intuitive grasp of situations • Performance is fluid and flexible. • Highly proficient and responds automatically

Source: Adapted from Patricia Benner, "Benner's Five Levels of Nursing Expertise," From Novice to Expert: Excellence and Power in Clinical Nursing Practice. Copyright © 1984 by John Wiley & Sons, Inc.

The length of time one is exposed to care activities promotes changes in skill level. Differences in skill levels reflect changes in three aspects of skill performance. These include:

1. Moving from relying on context-free rules that are applied universally to using past concrete experiences to guide care actions
2. Change from viewing situations as separate pieces to a holistic view and perspective of the whole
3. Movement from a passive observer, one outside of the situation, to an involved performer, actively engaged and participating

Critical thinking in nursing encourages nurses to be:

> habitually inquisitive, well-informed, trustful of reason, open-minded, flexible, fair-minded in evaluation, honest in facing personal biases, prudent in making judgments, willing to reconsider, clear about issues, orderly in complex matters, diligent in seeking relevant information, reasonable in the selection of criteria, focused on inquiry, and persistent in seeking results which are as precise as the subject and the circumstances of inquiry permit. (Facione, 1990, p. 2)

Critical thinking serves as a foundation for sound clinical judgment in the healthcare setting. These judgment decisions ultimately affect patient outcomes. There are **cognitive skills** and traits/dispositions of critical thinkers (American Philosophical Association, 1990). These are identified in Table 8.2.

TABLE 8.2 Cognitive Skills and Traits/Dispositions of Critical Thinkers

Cognitive Skills	Traits/Dispositions
• Interpretation—categorization, decoding significance, clarifying meaning • Analysis—examining ideas, detecting, and analyzing arguments • Evaluation—assessing claims and arguments • Inference—querying evidence, conjecturing alternatives, drawing conclusions • Explanation—stating results, justifying procedures, presenting arguments • Ability to self-monitor—self-examination and correction • Ability to seek information, discriminate, predict, apply standards, use logical reasoning	• Is truth-seeking—courageous about asking questions, honest and objective in pursuing inquiry • Is open-minded—sensitive to own bias, respects the rights of others to hold differing opinions • Is analytical—alert to potentially problematic situations • Is systematic—organized, orderly, focused, able to inquire diligently • Is self-confident—has trust in own reasoning • Is inquisitive—has intellectual curiosity, values being well informed • Is mature—disposed to make reflective judgments • Is able to reflect, persevere, have contextual perspective, be creative, be flexible, use intuition

Source: Adapted from Barbara K. Scheffer & M. Gaie Rubenfeld, "A Consensus Statement on Critical Thinking in Nursing," Journal of Nursing Education, vol. 39, no. 8, pp. 352-359. Copyright © 2000 by Slack, Inc.

When applying critical thinking, it is important to not rely just on the initial information received (i.e., anchoring a decision to this over other information) or favor information that supports a preconceived notion (i.e., confirmation bias). Adopt a systematic approach that allows one to be open-minded, flexible, and willing to revise assessments and nursing diagnoses as new information emerges during the patient's encounter. This will enhance the ability to identify the root causes of a patient's problem. This promotes the delivery of evidence-based, patient-specific solutions.

To see how you add up as a critical thinker, answer the questions in Table 8.3. Rate your use of each component as poor, good, or excellent. For those areas that you rate as poor, develop a plan to increase your proficiency and use of this component in your everyday life, which will transfer to nursing.

TABLE 8.3 Critical Thinking Self-Assessment

Component	Yes	Sometimes	No
1. I can work with change in a situation by making a logical plan for a successful outcome.			
2. I can tell the difference between fact and opinion when coming to a decision.			
3. I can evaluate evidence for use in making a decision.			
4. I recognize biases in myself and others.			
5. I value the opinion of others.			
6. I change my opinion when I find evidence that verifies that I am not correct.			
7. I recognize and can work within my own limitations.			
8. I am comfortable with the idea that there may be more than one answer or solution to a problem.			
9. I look at a situation from different directions or perspectives.			
10. I am organized and orderly in my approach to solving a problem.			
11. I use knowledge from previous situations in making decisions regarding current situations.			
12. I try to learn from my mistakes.			

The key to developing critical thinking is continuous learning. Through the use of lifelong learning activities, you can increase your knowledge and improve the depth of your clinical judgment. A self-assessment is a good place to start the critical-thinking process.

The Nursing Process

The ***nursing process*** is a structured mechanism used by nurses to guide them through steps to critically solve problems in professional practice. This method of problem-solving uses a series of techniques to address an issue in patient management. This process is a cycle that moves fluidly from one step to the other (see Figure 8.1). Movement through the cycle allows for individualized care administration and consideration of varied alternatives for outcome generation by experienced nurses. Each step involves critical thinking and clinical judgment to ensure that the best possible solution to the patient problem is identified and implemented. This dynamic, interactive process includes a reciprocal interpersonal relationship between patients and nurses. Nurses often engage with one patient in numerous activities that are at various steps in the process simultaneously; for example, nurses may be at the assessment step for a projected ambulation activity and at the step of implementation for a patient teaching activity. The nursing process is also flexible and can be used in any healthcare setting with patients of any age or at any developmental level.

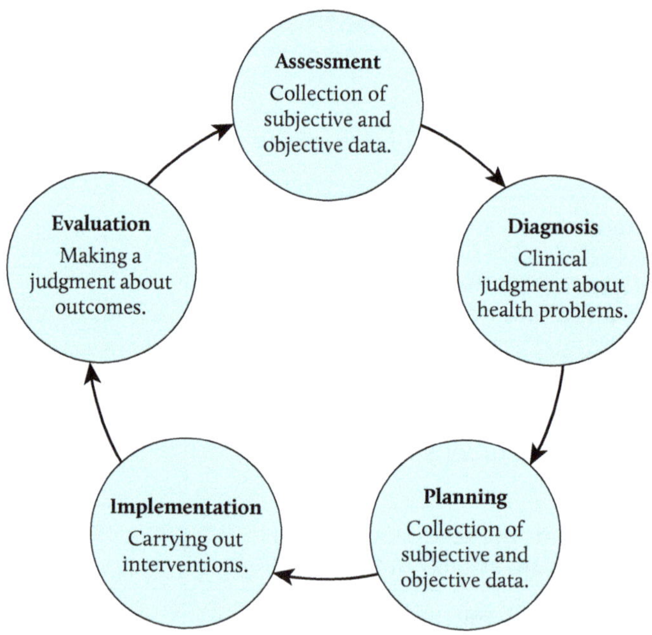

FIGURE 8.1 The Nursing Process

Step 1: Assess the Patient

Assessment starts the process of responding to actual (i.e., what is happening now) or potential (i.e., what could happen) patient problems. It involves collecting information from patients, family members, or other individuals who may have an impact on the patient's health status. Information is collected regarding immediate health issues, historical information regarding health issues, insurance status, and pharmacological history. Holistic information is retrieved from developmental, physiological, psychological, sociological, cultural, spiritual, and environmental perspectives. This information is input electronically as data and made a permanent part of the patient record.

Collecting Patient Data

Data are collected through an interview (see Figure 8.2) and physical examination. The interview starts the process and sets the stage for the development of trust between patients and nurses. Usually, this is done face to face upon patients' entry to a care setting. Occasionally, it may be done by phone or collected electronically. Even if other methods are used, a face-to-face validation session will occur between patients and nurses. Interviewing is a vital skill in beginning a trusting relationship and collecting key information upon which to base future care activities. Following are tips for conducting an interview that promotes a positive patient outcome:

- Clearly articulate the purpose of the interview as well as all questions.
- Choose an interview location that allows for comfort and privacy.
- Attempt to be on the same level as the patient (do not stand over the patient, as this may impede communication).
- Use various question types to encourage communication of information, such as:
    - Open questions that encourage verbalization (e.g., "What brought you to the clinic today?")
    - Closed questions that promote one- or two-word responses of factual information (e.g., "How old are you?")
- Do not combine multiple issues when asking questions (e.g., "Do you have heart disease, hypertension, or diabetes?").
- Do not use questions that may lead the patient to answer in a specific way (e.g., "You don't have any heart disease in your family, do you?" This could give the impression that heart disease is bad and may prompt the patient to answer "No" incorrectly).
- Listen attentively to responses. Actively listen and allow pauses to allow the patient time to think and respond.

Patient information is organized as it is being collected as much of this information will immediately be input into a computerized template and made part of the data in the permanent patient record.

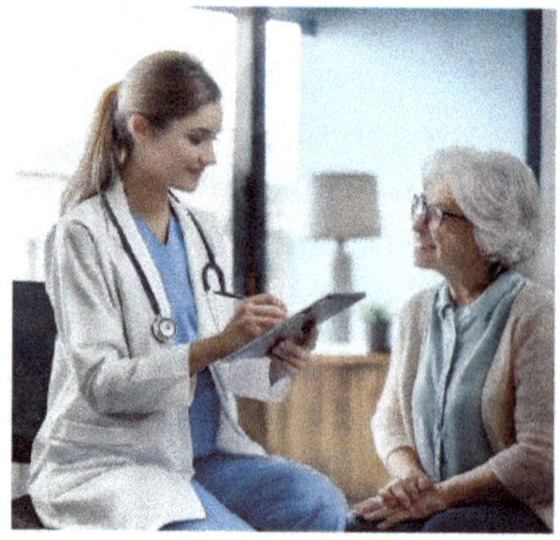

FIGURE 8.2 Interviewing starts the nursing process and lays the foundation for care delivery.

Information is also retrieved by physical examination of patients. Assessment techniques include inspection, palpation, percussion, and auscultation to obtain information that expands the base of patient data. This allows for investigation of body systems and functions to further validate other information collected from patients or other sources. This promotes movement to subsequent areas of the nursing process.

Types of Data

Two types of patient data are collected: subjective and objective. ***Subjective data*** include information supplied by the patient in the form of complaints and descriptions about their current health issue. These are referred to as the *chief complaint* and are the first step in identifying the reason for seeking medical intervention. In other words, it is what patients say or actually tell you is wrong. Examples include "I have a pain in my leg," "My wrist hurts when I try to pick up something," and "I have been vomiting since yesterday." If patients are unable to respond, a significant other or knowledgeable person who came with them may give the reason why they are seeking medical care. Symptom characteristics are important to gather at this time. Mnemonics that can be used to remember clues to symptom collection information during the interview include the OPQRST (List 8.1) and OLDCARTS lists (List 8.2).

List 8.1
***OPQRST* Mnemonic**

- **O**nset
- **P**recipitating and **P**alliating factors
- **Q**uality
- **R**egion or **R**adiation
- **S**everity
- **T**iming or **T**emporal characteristics

List 8.2
OLD CARTS Mnemonic

- **O**nset
- **L**ocation
- **D**uration
- **C**haracter
- **A**ggravating or **A**lleviating factors
- **R**adiation
- **T**iming
- **S**everity

Objective data are signs that can be observed, measured, and verified through the senses. They can be collected through observation or examination. These data can be retrieved through measurement techniques such as temperature, heart rate, respiration, blood pressure, laboratory findings, and radiological results. Another term for these data is *signs*. They are a sign of something that is going on with the patient. Examples of physiological findings of this type of data include red swollen joints, a patient grimacing when a joint is moved, an open and bleeding wound, or a patient holding their stomach in pain.

These two types of data can be used to validate each other and should have agreement between them. If a patient described having a painful ankle after a fall (subjective data) and their ankle was swollen and showed evidence of bruising (objective data), these two pieces of information would be in agreement. If the patient complained of a painful ankle (subjective) and there was no sign of swelling or bruising (objective data), these two pieces of information would not be in agreement. Information that is not in agreement may require a more intensive investigation as it could be a secondary finding for a primary situation. It may also indicate that the problem is not physiological but rather psychological in nature. Through the use of astute nursing interviewing skills, other problems may be identified that may require medical intervention.

Sources of Patient Data

Information may be obtained from three sources: primary, secondary, or tertiary. The primary data source includes the patient and any information collected directly from this individual. Secondary sources include family, friends, or nurses' own knowledge from prior interactions or observations. Tertiary sources are sources that compile or digest other sources (primary and secondary source information), such as patients' medical record, which is a compilation of care delivery over time. These sources present summaries of activities and interventions that can be used for current care decision-making.

Confidentiality of Patient Information

Information collected by nurses may include extremely personal and confidential types of data. It is important to maintain the strictest confidence for this information. Establishing a trusting relationship means that nurses have a legal and ethical obligation to guard this information from inadvertent disclosure. It is important to remember that patient information is confidential and comes under the Health Insurance Portability and Accountability Act of 1996 (HIPAA) ruling for disclosure on a need-to-know basis. This may be difficult when information is collected in partially open areas. Every effort must be made to prevent others from inadvertently overhearing this information (e.g., lowering voices, closing doors, or pulling curtains to reduce vocalizations). Electronic information should not be accessed out of curiosity or personal interest. Electronic access or data retrieval is acceptable to be retrieved in an organization only by healthcare providers who have direct care responsibilities for a patient. This means that no discussion of a patient should occur in the cafeteria or elevator. Even if no identifying information is disclosed, it may not be difficult for others who work in an area to clearly identify an individual from the smallest piece of information. Informational discussions between members of the interdisciplinary team should also be done in an area that promotes privacy and eliminates the probability of inadvertent disclosure of information to another person.

Step 2: Formulate the Nursing Diagnosis

Based on the information collected and organized in the assessment phase, a process of reasoning is used to identify problems and develop **nursing diagnoses**. Information should be organized into groups in order to facilitate analysis and identification of problems related to each specific group (see Figure 8.3). Systematic organization allows easy review, analysis, and identification of nursing diagnoses related to each body system (e.g., neurological system, cardiovascular system, gastrointestinal system).

Nursing diagnoses differ from **medical diagnoses** as the former focus on patient problems that nurses identify that describe objectives and interventions related to health problems that nurses are capable of managing (Thomas, 2024). A nursing diagnosis is a human response to "actual or potential health problems which nurses, by virtue of their education and

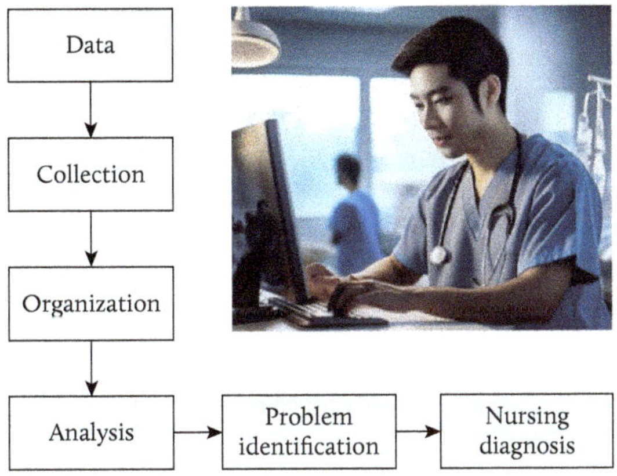

FIGURE 8.3 Process of Nursing Diagnosis Formulation

experience are capable and licensed to treat" (Gordon, 1976, p. 1299). They may be related to the individual, family, or community. They focus on the human response and may address patients' physical, sociocultural, psychological, and/or spiritual response to an illness or health problem. Through the nursing diagnosis process, nurses assign meaning to patient data (Cachón-Pérez et al., 2021). Nurses are responsible and accountable for the outcomes of a nursing diagnosis. A medical diagnosis is specific and related to a pathological disease process. It is a diagnosis that requires medical or surgical intervention.

Nursing diagnoses are standardized by a professional organization known as ***NANDA International*** (**NANDA-I**; formerly called the North American Nursing Diagnosis Association; https://www.nanda.org). This organization facilitates the development, refinement, dissemination, and use of standard terminology for nursing diagnoses. It promotes a global network of nurses who are committed to their improving care quality and improving patient safety through the use of evidence-based practice. The organization funds research to establish evidence-based nursing diagnoses for use in nursing practice in order to identify interventions and outcomes that contribute to safe clinical decisions. It continues to develop and refine nursing diagnoses with input from nurses internationally.

Many nursing programs use nursing diagnoses in identification and development of care plans or plans for care in managing patient interventions. These can be developed with help from the list of NANDA-I-approved nursing diagnoses. The initial part of the nursing diagnosis is the label, which is the concise term or phrase that represents a pattern of related cues. This is essentially the name of the specific diagnosis in the NANDA-I list. This information is followed consecutively by the (a) definition or term/phrase that delineates meaning and differentiates it from other similar diagnoses; (b) defining characteristics that are observable components such as things the nurse can see, hear, touch, or smell; (c) factors that increase the individual's, family's, group's, or community's vulnerability to an unhealthy event; and (d) related factors that precede, are associated with, or relate to the diagnosis.

One format for writing nursing diagnoses is the **PES** format. This includes a **P**roblem, **E**tiology, and **S**igns and symptoms component (see Figure 8.4).

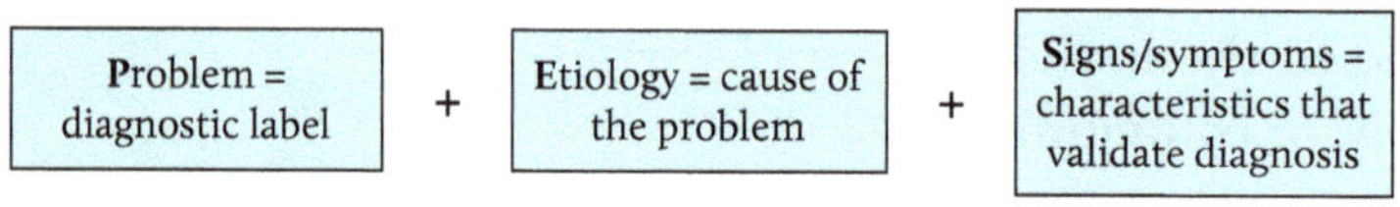

FIGURE 8.4 PES Nursing Diagnosis Format Example

The nursing diagnosis would be constructed based on the format seen in Figure 8.5.

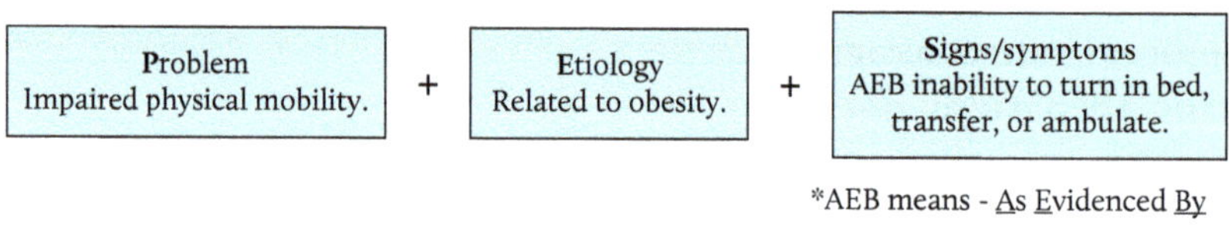

FIGURE 8.5 Nursing Diagnosis Construction

The nursing diagnosis in Figure 8.5 would be written as "Impaired physical mobility related to obesity AEB inability to turn in bed, transfer, or ambulate." All nursing diagnoses using this format would follow this construction format. Now use the activity in Table 8.4 to test your knowledge of nursing versus medical diagnoses. Select the correct category for each diagnosis in the table. The correct answers can be found in the appendix at the end of the chapter.

TABLE 8.4 Activity to Identify Nursing Versus Medical Diagnoses

Diagnoses	Nursing Diagnosis	Medical Diagnosis
1. Ineffective airway clearance		
2. Asthma		
3. Hypertension		
4. Activity intolerance		
5. Sleep pattern disturbance		
6. Diabetes		
7. Fluid volume excess		
8. Congestive heart failure		
9. Pain, acute		
10. Skin integrity, impaired		

Correct answers can be found in the appendix at the end of this chapter.

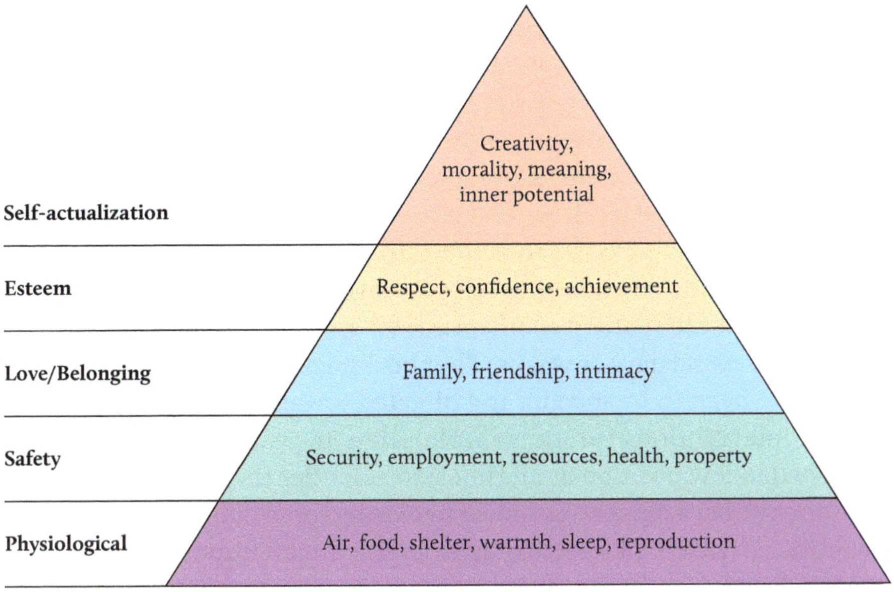

FIGURE 8.6 Maslow's Hierarchy of Needs

Following identification of nursing diagnoses, it is important to prioritize these based on patient safety and harm that may occur. **Maslow's hierarchy of needs** may also be used to prioritize these (see Figure 8.6; Hayre-Kwan et al., 2021). Lower needs are more fundamental and necessary for survival (physiological and safety). Nursing diagnoses that fit into these two categories should be addressed first and, in the order, presented in the diagram, with physiological needs taking priority over safety-related needs.

A nursing diagnosis that deals with a situation that threatens a physiological need would be addressed first by the nurse. This would mean that a nursing diagnosis of "ineffective airway clearance" would be dealt with before "sleep pattern disturbance." When possible, nurses should involve patients in their care by working with them to identify and prioritize nursing diagnoses. This interaction promotes patient-centered collaborative care. They can assist in identifying those symptoms that do not relate to life-threatening situations but rather to feelings of self-worth and knowledge on a specific topic. These may then be addressed through patient education and promote self-care and ownership in personal care outcomes.

Step 3: Plan for Provision of Patient Care

The third step in the nursing process is planning for patient care. At this step, problems that have been prioritized are taken further and worked through stages needed to accomplish a successful outcome. All needs cannot be addressed simultaneously. The first stage is to identify which needs are immediate and which can be delayed. Those needs requiring immediate attention, such as those that are life-threatening, are addressed first. In the second stage, goals or outcome statements for planning nursing actions will need to be established. Patient goals may be long- or short-term. Long-term goals require weeks to months to achieve, whereas short-term goals can be achieved in hours or days. It is good to have both types of goals. Long-term goals keep patients working to achieve their maximum potential. Short-term goals provide a sense of accomplishment and promote self-esteem. These can maintain patient momentum for goals that do not demonstrate change over several days or weeks. The third stage is to determine interventions. These need to be specific and directed toward realistic outcomes for patients. Interventions can range from safety measures (e.g., bedside rails up and bed in low position at all times) to activities that promote sleep and rest (e.g., promote a quiet atmosphere by closing room door and coordinating disruptive activities). In selecting appropriate interventions, it is important to remember that they must be:

- Safe for intervention
- Appropriate for patients' age and overall health
- Consistent with patients' values, beliefs, and culture
- Compatible with collaborative therapies of other healthcare professionals
- Within established standards of nursing care
- Based on nurses' knowledge and experience
- Evidence-based

Planning should be focused on meeting one of the three types: initial planning, ongoing planning, and discharge planning. These are not mutually exclusive but can occur simultaneously. Initial planning is important for retrieving historical information and addressing immediate needs (e.g., postsurgical patient admission). Ongoing planning occurs throughout the interactive nurse-patient period of involvement over a given period of time (e.g., shift of work). This is necessary to determine appropriate care necessary to address patient care. Discharge planning is necessary to promote self-care and prepare the individual to address issues related to health following discharge from the facility. This should start on admission in order to allow time for learning to occur. Continuous feedback promotes learning and builds confidence in performing self-care activities.

Nursing interventions can be independent, dependent, or collaborative. Independent interventions are those that can be initiated by nurses, such as physical care and ongoing assessment of patients. Dependent interventions are those that are carried out under the specific order of a physician (e.g., administration of medication or special dressing management post-surgical intervention). Collaborative interventions are actions that nurses carry out in a cooperative manner with other healthcare professionals, such as managing the pulmonary status of a patient in collaboration with the respiratory therapist.

Step 4: Implement Plan of Care

Implementation of nursing actions identified in the plan is the fourth step in the nursing process. This is where the plan is actually put into action through the implementation of nursing activities. Before the plan is implemented, it is important to (a) review and validate it to make any modifications that may be required, since the plan may be written hours or days before it is actually implemented; (b) assess and correlate the current level of knowledge and skills compared with the actual knowledge and skills needed to implement the plan and request assistance as needed; (c) prepare patients for nursing actions and expectations; and (d) prepare the environment for implementation activities (Institute of Medicine (U.S.) Committee on the Work Environment for Nurses and Patient Safety, 2004).

These activities should be nursing-focused and patient-centered. Care activities should be individualized to meet current health care needs. Activities should be focused toward successful achievement of goals and objectives. Competent, safe nursing interactions will be needed to address all needs identified in the plan. Care activities should be carried out efficiently in order to conserve energy and promote healing for the patient. As activities are implemented, nurses should continue to evaluate patients' response in order to make any adjustments to the plan during care activities. Other activities may also alter the patient care plan. For example, a nursing intervention may be identified that states a patient is to be ambulated for 30 minutes based on a predetermined schedule; however, following an interventional procedure (e.g., lumbar puncture, also called a *spinal tap*), this activity may need to be altered to allow for a restricted reclining position for a designated period of time based on physician orders. Additional measures may need to be implemented based on the patient's physical condition prior to the procedure, which were not in the original plan for the patient. These may include increased rest for 24 hours and reduction of activities, including ambulation and exercise, for a period of time.

This phase also requires documentation of activities performed and patients' response. Documentation should be sequential based on time of activity implementation. Do not chart activities done at 2 p.m. before activities completed at 12:30 p.m. It is good to chart as close to an activity as possible in order to accurately reflect all parts of the activity—including nursing activity and patient response. Organizations have electronic charting, which allows for immediate documentation since computer stations are in the patient room, on mobile carts, or centrally located close to patient care rooms. Charting is a legal responsibility of nurses and part of the permanent patient record.

Step 5: Evaluate Outcome

The fifth step in the nursing process is evaluation. At this time, nurses systematically compare patients' health status with identified goals and expected outcomes. This step involves the nurses, patients, and other members of the healthcare team. During this step, patients' status, progress toward goal, and outcome achievement and effectiveness of nursing strategies are evaluated.

Using the nursing diagnosis of "Fluid volume deficit related to fluid loss from vomiting and diarrhea AEB signs of dehydration and loss of 10 pounds over seven days," the expected outcome may state: The patient will maintain normal fluid balance and increased weight by discharge AEB the following:

- Increased body weight
- Normal skin turgor (elasticity of the skin)
- Moist mucous membranes
- Stable vital signs (blood pressure, heart rate, and respiratory rate) while supine, sitting, and standing
- No episodes of vomiting or diarrhea

Evaluation would validate that the patient had gained 3 pounds since admission and had normal skin elasticity with moist and pink mucous membranes. Vital signs were stable in all positions with no significant changes, and there had been no episodes of vomiting or diarrhea in 72 hours. In this situation, the goal was met. There may be two other outcomes for patients related to goal achievement. Goals may be partially met or not met. For goals that are achieved, a patient's problem is resolved, or a potential problem was prevented. If the goal was achieved but the patient's problem persisted, there may have been a mismatch between the stated goal and the patient's current condition. This will require revision of the care plan. Regardless of the outcome, charting should occur. For goals that are not met or partially met, there should be a reassessment of the situation, with revisions of the plan for patient care. Evaluation should identify why goals were partially achieved or not achieved. Some reasons might include the following:

- There was a mismatch between the client's capabilities and the goal, making the goal unrealistic.
- The nursing diagnosis was not accurate and did not correctly reflect the actual or potential problem.

- Nursing actions did not match the goal or achieve a level sufficient to address the goal.
- Medical intervention and/or orders changed, affecting nursing and patient priorities.
- The patient's condition changed, which required a change in health care interventions from the interdisciplinary team, including nursing.
- The patient and/or family decided to alter the plan due to a change in the direction of desired care (e.g., change in the patient's advanced directive for health care).

Evaluation is part of this continuous process for nursing and allows for measurement of quality, appropriateness, and effectiveness of care. Actual care delivered should correlate to the plan of care and promote the achievement of collaborative goals.

Clinical Reasoning and Critical Inquiry in Nursing

The nursing process is a problem-solving technique that requires practice, just the same as any other skill in nursing (Papathanasiou et al., 2014). The process provides a framework for responsible and accountable nursing care. Using this process in a nonlinear format may promote **clinical reasoning** in patient management (Banning, 2008). This is done more efficiently by experienced nurses, who do not visualize the process as moving from one step to the next and only in a forward direction but move between the steps, repeating and revising them as necessary prior to arriving at a solution.

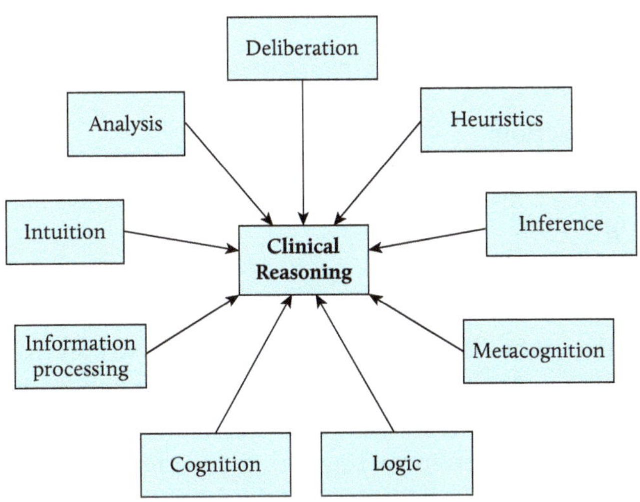

FIGURE 8.7 Attributes of Clinical Reasoning

Clinical reasoning is a critical skill that allows nurses to formulate wise decisions. This thinking process promotes the performance of the best-judged action in a specific situation. It is a combination of several attributes (see Figure 8.7) that result from formal and informal thinking processes. It is dynamic and allows nurses to retrieve information, analyze it for relevance, and elect to use or discard the information or reserve it for later use. Information continuously goes through this process, integrating organizational policies, the level of patient care needed, the collaborative level required for implementation, and the level of experience needed to carry out necessary interventions.

Critical thinking and clinical reasoning are closely aligned in that they both are techniques used for problem-solving. *Clinical reasoning* is a cognitive process and "encompasses health professionals thinking and acting in assessment, diagnostic, and management processes in clinical situations taking into account the patient's specific circumstances and preferences." (Huesmann et al., 2023, p. 996). Clinical reasoning is established as nurses gain knowledge and expertise (Hong et al., 2021; Simmons, 2010). It has as its primary objective to promote decisions that resolve problems. These decisions are developed by experienced nurses through the use of predictive reasoning based on knowledge and prior exposure to the situation with other patients, backward reasoning by searching for previous data that explain a clinical suspicion, and forward reasoning, which incorporates new data into the developed plan of care in an effort to make clinical decisions for the best patient outcome.

Clinical reasoning depends on nurses collecting critical information. The following were identified by Levett-Jones and colleagues (2010) as the five rights of clinical reasoning:

1. The right cues
2. The right action
3. The right patient
4. The right time
5. The right reason

Use of the five rights is just one strategy the nurse can use to promote clinical reasoning in developing a decision for patient management. ***Critical inquiry*** is also a process of examining existing assumptions, knowledge, and questions. Nurses can then move to gaining and creating new information needed to address a patient care issue. This leads to gaining new perspectives, critically analyzing, sharing what was learned, taking action, and reflecting.

This process allows nurses to identify a problem, propose a solution, locate evidence for validation (for or against proposed solutions), and evaluate solutions based on the evidence. Nurses examine and challenge current situations used for patient management and identify potential evidence-based solutions (Jennings & Potter-Smith, 2002).

There can be challenges in applying clinical reasoning and critical inquiry in practice. One common challenge is time constraints. In areas that are fast-paced, such as emergency rooms and intensive care units, nurses need to make quick decisions with limited information. If nurses are not fully able to engage in the critical inquiry process, they may make errors in decisions regarding the implantation of care activities. If nurses lack sufficient knowledge or experience, making decisions regarding complex patient situations may also be difficult.

Ambiguous clinical situations may pose challenges. There are times when patients present with vague symptoms or conflicting information or have poor historical information recall. It may be difficult to identify the specific pieces of information on which to focus for nursing diagnosis determination. In this case, it is important to collaborate with other healthcare professionals to collect additional information to make a nursing decision and implement appropriate interventions.

Barriers in communication can occur between members of the healthcare team, which can impede clinical reasoning. It is important to be an active member of a patient's care team, engaging and communicating to collect information from various perspectives. Discussing care requirements collectively promotes a holistic approach in addressing patient needs. It provides clarity and facilitates cohesion between team members, which serves to promote a safe, high-quality, evidence-based patient outcome.

Interdisciplinary Collaboration in Patient Management

Patient care involves many healthcare professionals, including nurses, physicians, therapists, social workers, pharmacists, and other professionals. Effective patient management requires a team approach, with input from all in order to create a holistic care plan and promote an effective outcome. The physician may focus on medical interventions, the pharmacist ensures appropriate medication management, and the social worker addresses psychosocial concerns. The focus of each is different but interconnected for nurses. They synthesize this information and integrate it into a comprehensive patient care plan. This plan is then implemented, and nurses monitor the response to treatment. Collaboration reduces the probability of errors and improves patient outcomes.

Interdisciplinary collaboration promotes a culture of mutual respect and shared decision-making. This ultimately enhances patient safety and satisfaction. Effective collaboration allows for anticipatory complication identification. Various perspectives and views support the identification of gaps in care and promote continuity across all care delivery settings.

Summary

Critical thinking and problem-solving are at the core of effective nursing practice (Ennis, 1962; Locsin, 2001). They enable nurses to navigate the complexities of patient management. There is no one technique or strategy used by nurses in clinical settings to arrive at solutions for clinical problems. Nurses may use several strategies for the development of clinical expertise and promotion of problem-solving techniques that promote the best patient outcome. Mind actions may occur in various combinations to achieve an outcome. Clinical reasoning and critical inquiry are only two strategies that incorporate recognition of a situation that requires intervention, reflection on the known information to make a wise decision, interpretation of that information, and action or movement toward an outcome. Applying critical-thinking techniques, using problem-solving processes, and overcoming challenges in clinical reasoning will allow nurses to deliver high-quality, evidence-based, patient care. It is important for nurses to know how to incorporate these methods into thinking on their feet as they move from situation to situation. These form a foundation that nurses can use to promote effective communication to collaboratively enhance processes that ensure that all aspects of patient care are addressed through a team-based approach.

References

Alfaro-LeFevre, R. (2019). *Critical thinking and clinical judgment: A practical approach* (7th ed.). Elsevier.

American Association of Colleges of Nursing. (2021). *The essentials: Core competencies for professional nursing education.* https://www.aacnnursing.org/Portals/0/PDFs/Publications/Essentials-2021.pdf

American Nurses Association. (2024, February 9). *Critical thinking in nursing: Tips to develop the skill.* https://www.nursingworld.org/content-hub/resources/nursing-leadership/critical-thinking-nursing/

American Philosophical Association. (1990). *Critical thinking: A statement of expert consensus for purposes of educational assessment and instruction: Delphi report.* California Academic Press, ED 315–423. https://www.qcc.cuny.edu/socialSciences/ppecorino/CT-Expert-Report.pdf

Banning, M. (2008). Clinical reasoning and its application to nursing: Concepts and research studies. *Nurse Education in Practice, 8*(3), 177–183. https://doi.org/10.1016/j.nepr.2007.06.004

Benner, P. (1984). *From novice to expert*. Addison-Wesley.

Cachón-Pérez, J. M., Gonzalez-Villanueva, P., Rodriguez-Garcia, M., Oliva-Fernandez, O., Garcia-Garcia, E., & Fernandez-Gonzalo, J. C. (2021). Use and significance of nursing diagnosis in hospital emergencies: A phenomenological approach. *International Journal of Environmental Research and Public Health, 18*(18), 9786. https://doi.org/10.3390/ijerph18189786

Ennis, R. H. (1962). A concept of critical thinking. *Harvard Educational Review, 32*(1), 81–111.

Facione, P. A. (1990). *Critical thinking: A statement of expert consensus for purposes of educational assessment and instruction—The Delphi report*. California Academic Press.

Elder, L., & Paul, R. (2010). Critical thinking: Competency standards essential for the cultivation of intellectual skills, Part 1. *Journal of Developmental Education, 34*(2), 38–39.

Foundation for Critical Thinking. (2019). *Defining critical thinking*. https://www.criticalthinking.org/pages/defining-critical-thinking/766

Gordon, M. (1976). Nursing diagnosis and the diagnostic process. *American Journal of Nursing, 76*(5), 1298–1300.

Hayre-Kwan, S., Quinn, B., Chu, T., Orr, P., & Snoke, J. (2021). Nursing and Maslow's hierarchy: A health care pyramid approach to safety and security during a global pandemic. *Nurse Leader, 19*(6), 590–595. https://doi.org/10.1016/j.mnl.2021.08.013

Hong, S., Lee, J., Jang, Y., & Lee, Y. (2021). A cross-sectional study: What contributes to nursing students' clinical reasoning competence? *International Journal of Environmental Research and Public Health, 18*(13), 6833. https://doi.org/10.3390/ijerph18136833

Huesmann, L., Sudacka, M., Durning, S. J., Georg, C., Huwendiek, S., Kononowicz, A. A., Schlegel, C., Hege, I. (2023). Clinical reasoning: What do nurses, physicians, and students reason about? *Journal of Interprofessional Care, 37*(6), 990–998. https://doi.org/10.1080/13561820.2023.2208605

Institute of Medicine (U.S.) Committee on the Work Environment for Nurses and Patient Safety. (2004). *Keeping patients safe: Transforming the work environment of nurses*. National Academies Press (U.S.). https://pubmed.ncbi.nlm.nih.gov/25009849/

Jennings, L. B., & Potter-Smith, C. (2002). Examining the role of critical inquiry for transformative practices: Two joint cases of multicultural teacher education. *Teachers College Record, 104*(3), 456–481. https://doi.org/10.1111/1467-9620.00169

Levett-Jones, T., Hoffman, K., Dempsey, J., Yeun-Sim Jeong, S., Noble, D., Norton, C.A., Rouche, J., & Hickey, N. (2010). The 'five rights' of clinical reasoning: An educational model to enhance nursing students' ability to identify and manage clinically 'at risk' patients. *Nurse Education Today, 30*(6), 515–520. https://doi.org/10.1016/j.nedt.2009.10.020

Locsin, R. C. (2001). The dilemma of decision-making: Processing thinking critical to nursing. *Holistic Nursing Practice*, *15*(3), 1–3. https://doi.org/10.1097/00004650-200104000-00003

Papathanasiou, I. V., Kleisiaris, C. F., Fradelos, E. C., Kakou, K., & Kourkouta, L. (2014). Critical thinking: the development of an essential skill for nursing students. *Acta Informatica Medica*, *22*(4), 283–286. https://doi.org/10.5455/aim.2014.22.283-286

Scheffer, B. K., & Rubenfeld, M. G. (2000). A consensus statement on critical thinking in nursing. *Journal of Nursing Education*, *39*(8), 352–359. https://doi.org/10.3928/0148-4834-20001101-06

Simmons, B. (2010). Clinical reasoning: Concept analysis. *Journal of Advanced Nursing*, *66*(5), 1151–1158. https://doi.org/10.1111/j.1365-2648.2010.05262.x

Thomas, A. (2024, September 4). *Nursing diagnosis: A complete guide for students and professionals*. SimpleNursing. https://simplenursing.com/nursing-diagnosis-guide/

Image Credits

Fig. 8.2: Generated using Adobe Firefly.

Fig. 8.3a: Generated using Adobe Firefly.

Fig. 8.7: Barbara Simmons, "Attributes of Clinical Reasoning from 'Clinical Reasoning: Concept Analysis,'" Journal of Advanced Nursing, vol. 66, no. 5. Copyright © 2010 by John Wiley & Sons, Inc.

Appendix

KEY: TABLE 8.4 Activity to Identify Nursing Versus Medical Diagnoses (Correct Responses)

Diagnoses	Nursing Diagnosis	Medical Diagnosis
1. Ineffective airway clearance	X	
2. Asthma		X
3. Hypertension		X
4. Activity intolerance	X	
5. Sleep pattern disturbance	X	
6. Diabetes		X
7. Fluid volume excess	X	
8. Congestive heart failure		X
9. Pain, acute	X	
10. Skin integrity, impaired	X	

CHAPTER 9

Ethical Aspects of Nursing

Objectives

Upon completion of this chapter, the learner will be able to do the following:

1. Define fundamental ethical principles in nursing.
2. Analyze the role of integrity and accountability in maintaining trust, ethical practice, and professionalism in nursing.
3. Formulate strategies for effectively addressing ethical patient challenges.
4. Discuss ethical theories that may underlie ethics in nursing.

Key Chapter Terms

- Ethics
- Ethical dilemmas
- Morals
- Moral principles
- Code of Ethics for Nurses
- Autonomy
- Beneficence
- Nonmaleficence
- Fidelity
- Justice
- Veracity
- Deontology
- Virtue ethics
- Principlism
- Consequentialism
- Utilitarianism

Ethical Aspects of Nursing

Ethics is an extremely complex issue and may have no clear right or wrong answers based on the scenario. ***Ethical dilemmas*** are situations created by societal changes, technological advances, and changes in laws, regulations, and reimbursement. Decisions are further complicated by conflicts in patients' wishes and family members' desires. Nurses face these situations daily as they strive to balance patient advocacy, moral philosophies, and personal values. These conflicts can cause nurses psychological distress. It is important for nurses to be knowledgeable about how to incorporate all these issues into a decision that represents balance.

Ethics and Morals

Nursing literature interchanges the terms *ethics* and *morals*; however, they are not the same. ***Morals*** are principles or standards of conduct regarding behaviors or beliefs that are acceptable or unacceptable regarding a situation. These established rules of conduct are used in situations in which right-and-wrong decisions are needed relative to what is done. An individual's personal standards may serve as a thermometer for these decisions. The basis of these decisions is from societal attitudes and norms that are conveyed through customs, tradition, and religion. Recognition with individual reference groups may also be used. These reference groups may be based on age, gender, profession, and ethnicity, among others. Group references may overlap and promote stability in making a decision or cause an imbalance if references do not match on a specific situation. Morals may be learned through exposure to situations that require choices. Selection of the right choices may be facilitated through exposure to parental controls, formal education of policing laws, and culture. Peer and societal expectations as well as personal values also affect choices regarding moral issues.

Ethics are **moral principles** that govern an individual or group's behavior. Ethics involve critical analysis of a situation to identify what should be done based on habits or customs. This requires consideration of all possible known actions in order to make the best ethical decision in a given situation. Codes of behavior may also be used to guide these decisions. In nursing, this is the American Nurses Association's (ANA) **Code of Ethics for Nurses** (see Box 9.1).

The International Council of Nurses (ICN) also developed a Code of Ethics for Nurses in 1953. The ICN is an organization that includes more than 130 national nursing associations and represents nurses worldwide. Its purpose is to represent nurses worldwide and serve as the voice of nursing internationally (ICN, 2023, p. 4).

Code of Ethics for Nurses

Provision 1. The nurse practices with compassion and respect for the inherent dignity, worth, and unique attributes of every person.

Provision 2. A nurse's primary commitment is to the recipient(s) of nursing care, whether an individual, family, group, community, or population.

Provision 3. The nurse establishes a trusting relationship and advocates for the rights, health, and safety of recipient(s) of nursing care.

Provision 4. Nurses have authority over nursing practice and are responsible and accountable for their practice consistent with their obligations to promote health, prevent illness, and provide optimal care.

Provision 5. The nurse has moral duties to self as a person of inherent dignity and worth, including an expectation of a safe place to work that fosters flourishing, authenticity of self at work, and self-respect through integrity and professional competence.

Provision 6. Nurses, through individual and collective effort, establish, maintain, and improve the ethical environment of the work setting that affects nursing care and the well-being of nurses.

Provision 7. Nurses advance the profession through multiple approaches to knowledge development, professional standards, and the generation of policies for nursing, health, and social concerns.

Provision 8. Nurses build collaborative relationships and networks with nurses, other healthcare and nonhealthcare disciplines, and the public to achieve greater ends.

Provision 9. Nurses and their professional organizations work to enact and resource practices, policies, and legislation to promote social justice, eliminate health inequities, and facilitate human flourishing.

Provision 10. Nursing, through organizations and associations, participates in the global nursing and health community to promote human and environmental health, well-being, and flourishing.

Source: American Nurses Association, "Code of Ethics for Nurses." Copyright © 2025 by American Nurses Association. Reprinted with permission.

The organization has continued to revise the ICN code with updates based on the world's ever-evolving and changing social perspectives, which affect nursing's professional focus in response to these situations (e.g., telehealth, telenursing). The most recent revision was in 2023. The *ICN Code of Ethics for Nurses* has four principal elements: (a) a nurse's responsibility to provide care to all individuals; (b) a requirement for personal responsibility

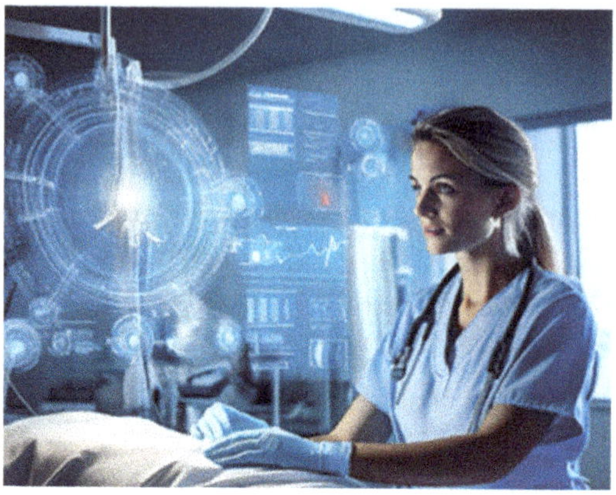

FIGURE 9.1 Potential Future Technology in Patient Care

and accountability to maintain competence in practice; (c) the assumption of a key role in identifying and implementing acceptable standards of clinical nursing in all areas, which include practice, management, research, and education; and (d) the sustainment of a supportive relationship with peers and colleagues.

Ethical dilemmas are complex situations that result from a debate between two moral principles. In this situation, both sides have responses that may be reasonable to consider. Technological advances can be one source of these dilemmas. Advances have served to prolong life for individuals who, prior to technology, would not have survived. Future technologies will undoubtably expand life expectancies across the globe (see Figure 9.1).

Devices such as ventilators for respiratory support and left ventricular assist devices to promote the workings of a defective heart may prolong the life of individuals who have no identifiable brain activity as evaluated by physical assessment or machine (an electroencephalogram can be used to detect brain wave activity). The mismatch of these signs of life and death generate questions related to quality of life and patient rights. Nurses must use ethics on a daily basis to arrive at decisions and ways to manage these type of patient care situations.

Basic Ethical Principles

Autonomy

Autonomy is the principle that states individuals have the right to make their own decisions and subsequently control their own lives. This principle is generally valued by individuals (Entwistle et al., 2010). It is often correlated to the concepts of being one's own person and shaping one's own life. For patients, this principle focuses on situations in which decisions are required for health care interventions. It is important that patients be offered options and allowed to make voluntary choices about these potentially life-changing decisions.

Autonomy is the ability of self-determination and the moral foundation for informed consent. Patients' choices must be made without coercion or undue influence. This includes not using techniques such as gaining the assistance of outside influences to convince patients, applying consequences, or coaxing. Respect for patients' autonomy acknowledges their right to hold views, make choices, and take actions based on personal values and beliefs. Each person is unique and deserves to have their life experiences respected because only they are aware of the emotions, motivations, and physiological issues that govern their decisions. This requires that healthcare professionals respect individuals and their decisions (Ganzini et al., 2003). It is important that individuals are identified as old enough and competent to make these decisions. This means that they have the ability to make decisions regarding their own care and treatment based on information obtained from healthcare professionals as well as to refuse treatment regardless of the opinions of care providers.

A situation that challenges autonomy is one that involves compulsory or forced treatment. This can result in a battle of wills between the patient, who is determined to maintain autonomy, and the care provider, who is determined to treat the patient's illness. For example, a geriatric patient who is alert and oriented but in poor health and significant pain refuses to eat or drink. There is an alternative health care therapy called *nasogastric tube feeding*. According to this method of feeding, a tube is inserted through the nose (usually) directly into the stomach in order to give the patient nutritional substances. However, this procedure is considered invasive, requires collaborative management (e.g., medical, nursing, and nutritionist), and can be associated with complications. As with many ethical situations, there are several ethical principles involved in this scenario. Not only is autonomy an issue to be considered, but so are beneficence, nonmaleficence, and justice. These are explained in the following sections. Think of this scenario as you explore these ethical principles.

Beneficence

The principle of ***beneficence*** is one that is fundamental to nursing. When asked, many nursing students and professionals would say they desired to be a nurse in an effort to help people. This directly reflects healthcare professionals' responsibility to contribute to patients' welfare. It means to do good, be proactive in helping others, and avoid engaging in activities that risk harming other persons. It requires that benefits and risks are balanced for patients. Beneficence is the basis of the intent to work for patients' best interests (Varkey, 2021). It is patient-centered and draws on care providers' knowledge (Chou & Frazier, 2020).

Questions arise from definitions of the term *good*. When considering a definition for *good*, it is important to consider the following questions:

- Who defines what is "good" for a patient?
- Is all life "good"?
- How does quality of life fit into what is "good" for a patient?
- Can a "good" death be better than a not-so-"good" life for patients with terminal illnesses?

Answers to these questions are not the same for all patients. Many factors can affect patients' answers, including personal importance of their place in society, feelings of obligation to family and friends, and perceived burden on others (e.g., physiological, psychological, emotional, and financial).

Nonmaleficence

Nonmaleficence is the principle that requires that healthcare providers do no harm (Varkey, 2021). It reflects both the idea of not inflicting intentional harm and not engaging in activities or actions that risk harm to others. In health care, nonmaleficence includes avoiding negligent and harmful care. If, as the nurse, you fail to turn a patient every two hours and take precautions to prevent skin breakdown and the patient develops a decubitus ulcer, this would be a principle violation. This is because not turning the patient and taking precautions to prevent skin breakdown is negligent care, and as a result, the patient was harmed through the development of a decubitus ulcer. This situation is very clear in its violation, but often this is not the case. Some treatments cause temporary "harm" in an effort to give the possibility of a better life. This is the case with cancer treatment, which can include surgery, chemotherapy, radiation therapy, targeted drug therapy, and immunotherapy. Some potential side effects include anemia (reduced red blood cells), appetite changes, bleeding problems, hair loss, fatigue (feeling tired), memory loss, mouth and throat changes that can affect the ability to eat, nausea and vomiting, pain, skin and nail changes, swelling (fluid retention), and urination changes. These can cause significant discomfort throughout the process of cancer treatment. The end result of this treatment may be partial or complete remission. Partial remission would mean that a large percentage of the signs and symptoms of cancer are gone but some still remain. Total remission would mean that there are no signs or symptoms of cancer. When caring for patients experiencing these types of symptoms, it is difficult to view the treatment as not causing harm. It is important to remember that treatment was a decision made by these patients. The intent of the treatment is not to cause harm but rather as a potential to improve quality and length of life (Chou & Frazier, 2020).

Fidelity

The ethical principle of ***fidelity*** is the obligation to be loyal, be faithful, and honor commitments. Patients should be able to trust their healthcare provider and have faith in the therapeutic relationship. It is important for healthcare team members to be faithful or loyal to agreements and responsibilities as part of their professional foundation (Chou & Frazier, 2020). Not adhering to these important actions could threaten the therapeutic relationship between patients and care providers.

Fidelity supports the concept of accountability. Patients expect nurses to maintain fidelity when managing their care. This is reinforced by the organization when nurses report to duty. Patient assignments are made that identify nurse-patient care responsibility. Nurses are given a report on each patient to promote continuity of care, and they accept responsibility for the delivery of safe, professional care for a designated period of time. Throughout this period, nurses are accountable for delivery of care that complies with the ANA Code of Ethics and is within the scope of state nursing practice. Organizational policies and procedures also serve as a foundation for fidelity. Just as with other ethical principles, it is important to identify circumstances that would affect fidelity and its consequences.

Justice

Justice is the principle that states there should be social distribution of benefits and burdens (Chou & Frazier, 2020). This means that decisions should be fair for all people (Varkey, 2021). Everyone should be treated equally regardless of race, sex, religious beliefs, or life status (e.g., marital status, medical diagnosis, economic level). This principle underlies Provision 1, the first statement in the ANA's Code of Ethics, which states that "the nurse practices with compassion and respect for the inherent dignity, worth, unique attributes of every person" (ANA, 2015, p. 1). Justice is the promotion of equity or fairness in all nursing situations. This means that the allocation of nursing resources is done fairly; that would require nurses to engage in standards or criteria for ensuring equity for a staffing mix that addresses patient needs. It is also used by nurses when managing patient situations. Patients who are in need of immediate treatment are addressed first for care (e.g., responding to a bed alarm, which would signal to a nurse that a patient on fall alert needed attention).

Another principle has its basis in justice. It is called *distributive justice* and addresses the allocation of benefits. This expands on the justice principle by including a clause that defines *justice* as equal rights for everyone and states that the greatest benefit is to be given to the least advantaged persons or individuals with the greatest need. Evidence of this can be seen on the medical-surgical unit, where patients who are in pain have their needs addressed before a patient who is inquiring about discharge information.

Veracity

Veracity is the principle of truth-telling (Amer, 2019; Graf et al., 2020). It is grounded in respect for persons and autonomy. This principle requires that healthcare providers give patients the information necessary to make a rational decision based on available choices. The information delivered needs to be clear, internally consistent, coherent, comprehensive, and simple. Truth-telling can be violated by healthcare providers if they (a) do not tell the truth or deliberately give the patient erroneous information or (b) withhold information by omitting facts or deliberately using jargon that the patient cannot understand.

Informed consent is a significant part of this principle. Patients and families rely on information from caregivers in order to make informed choices regarding their health care (Varkey, 2021). They expect to be told the truth even if it is to disclose a care provider error. Truth-telling is expected regarding all forms of care activities.

Caregivers should be honest in their dealings with all individuals in addition to patients and their families. Truthfulness is expected in all patient and community interactions and activities. Care providers should be honest in all forms of documentation, review of peers for professional activities, compliance with standards of care and organizational policies and procedures, communications and transactions with community individuals, and regulatory reporting, to name several.

Ethical Theories

Deontology

Deontology is a duty-based theory with a central moral concept of duty. It holds that some feature of an act, other than the consequences, makes it right or wrong. Actions are based on a duty to perform certain activities. According to this theory, the most important aspects of our lives are governed by certain unbreakable moral rules. These rules may not be broken even if breaking them would improve the outcome. Using this theory means that ethical decision-making is based on rules and principles regardless of the consequences.

The ethical theory of deontology focuses on what is right. Rights are governed by set rules that cannot be changed regardless of the consequences, even in healthcare situations. Using this theory results in predictable decisions because decisions are based on individuals' set duties and not patient consequences or outcomes. This is an example of a nonconsequentialist theory, which means that it is based on something other than the rightness or wrongness of the consequences. This type of theory judges rightness and wrongness based on properties fundamental to the action and not based on the consequences.

The theory contends that individuals have a duty to do certain things and to refrain from doing others. Based on this theory, one would never tell a lie regardless of the consequences of this action. An example would be a patient who requested that their family members not be told about their cancer diagnosis. Based on deontological theory, if the patient's family members asked, the caregiver would be required to tell the truth and provide some information even against the patient's wishes. They would be required to respond in a manner that would not violate confidentiality. To tell the truth under any circumstances could be a significant constraint for this theory. The constraints caused by this theory are freely accepted by individuals who are bound to this theory, the using of which requires looking at the act itself, not the consequences.

Virtue Ethics

Virtue ethics identifies that an individual does the right thing knowingly and willfully. It does not take into account the reason for the action but instead emphasizes the importance of personality traits in the response. This ethical theory can be found in the works of Plato and Aristotle (Begley, 2006; Carr, 1988; Ross, 2021; Vardy, 1999). These Greek philosophers identified that virtue ethics was a collection of normative ethical philosophies that emphasized *being* rather than *doing*. To them, moral virtues represented excellence of character and were displayed in characteristics such as courage, temperance, or excellence. Aristotle identified that virtues of character were acquired by practicing them and not through just one exposure or situation. These take time to develop and internalize. According to Aristotle (c. 384 B.C.), the virtue of honesty could not be developed by performing one honest act (Ross, 2021, Urmson, 1998). One act alone did not represent internalization of the virtue. Plato (c. 427 B.C.) identified that virtue was based on knowledge or wisdom. Both philosophers focused their questions of character around what type of person an individual should be.

Virtue ethics deemphasizes rules, consequences, and specific acts and places the focus on the type of person who is acting. It is not necessarily based on a right intention or whether a specific rule is followed, but rather on whether the person is expressing good character or not. This theory sees a person as the total sum of their virtues or character traits. These traits can range on a continuum from good to bad and are deeply entrenched in their person. Some character traits include being attentive, confident, cooperative, efficient, honest, polite, reliable, thoughtful, and trustworthy, among many others.

Individuals develop character traits by habits of perception, motivation, and action. As a result, the individual who practices this ethical theory will act in a good way, not because of principle or duty, but rather because they are good.

Virtue ethics is used in one's personal and professional dealings with individuals. As an internalized part of the person, no distinction is made between personal and professional use of the virtue. Responding in such a way to take virtue ethics into consideration does not guarantee that an individual will engage in the correct behavior, but it does predispose them to the correct action.

Principlism

Principlism is a system of ethics that uses principles in place of theory and moral rules and ideals in addressing ethical situations. It is based on four ethical principles: autonomy (free will), beneficence (to do good), nonmaleficence (to do no harm), and justice (the social distribution of benefits and burdens) (Chally, 1998). The four-principles approach of principlism is a generalist approach to addressing various ethical situations. Individuals who are proponents of principlism state that these four moral principles are evident in decisions of the past and are compatible with many intellectual individuals, religions, and cultural beliefs. This makes principlism a unified moral approach, in which each principle assists in arriving at an ethical decision. The goal is to balance each principle, giving importance to each but not ranking them, as there is no intrinsic priority for these principles. This allows each one to be used as an attribute to unify the decision-making process when dealing with ethical situations. This does not mean that one principle may be more influential than the other in a given situation. Awareness of this change in balance allows the principlism user to work toward balance. This allows the decision-maker to obtain the maximum benefit from each principle.

The four principles of autonomy, beneficence, nonmaleficence, and justice are role-specific duties that are always in effect when administering care. There can be a dilemma for caregivers in using this system of ethics (Kennedy, 2004). For example, if a patient desires to discontinue taking a medication needed for healthcare management, nurses may feel obligated to respect the patient's autonomy but compelled to promote patient wellness, which is the ethical role of beneficence (to do good). It is important for the principlism user to be aware of potential balance conflicts in using this system in managing ethical situations (Lindridge, 2017).

Consequentialism

In ***consequentialism***, an action is right if it promotes the best consequences. This theory is result-based and focuses on the right act. An act is better or more right if it produces more good consequences. This means that an ethical decision would be based on which act resulted in the best consequences for the patient. In consequentialism, an action should be chosen that maximizes good consequences. This theory is designed to maximize the good for a given situation. Based on consequentialism, lying would be wrong because it usually produces bad consequences. Utilitarianism is one form of consequentialism.

Utilitarianism

Utilitarianism looks at right and wrong from the perspective of promoting the greatest good for the greatest number of individuals (Williams, 2009). It seeks an answer to an ethical situation through the perspective of an answer to the question, what is the greatest good for the greatest number of people? In addition to this question, there is the premise of increasing human well-being or welfare, which is called *utility*, the derivative term for the theory. In this theory, well-being for humans consists of pleasure.

Utilitarianism focuses on outcomes and not on intentions for that outcome. This theory promotes no independent sense of right and wrong. According to Pollock (2004), good for many individuals outweighs a negative situation for one individual. This is very evident in disaster management (Vearrier & Henderson, 2021). In a situation in which hundreds of individuals are injured, some of them critically, time distribution for care management would be focused on helping as many individuals as possible instead of focusing numerous hours on the treatment of one person. Decision actions are judged and evaluated based on the achieved goal or outcome, which should result in a general good for the majority of individuals. This is also used by healthcare programs and other organizations in determining the distribution of healthcare dollars. With limited monies available to a program or an organization, they could use this theory to make a decision aimed at spending these dollars on immunizations for numerous individuals in the community as opposed to paying for a liver transplant for one individual. What makes this action right is the fact that it produced the most positive consequences.

Ethical Dilemmas

An *ethical dilemma* is a moral problem or situation that can have two or more mutually exclusive—yet morally correct—courses of action. Successful resolution is a complex process and requires care providers to consider many competing alternatives and variables prior to taking action. Situational circumstances may be unpleasant based on the involvement of other individuals. Situations that involve promoting advocacy through patient protection, confronting a peer, or reporting situations to authorities can cause feelings of confusion, anxiety, doubt, and even anger about being involved or placed in such a situation. It is important to be knowledgeable about organizational policies, professional codes, and personal ethical principles and concepts. Nurses must be prepared to think critically in arriving at a resolution to ethical situations.

Framework for Arriving at Ethical Decisions

It is imperative that nurses have the ability to make ethical decisions. Educational programs strive to facilitate this in an effort to produce graduates—and, subsequently, nurses—who are morally informed, knowledgeable, and accountable. Frameworks for ethical decisions are designed to be used in an effort to enhance the process. They are not designed to be an absolute to decision-making, since many factors must be used in reaching an ethical decision. There is no one model or foolproof method that can account for all of these factors in arriving at the right decision. An ethical decision involves integration of an individual's personal beliefs and values, use of ethical concepts relative to the nursing profession, and incorporation of standards or codes of behavior. All of these affect the ultimate outcome, and the weight of each may vary considerably based on the situation. In one situation, personal beliefs and values may dominate the equation, whereas in another, the standards or codes of behavior take the front-row seat in the equation. Differences in

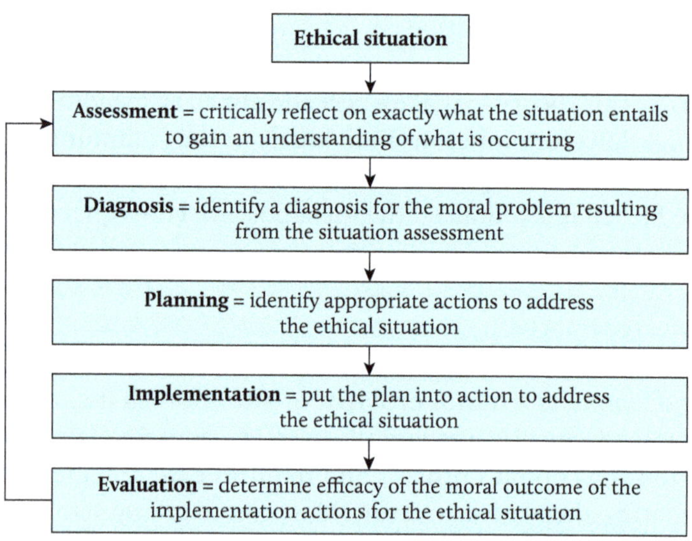

FIGURE 9.2 Nursing Process as a Model for Ethical Decisions

patient care situations will require different approaches to solving ethical problems. These differences are affected by the values of the decision-maker (the patient or patient-designated decision-maker), the nurse, and other care providers involved in the situation.

Use of the nursing process can effectively be one model for arriving at ethical decisions. This model can be adapted to incorporate ethical components in place of patient care activities and might look like Figure 9.2. Key questions for each process step can also assist with arriving at an ethical decision (see Table 9.1).

TABLE 9.1 Key Questions for Using the Nursing Process in Ethical Decision-Making

Nursing Process	Key Questions
Assessment	1. What is the client's mental status? 2. Has the patient been given any medication that would obscure decision-making ability? 3. Is anyone at risk for physical harm? 4. What are my values, feelings, and reactions to the client's situation?
Nursing Diagnosis	1. What ethical principles are involved? a. Which principle is most important? b. Which principle is least important? 2. What ethical theories are involved? a. Which theory is most important? b. Which theory is least important?
Planning	1. What do the policies, principles, and codes say about this situation? 2. Does this situation require consultation with others? 3. What actions can be taken in this situation? 4. What actions comply with the most important ethical principle? 5. Which actions comply with the most important ethical theory?
Implementation	1. Does this plan feel right as it is being put into action? 2. Is this causing more distress for any persons involved as it is being put into action?
Evaluation	1. What were the ethical, legal, emotional, or therapeutic consequences for the patient? 2. What were the ethical, legal, emotional, or therapeutic consequences for the patient's family and/or significant others? 3. What were the ethical, legal, emotional, or therapeutic consequences for the healthcare professional?

Ethical Situation

Scenario: A 36-year-old woman is admitted to the hospital for evaluation of a left breast lesion identified on her mammogram. As suspected, it is found to be malignant, and she is given the results. She is scheduled for a mastectomy the next afternoon. The patient is visibly distraught and crying. During the day of surgery morning report, the off-going nurse reports that the patient cried most of the previous day and did not sleep during the night. She has also been asking about other options or treatments for her situation. The night nurse informs you that she recommended to the patient that she discuss any issues and questions with her surgeon. She noted that the patient had a list of questions that she worked on throughout the night. When you make morning rounds, the patient asks you about other treatments as well. You reinforce that she needs to speak with her surgeon and that they would be in later in the morning.

When the surgeon comes in to explain the procedure and get the surgical consent form signed by the patient, he is astonished by the volume of questions the patient has and is disturbed that nurses encouraged the patient to speak with him about these questions. He is not prepared to address all her questions and fails to explain to her satisfaction why surgery is the best option. She decides against the surgery for a few days in order to give herself time to investigate other options. The physician is angry and tells the nurses that this situation is "all their fault." He relays that because of them, the patient may not have the best outcome because she delayed the surgical procedure.

Both nurses meet to discuss this situation in terms of ethical decision-making, and they use the nursing process grid from Table 9.1. Their responses are in underlined caps in Table 9.2.

Collaborative completion of this tool served to validate for each nurse that they did the right thing for the patient. If you look at this situation, you may identify different principles and theories. As a result, you may use this tool a bit differently. This is because part of the equation in ethical problem-solving is based on nurses' personal decisions. Neither you nor the nurses in this scenario are wrong—the decisions are just different.

TABLE 9.2 Responses to Key Questions for the Nursing Process in Ethical Decision-Making for the 36-Year-Old Patient With a Left Breast Lesion

Nursing Process	Key Questions
Assessment	1. What is the client's mental status? THE PATIENT IS ALERT AND ORIENTED. 2. Has the patient been given any medication that would obscure decision-making ability? NO. 3. Is anyone at risk for physical harm? NO. 4. What are my values, feelings, and reactions to the client's situation? NEED TO ACT AS A PATIENT ADVOCATE AND PROMOTE AN INFORMED DECISION.
Nursing diagnosis	1. What ethical principles are involved? AUTONOMY, BENEFICENCE, FIDELITY, AND VERACITY. a. Which principle is most important? AUTONOMY. b. Which principle is least important? BENEFICENCE. 2. What ethical theories are involved? DEONTOLOGY, VIRTUE ETHICS, AND CONSEQUENTIALISM. a. Which theory is most important? DEONTOLOGY. b. Which theory is least important? CONSEQUENTIALISM.
Planning	1. What do the policies, principles, and codes say about this situation? USED THE ANA CODE OF ETHICS FOR NURSES AND THE ICN CODE OF ETHICS. 2. Does this situation require consultation with others? NO. 3. What actions can be taken in this situation? PROMOTE AUTONOMY USING THE THEORY OF DEONTOLOGY. 4. What actions comply with the most important ethical principle? ENCOURAGE THE PATIENT TO SPEAK FURTHER WITH THE SURGEON TO GAIN INFORMATION FOR AN INFORMED DECISION. 5. Which actions comply with the most important ethical theory? ENGAGE IN ACTIVITIES THAT PROMOTE PATIENT AUTONOMY.
Implementation	1. Does this plan "feel right" as it is being put into action? YES. 2. Is this causing more distress for any persons involved as it is being put into action? NO.
Evaluation	1. What were the ethical, legal, emotional, or therapeutic consequences for the patient? RIGHT TO HAVE ANSWERS TO PROMOTE AN INFORMED CONSENT TO PROCEDURES AND INTERVENTIONS. 2. What were the ethical, legal, emotional, or therapeutic consequences for the patient's family and/or significant others? INCREASED PSYCHOLOGICAL AND FINANCIAL DISTRESS, WHICH COULD LEAD TO FAMILY DYSFUNCTION. 3. What were the ethical, legal, emotional, or therapeutic consequences for the healthcare professional? PSYCHOLOGICAL STRESS OF NOT ACTING IN THE BEST INTEREST OF THE PATIENT.

Summary

It is important to consider ethical principles and theories in arriving at ethical decisions. Managing ethics requires strategic combinations and integration of these principles and theories with understanding in order to arrive at a balance. It involves an integration of knowledge and life skills. Fulghum (1990) said it best: "Live a balanced life—learn some and think some and draw and paint and sing and dance and play and work every day some. ... When you go out into the world, watch out for traffic, hold hands, and stick together. ... Everything you need to know is in there somewhere" (pp. 6–7).

Making ethical decisions is an inevitable part of nursing. These decisions will be independent and interdependent. Patients and families are an integral part of the decision-making process. Nurses must gain theoretical knowledge and work to develop the necessary skills to form a foundation for engaging in the practice of right actions regarding ethics and its consequences on patients, families, and self.

References

Amer, A. B. (2019). The ethics of veracity and it is importance in the medical ethics. *Open Journal of Nursing*, *9*, 194–198. https://doi.org/10.4236/ojn.2019.92019

American Nurses Association. (2015). *Code of ethics for nurses with interpretative statements*. https://www.nursingworld.org/practice-policy/nursing-excellence/ethics/code-of-ethics-for-nurses/

Begley, A. M. (2006). Facilitating the development of moral insight in practice: Teaching ethics and teaching virtue. *Nursing Philosophy*, *7*(4), 257–265. https://doi.org/10.1111/j.1466-769X.2006.00284.x

Carr, D. (1988). The cardinal virtues and Plato's moral philosophy. *Philosophical Quarterly*, *38*(151), 186–200. https://doi.org/10.2307/2219923

Chally, P. S., & Loriz, L. (1998). Ethics in the trenches. Decision making in practice. *American Journal of Nursing*, *98*(6), 17–20.

Chou, T., & Frazier, S. L. (2020). Supporting ethical practice in community-engaged research with *4R*: Respond, Record, Reflect, and Revise. *Ethics & Behavior*, *30*(5), 311–325. https://doi.org/10.1080/10508422.2019.1645665

Entwistle, V. A., Carter, S. M., Cribb, A., & McCaffery, K. (2010). Supporting patient autonomy: The importance of clinician-patient relationships. *Journal of General Internal Medicine*, *25*(7), 741–745. https://doi.org/10.1007/s11606-010-1292-2

Fulghum, R. (1990). *All I really need to know I learned in kindergarten*. Villard Books.

Ganzini, L., Goy, E. R., Miller, L. L., Harvath, T. A., Jackson, A., & Delorit, M. A. (2003). Nurses' experiences with hospice patients who refuse food and fluids to hasten death. *New England Journal of Medicine, 349*(4), 359–365. https://doi.org/10.1056/NEJMsa035086

Graf, W. D., Epstein, L. G., & Pearl, P. L. (2020). Practical bioethics during the exceptional circumstances of a pandemic. *Pediatric Neurology, 108*, 3–4. https://doi.org/10.1016/j.pediatrneurol.2020.04.011

International Council of Nurses. (2023). *Constitution*. https://www.icn.ch/sites/default/files/2023-09/ICN%20Constitution%202023_0.pdf

Kennedy, W. (2004). Beneficence and autonomy in nursing. A moral dilemma. *British Journal of Perioperative Nursing, 14*(11), 500–506. https://doi.org/10.1177/175045890401401103

Lindridge, J. (2017). Principlism: When values conflict. *Paramedic Practice, 9*(4). https://doi.org/10.12968/jpar.2017.9.4.158

Pollack, J. (2004). *Ethics in crime and justice: Dilemmas and decisions* (4th ed.). Wadsworth.

Ross, D. (2021, March 27). *The Nicomachean ethics of Aristotle.* https://www.gutenberg.org/files/8438/8438-h/8438-h.htm

Urmson, J. O. (1998) *Aristotle's ethics*. Blackwell.

Vardy, P., & Grosch, P. (1999). *The puzzle of ethics*. Fount.

Varkey, B. (2021). Principles of clinical ethics and their application to practice. *Medical Principles and Practice, 30*(1), 17–28. https://doi.org/10.1159/000509119

Vearrier, L., & Henderson, C. M. (2021). Utilitarian principlism as a framework for crisis healthcare ethics. *HEC Forum, 33*(1–2), 45–60. https://doi.org/10.1007/s10730-020-09431-7

Williams, D. (2009). Forensic nursing and utilitarianism: The quest for being right. *Journal of Forensic Nursing, 5*(1), 49–50. https://doi.org/10.1111/j.1939-3938.2009.01031.x

Image Credits

Fig. 9.1: Generated using Adobe Firefly.

CHAPTER 10

Legal Aspects of Nursing

Objectives

Upon completion of this chapter, the learner will be able to do the following:

1. Describe the key laws, regulations, and standards that govern nursing practice.
2. Identify nurses' legal responsibilities in patient care, which include duty of care, documentation, informed consent, and potential liabilities associated with malpractice or negligence.
3. Define common legal terminology.
4. Identify delegation and its responsibilities for nurses making empowering act decisions.
5. Summarize Health Insurance Portability and Accountability Act of 1996 (HIPAA) Security Rule safeguards and specifications.

Key Chapter Terms

- Common law
- Statutory law
- Administrative law
- Civil law
- Criminal law
- Civil law violations
- Criminal law violations
- Good Samaritan act
- Good Samaritan statute
- Nursing malpractice
- Torts
- Negligence
- Delegation
- Assault and battery
- Informed consent
- Abandonment
- Confidentiality
- Health Insurance Portability and Accountability Act (HIPAA)

- Health Information Technology for Economic and Clinical Health (HITECH) Act
- HIPAA Security Rule
- Licensure
- Nurse Licensure Compact
- Professional liability insurance

Legal Aspects of Nursing

Nurses are faced with decisions that are affected by legal and ethical issues in their lifetime. Both of these areas of nursing are important for nurses to know and understand. As health care evolves and society changes in both its healthcare dilemmas and pattern of health issues, these areas are constantly changing. Technological innovations only add to the complexity of decisions nurses will make regarding care and outcome or quality of life. This chapter highlights both of these important and complex issues that nurses will face on an ever-increasing basis as time moves health care to a more complex interdisciplinary method of care delivery and management.

Laws

Laws in this country originate from the U.S. constitution, which was adopted in 1787 and is the framework for government organization. This document has as its purposes to (a) establish justice, (b) provide for the common defense, (c) promote the general welfare, and (d) secure liberty. Laws are rules of conduct that are developed for these purposes and provide mechanisms to promote conformity to these stated purposes. There are three major types of laws in the United States: **common law**, **statutory law**, and **administrative law**.

Common law is also known as *case law*. This type of law is developed by judges from court decisions. In this type of law, judges use their knowledge of how similar cases have been managed in the past to make legal decisions for current and future cases. The court is bound to maintain the precedent of prior decisions when resolving similar disputes. This allows for similar cases to be decided using consistent principles or rules so that they will have similar results. This type of law is widespread and used in many other countries outside of the United States.

Statutory law is also known as *statute law*. This type of law is written and formally set down by the legislature at a state or federal level. These develop general propositions of law that courts apply to specific situations when making decisions. A statute may forbid a certain act, direct a certain act, make a declaration, or identify specific government mechanisms to aid society at large. These laws or statutes may be changed or repealed by lawmakers or overturned by a court. Statutes may be time-limited and may automatically terminate or be required to be reapproved for continuation.

Administrative law is a group of laws that govern the activities of administrative state and federal government agencies. This law delegates authority to specific agencies for the purpose of creating laws that meet statute intent. Actions of these government agencies include rulemaking or the enforcement of a regulatory agenda. These laws may be state or federal. They can address police issues, international trade, immigration, or manufacturing, for example. Administrative laws increase when necessary to address societal, political, or economic issues that evolve over time.

Violation of Laws

There are two general violations that can occur when referring to the law. These include **civil law violations** and **criminal law violations**.

Civil law deals with the resolution of noncriminal disputes, such as disagreements over property ownership, contractual components, and personal and property damage. Divorce and child custody are also under this type of law. Civil law serves to resolve these types of situations. These disputes may occur between individuals, organizations, specific parties of people, or a combination of any of these. There is usually a plaintiff, who is the person or persons complaining about the dispute, or the defendant, who is the person or persons defending themselves against identified accusations. These situations may be resolved without the aid of legal representation in a court of law. Resolution may occur based on state or federal statutes. In other situations, civil law may be based on a court ruling. If no statute exists, the decision in a civil law case may create new laws.

Criminal law is also called *penal law* as this body of law relates to crime. This law relates to conduct that is prohibited or unlawful because it may cause harm or endanger public safety and welfare. This law also identifies punishment that may be imposed if individuals breach these laws as well. These punishments or sanctions are imposed based on the severity of the violation and can include imprisonment for a designated period of time to loss of one's life for severe crimes against humanity. Elements of criminal law may include punishment of the individual and a requirement for that person to give back to those who have been harmed (restitution). Some criminal law can extend to include rehabilitation and allow the individual to gain an education and receive psychological help in order to encourage civil obedience after being released from the prison system (parole).

The Nurse and the Law

The nursing profession holds individuals working within its borders to standards that promote trust by society. These include requirements to practice within the guidelines of the State Nurse Practice Act and civil law. The ever-expanding role of nurses and increasing demands leave patients open to healthcare outcomes that may not be desired by the patients or providers. It is important for nurses to be knowledgeable about terms such as *malpractice*, *assault and battery*, *delegation*, *informed consent*, and *patient confidentiality*. Even though the chances of nurses being involved in legal proceedings are small; by exercising one's right to know, they take the first step toward prevention of poor patient outcomes and subsequent legal issues (Khalili & Heydari, 2022).

Good Samaritan Act

The ***Good Samaritan Act*** relates to individuals with healthcare backgrounds who respond to emergency situations and render medical care to accident victims. The law protects healthcare providers from claims of malpractice unless there is proof of gross negligence or willful misconduct (Kim et al., 2021).

A *good Samaritan* is an individual who voluntarily renders aid in an emergency to an injured individual (McCoy, 2024; West & Varacallo, 2022). Even when responding to this type of situation, nurses are responsible for administering reasonably safe care. In most states, no individual is required to perform first aid unless it is part of a job description. Some states consider it an act of negligence if no assistance is given (e.g., calling 911). Some states offer immunity to good Samaritans, which includes protection for errors during the administration of prudent care. This type of statute does not protect acts that are willful and reckless in the administration of assistance. Good Samaritan laws do not apply to individuals performing first aid as part of their duty or job position (e.g., nurses performing first aid in a hospital or clinic). To fall under a good Samaritan act, assistance must be given at the scene of the accident or incident, and the volunteer must be administering aid without anticipated reward or compensation. Following is an example of a **Good Samaritan statute** that applies to nurses:

> When any doctor of medicine or dentistry, nurse, member of any organized rescue squad, member of any police or fire department, member of any organized volunteer fire department, emergency medical technician, intern or resident practicing in a hospital with training programs approved by the American Medical Association, state trooper, medical aidman functioning as a part of the

> military assistance to safety and traffic program, chiropractor, or public education employee gratuitously and in good faith, renders first aid or emergency care at the scene of an accident, casualty, or disaster to a person injured therein, he or she shall not be liable for any civil damages as a result of his or her acts or omissions in rendering first aid or emergency care, nor shall he or she be liable for any civil damages as a result of any act or failure to act to provide or arrange for further medical treatment or care for the injured person. (USLegal.com, n.d.)

Nursing Malpractice

Nursing malpractice can occur when a nurse fails to properly treat a patient regardless of setting. This covers actions that are acceptable when compared with other professionals as well. Nursing malpractice is possibly the number one fear of many practicing nurses. Malpractice can cover failure to observe vital signs, failure to monitor or report changes in a patient's condition, errors in patient treatment or care, medication errors that result in patient harm, or any number of care provision activities that are nurses' responsibility.

There are two terms that are important for nurses to understand when it comes to malpractice. These include ***torts***, which can be intentional and unintentional, and *negligence* (see Figure 10.1).

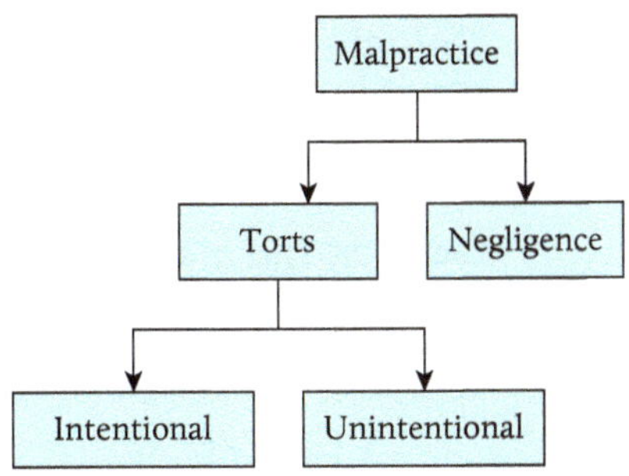

FIGURE 10.1 Connection of Legal Terminology

A *tort* is a harm done to someone else. In order for a tort to exist, physical, psychological, or economic harm must be the result. These civil wrongs may be intentional or unintentional. Intentional torts are willful acts. These can range from assault and battery to libel (see List 10.1).

Negligence is failure to exercise the care a reasonable and prudent person would in like circumstances. An example would include a medication error, such as a situation in which the patient was not given their medication at the correct time and a seizure resulted due to absence of this medication dose. A reasonable nurse would check for medication administration times and administer medications as ordered for the patient. *Malpractice* is a type of professional negligence. There are two prerequisite actions that must be in place before a patient can claim a malpractice action. These include the following: (a) The nurse performed a specialized action and used their skills,

List 10.1
Intentional Torts

- *Assault*: Verbal or an offensive contact (e.g., threatening to give an injection without patient consent)
- *Battery*: Any form of intentional touching without patient consent (e.g., actually giving the threatened injection)
- *Invasion of privacy*: Any form of intrusion (physical or electronic) or dissemination of private information
- *Intrusion upon seclusion*: Invasion of privacy
- *Appropriation of name*: Unauthorized use of an individual's name for some benefit
- *Publication of private or embarrassing facts*: The making public of facts that place a person in a shameful situation
- *Publicly placing one in a false light*: Dissemination of facts that cause one to view a person with an erroneous perspective
- *Defamation of character*: Publication of false statements that result in damage to a person's reputation
- *Malice*: Publication by a person who knows the information is false but publishes it anyway
- *Slander*: The making of a harmful statement in oral form
- *Libel*: The making of a harmful statement in written form

and (b) through the performance of these specialized actions and skills, the patient was harmed. These elements do not just pertain to nurses but to all professionals. In addition, for malpractice to be proven, the following four elements must exist: duty (the professional nurse assumed responsibility for the patient's care); breach of duty (the professional nurse failed to meet the standard of care); proximal cause (the professional nurse failed to meet the standard of care, which was the cause of patient harm); and harm (the harm or injury is provable).

Nurses with specialized training and extensive experience are held to a higher standard of patient care. This care would be correlated to what reasonable and prudent nurses with the same training and experience would have done in similar circumstances. Using this standard, critical care nurses would be expected to recognize the potential for as well as actual problems and assume responsibility for care. Nurses would be liable for tort if patient harm resulted from an inability to use their knowledge, skill, care, and diligence in nursing care delivery.

As nursing responsibility has increased in complexity, sophistication, and specialization, the role of nurses as legally accountable for their actions has also expanded, as have the expectations of society. Nurses are being held responsible and accountable for actions that promote safe patient care.

Delegation

Delegation is defined as "the act of empowering to act for another" (Johnson, 2024). This relates to one person acting for another in the nursing profession. Registered nurses (RNs) delegate as part of their responsibilities since they are licensed. As part of the scope of practice, they are endowed with this ability in order to accomplish designated care activities. Licensed practical nurses (LPNs) and vocational nurses are given delegation authority to assistive personnel as allowed by their state or jurisdiction.

Nurses make delegation decisions every day as part of their care responsibilities. These decisions must be based on the fundamental principle that the outcome will be the protection of public health, safety, and welfare. Effective delegation provides public protection and increases productivity of the nursing care area (Ugoani, 2020). It allows for efficiency and continuity of care activities by blending a team of individuals to accomplish specific goals within a designated time limit (Johnson, 2024).

It is imperative that nurses understand delegation. Even though activities are delegated, the ultimate responsibility rests with the nurses delegating the activity unless the individual who performs the act is also a licensed professional. It is imperative to identify whether the person being delegated the responsibility is capable and educated in such a manner to carry it out.

The National Council of State Boards of Nursing (NCSBN) and American Nurses Association (ANA) developed a joint position paper on delegation in 2019. The intent of this document was to standardize the nursing delegation process. There are five rights of delegation: the right task, the right circumstance, the right person, the right directions and communication, and the right supervision and evaluation. These rights reinforce the legal and ethical accountability of the nurse when delegating specific nursing care activities. These five rights with additional explanation are as follows:

1. **Right task:** Verify that the care task is one appropriate to delegate to the individual based on their knowledge and skill set.
2. **Right circumstance:** Verify that the patient setting is appropriate, resources are available, and all other relevant factors are considered in the situation.
3. **Right person:** Verify that the correct person with the appropriate knowledge, skill set, and competencies are identified and given the task.

4. **Right direction/communication:** Give clear, concise task details, description, and directions, which include task objectives, limitations, documentation, and expectations for completion.
5. **Right supervision and evaluation:** Appropriately monitor, evaluate, and intervene as necessary to accomplish the task in a safe manner. Give feedback to facilitate growth.

Because of the increased number of unlicensed individuals in healthcare organizations, nurses are finding themselves increasingly involved in situations in which delegation is a common occurrence and is mandatory in order to accomplish safe, efficient care. Responsibilities or delegation involve various personnel. These vary based on one's title, as identified in Box 10.1 for employer/nurse leader responsibilities, Box 10.2 for licensed nurse responsibilities, and Box 10.3 for delegatee responsibilities.

Box 10.1

Employer/Nurse Leader Responsibilities

1. Identify a leader for oversight of delegated responsibilities.
2. Determine the nursing responsibilities that may be delegated, to whom, and under what circumstances.
3. Develop the policies and procedures to identify specific responsibilities to be delegated and to whom.
4. Communicate delegation information to licensed and assistive personnel.
5. Validate the delegatee's knowledge and competency in performing delegation.
6. Evaluate the delegation process.
7. Promote a positive culture and work environment for delegation.

Box 10.2

Licensed Nurse Responsibilities

1. Determine when and what to delegate, which is determined by the practice setting, patient needs and conditions, state/jurisdiction provisions, and employer policies and procedures.
2. Communicate with the delegatee regarding patient care requirements.
3. Be available to the delegatee for guidance and questions.
4. Follow up with the delegatee and patient after delegated responsibilities are completed.
5. Provide feedback information to nurse leadership about the delegation process and any issues related to the delegatee's level of competence.

Box 10.3

Delegatee Responsibilities

1. Accept only delegated responsibilities that were appropriately trained and educated so that you can perform and feel comfortable about completing given the setting and patient condition circumstances.
2. Maintain competency for all delegated responsibilities.
3. Communicate with the licensed nurse in charge of the patient.
4. Verify acceptance of the delegated responsibility, carry out the responsibility correctly and in a timely manner, and accurately document the activity.

Nurses have significant responsibility as supervisors of delegated activities. Professional nurses retain legal liability for the actions of any unlicensed individual performing the activity. As nurses, it is important to know the job descriptions of the individuals being supervised. These will assist in identifying the abilities and approved activities that may be delegated to individuals in specific categories (e.g., LPNs, certified nursing assistants). Inappropriate delegation may be grounds for disciplinary action by a state Board of Nursing. As a result, nurses are required to refuse to perform tasks that are not within their scope of practice—regardless of the requesting individual or organization. This is not only a legal issue; it underlies ethics as well. In choosing to delegate, nurses should consider using a delegation process for decision-making. This process includes the following steps:

1. Assess the situation to identify patient needs, consider the circumstances and setting, and ensure availability of resources.
2. Plan for the specific task by ensuring that the individual who has been delegated the task has the knowledge and skills to perform it.
3. Ensure accountability and validate that the individual delegated the task accepts accountability for their portion of the assignment and understands the task to be performed.
4. Supervise by providing clear directions and validating that performance complies with standards of care and are within organizational policies. Intervene, if necessary, to ensure quality and safety.
5. Evaluate the entire process of delegation, which includes the patient, performance of the task, and feedback regarding quality.

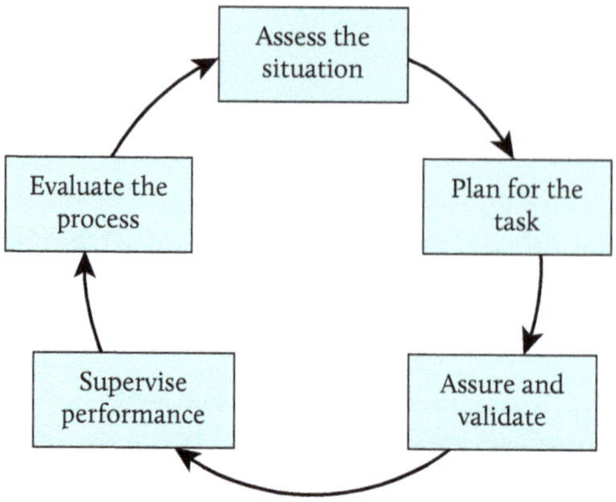

FIGURE 10.2 Delegation Decision-Making Process

This process is circular and allows continuous movement for activities delegated throughout the patient care regimen (see Figure 10.2).

Nurses may identify specific tasks within the nursing process, but accountability for the process itself is strictly held to RNs. It is important for nurses to know which tasks can be delegated within their realm of responsibility based on their specific state (National Council of State Boards of Nursing & American Nurses Association, 2019). When moving from delegation to evaluation, knowledge and expertise improve nurses' chances of effectively using this authority to accomplish safe patient care.

Legal Issues

Assault and Battery

Assault and battery is a tort that can result in legal action against a nurse. Assault occurs when there is a threat of bodily harm or an individual is put in fear of being touched without consent. *Assault* would occur even if there were an attempt to touch another person or a threat to enlist the assistance of others in performing an action against the patient's will. *Battery* occurs if there is actual physical impact on a person or when a person is actually touched without their permission (Ahrenstedt, et al., 1985). If a nurse pushed or slapped a patient, this would be considered battery. Forcing a person to eat or to take a medication is also a form of battery. As nurses, in order to avoid potential claims of assault and/or battery, it is important to:

1. Inform the patient about care activities prior to initiating them
2. Verify that the patient understands what the care activity entails
3. Take time to allow the patient to ask any questions about the activity and consent or refuse the care activity
4. Make sure that the patient fully understands what refusal means regarding the activity

5. Report refusal to the appropriate person (e.g., charge nurse, supervisor, physician) and chart all facts related to patient refusal
6. Never impose an activity for a patient against their wishes or desires

Informed Consent

Many nurses participate in the **informed consent** process. Informed consent can be written, verbal, or implied. In this process, patients have an opportunity to give permission for care activities. Regardless of the type of consent, informed consent must be (a) voluntarily given, (b) given by a competent individual, and (c) received after giving the patient enough information to allow an informed decision regarding the health care activity. Most often consent is in written form for invasive procedure validation in a format that can be maintained in a permanent record. These consents are required for situations such as surgery or invasive radiology. Prior to surgical intervention, it is the responsibility of the surgeon who is performing the surgical procedure to provide information and answer patient questions regarding the specific surgical intervention. It is the responsibility of the ordering physician of the invasive procedure to explain the procedure to the patient and answer all questions. Following explanation, it is the responsibility of the nurse to witness the patient's signature and act as the patient advocate to verify that the patient understands the intended surgical (i.e., any procedure requiring sedation or anesthesia) or procedural (e.g., insertion of a chest tube, biopsy, paracentesis, lumbar puncture, radiological procedures requiring contrast or dye) intervention. Verbal and implied consent is routinely sought by nurses when performing bedside procedures such as vital signs and inserting intravenous catheters. In the procedure explanation, patients have an opportunity to ask questions and understand the need for any procedure. Consent for routine care activities is also included in the provisions of the typical general consent for treatment signed by patients on admission to a healthcare institution.

The four elements of informed consent include capacity, competency, control, and disclosure. Typically, *capacity* requires that the person be considered an adult unless they have verification that they are an emancipated minor. *Competency* involves the ability to comprehend and process treatment options. This means that the person has not received medications or is not under the influence of alcohol or a street drug that would alter their ability to be alert and oriented. The patient must be able to assess the risks and benefits of the treatment option or intervention to which they are consenting and signing for and note its effect on their overall quality of life. For individuals who are cognitively impaired, mentally ill, or neurologically incapacitated and have a court-appointed guardian or person with power of attorney, they are approached for consent. Although family members may be at the bedside, they have no legal right to give or withhold consent for treatment for a competent patient. *Control* is the ability to actually give consent freely and without coercion. Coercion should not be perceived from any healthcare individual, family member, friend, or acquaintance. *Disclosure* means that the healthcare provider must give the patient sufficient information to allow them to make an informed decision. There is no court ruling that precisely states what information the patient should receive, but it must include information related to the nature, purpose, alternatives, and risks for the procedure or intervention. Explanations must be in the language understandable by the patient, and the provider must address any patient deficits (vision or hearing).

Informed consent (see Table 10.1) is intended to protect the patient's right to autonomy and self-determination as well as provide validation to the care provider that the patient has given consent for treatment. Decisions cannot be made by anyone other than the patient without verification that another person has legal responsibility and authority to make such a decision.

TABLE 10.1 Procedure for Obtaining Informed Consent

Responsible Individual	Task
Nurse	Obtain the consent form and have form procedural information completed prior to taking it to bedside.
Nurse, with or following physician explanation visit	Go to the patient bedside with the completed form.
Physician	Explain procedure to the patient and others identified by the patient to be in attendance. Respond to questions that the patient may have about procedure.
Nurse	Verify that all questions have been answered to the patient's satisfaction. Inform the physician if the patient has new concerns or objections prior to signing the consent form.
Nurse	Sign the form as witness to the patient's signature, validating authenticity, capacity, and voluntariness.
Nurse	Verify that the form has been placed in the patient's permanent record. Document that the form has been completed and all issues have been addressed in the nurse's notes.

Abandonment

Abandonment means failing to provide adequate patient care until the care of a specific patient is assumed by an approved licensed healthcare provider. In order for abandonment to occur, there must be two components:

1. The nurse has accepted and assumed responsibility for taking care of the patient (e.g., patient assignment was given and accepted).
2. The nurse-patient relationship has been severed without reasonable cause or notice to appropriate persons or arrangements made for care continuation.

These two components validate that the nurse has assumed responsibility for patient care and demonstrate that the care relationship has been severed by the nurse without reasonable notice. There are times when nurses are requested to extend their work hours beyond the regularly scheduled hours. These overtime hours can be consecutive upon completion of an already scheduled shift or in addition to days scheduled. Nurses are expected to exercise critical judgment regarding their ability to accept these hours. They must be able to offer safe care without evidence of sleep deprivation or excessive fatigue. Refusal to accept additional hours or shifts by nurses is not considered abandonment. Actions that constitute abandonment may vary from state to state, but all include patient safety as a critical factor in determining the nurse's responsibility in a specific situation. Some examples of abandonment may include (a) leaving the place of employment during an assigned patient care shift without proper notification and approval; (b) leaving an emergency patient situation, in which the nurse's absence constitutes a danger to the patient; (c) not addressing an acute patient situation in which the patient is in distress; (d) sleeping while on duty without approval; (e) providing insufficient patient observation contacts; (f) leaving an organization without giving proper report to the oncoming nurse or approved provider; and (g) failing to report to a facility or care area (e.g., private duty, home care) where the nurse is the sole provider of care without notification.

Confidentiality

Confidentiality requires that nurses safeguard any patient information obtained during care provision and is a fundamental concept in a trusting nurse-patient relationship. Confidential patient information identifies private individual identifiable health and personal information that is often collected in the course of patient historical data retrieval. This could include information related to diagnosis and treatment of past, present, or future physical or mental health situations. This includes identifiable information where there is a reasonable basis to believe that this information can be used to identify an individual.

The ANA's Code of Ethics for Nurses, Provision 3.1, recognizes that nurses have a duty to maintain confidentiality of patient information, stating:

> Nurses safeguard the right to privacy for individuals, families, and communities. The nurse advocates for an environment that provides sufficient physical privacy, including privacy for discussions of a personal nature. ... The nurse has a duty to maintain confidentiality of all patient information, both personal and clinical in the work setting and off duty in all venues, including social media or any other means of communication. ... These rights of privacy and confidentiality pertain to all information in any manner that is communicated or transmitted. ... The duty to maintain confidentiality is not absolute and may be limited, as necessary, to protect the patient or other parties, or by law or regulation such as mandated reporting for safety or public health reasons. (ANA, 2015)

This does not exclude discussion of information with another care provider who has a need to know. It is important to collaborate and share patient information in order to ensure safe, quality nursing care. However, this would not include a nurse or another caregiver who was not involved in the care of the person. Nurses should also only disclose patient information to family members with patient permission or evidence of legal documentation to do so.

Patients have a basic expectation that any information they disclose is held in confidence. It is the responsibility and duty of nurses to respect this expectation. There are state and federal statutes that address the principle of confidentiality. These statutes address privileged communication with individuals such as attorneys and priests. Nurses are not included under privileged communication. If a situation is brought forward in a court of law, nurses may be required to disclose patient information given to them without patient consent. Nurses should be familiar with their state Practice Act and know any limitations that may exist related to confidentiality in this document. Consistent use of and adherence to specific guidelines can promote safe legal practice by nurses, related to confidentiality.

Nurses, like other healthcare professionals, have a duty to report specific situations and to not hold this information in confidence. This requirement to disclose information or duty to report includes violations against professional codes, standards of care, and statutes. Professional codes such as the ANA's *Code of Ethics for Nurses with Interpretive Statements* (2025) and the International Council of Nurses' *Code of Ethics for Nurses* (2021) mandate that nurses take appropriate action to safeguard patients in their care against any action of a coworker that may cause patient endangerment. This includes abuse situations (child or elder); peer conduct, such as practicing while impaired (under the influence of any substance that does not allow care to be delivered with skill and reasonable judgment); and diversion of controlled substances (unauthorized removal of a controlled substance from a patient or facility) (Board of Registration in Nursing, 2000,). The duty to report statutes regarding patient situations include certain communicable diseases, gunshot wounds, homicide incidents (e.g. gunshot wounds, stabbings, etc.), and Occupational Health and Safety Administration violations that affect patient safety. All situations should be reported to the proper authority.

Health Insurance Portability and Accountability Act of 1996

HIPAA was enacted by U.S. Congress and provides federal protection for personal patient information (Cohen & Mello, 2018). This act covers all information held by any healthcare entity (e.g., hospital, nursing home, physician's office) and communicated in any format (e.g., oral, electronic, hard copy). Throughout its evolution timeline (see Table 10.2), several components have been added by other federal agencies.

TABLE 10.2 HIPAA Timeline

Year	Component	Explanation
1996	HIPAA	Enacted with two main goals, which were to improve the portability of health insurance and protect the security and privacy of health information. Ensuring that individuals could maintain health insurance coverage between jobs and establishing protections against healthcare fraud and abuse were original intents.
1999	Privacy Rule proposal	The U.S. Department of Health and Human Services (DHHS) proposed the HIPAA Privacy Rule in response to increasing concerns about patient privacy in an increasingly digital healthcare environment. Its aim was to regulate how healthcare providers, health plans, and other covered entities handled and protected patient information.
2000	Privacy Rule finalized	This finalized rule established national standards for the protection of health information and limited when and how this information could be used and disclosed. The rule required providers to take steps to safeguard personal health data and specified that a patient had the right to access their health records.
2003	Privacy Rule compliance deadline	Covered entities, which included healthcare providers, insurance companies, and their business associates, were required to comply with the Privacy Rule. This compliance meant adopting practices to protect patient information and providing patients with greater access to their own health data.

(Continued)

TABLE 10.2 (Continued)

Year	Component	Explanation
2005	Security Rule compliance deadline	This rule specifically addressed the protection of electronic protected health information (ePHI), making it mandatory. It required covered entities to implement administrative, physical, and technical safeguards to secure ePHI against unauthorized access.
2009	**Health Information Technology for Economic and Clinical Health (HITECH) Act**	The HITECH Act expanded HIPAA provisions over growing concerns about health information security and privacy with organizational adoption of electronic health records (EHRs). Tougher penalties were introduced for noncompliance, which required breach notifications and extended HIPAA obligations to business associates.
2013	Omnibus Rule	This rule further strengthened HIPAA's privacy and security protections as it brought major changes to the existing privacy, security, and enforcement rules. It mandated increasingly strict guidelines for data breaches and heightened the responsibilities of business associates. The Omnibus Rule also clarified patients' rights to obtain electronic copies of their health records and restricted the sale of PHI without patient consent.
2021 and beyond	Refinement in HIPAA guidelines	With ongoing technological advances and data-sharing practices, further refinements in HIPAA guidelines will be required. The DHHS has continued to issue guidance on topics such as telehealth, the use of mobile health applications, and patient data privacy in remote healthcare settings. The COVID-19 pandemic increased reliance on digital health services, which was an impetus for ongoing changes.

HIPAA has thus evolved significantly since its inception, adapting to new challenges in data protection and healthcare privacy in an increasingly digital and interconnected world (Alder, 2024). Its primary mission remains to protect patient information while allowing secure and lawful sharing within the healthcare ecosystem (Cooper, n.d.).

The **HIPAA Security Rule** is one of which to take note. The rule deals with compliance, addressing three types of security safeguards: administrative, physical, and technical. These standards must be adopted and administered by the organization, which identifies the best way to address specifications based on its unique healthcare situation. Implementation costs can include initiation of sophisticated technologies by many organizations. There was also an increase in required validation and verification, including repetitive charting and duplication of patient information entry. HIPAA safeguards and specifications are listed in Table 10.3.

TABLE 10.3 HIPAA Security Rule Safeguards and Specifications

Security Safeguard	Definition	Examples of Safeguard
Administrative safeguards	Policies and procedures designed to clearly demonstrate how compliance is achieved	• Written set of privacy procedures with a privacy officer responsible for development and implementation • Policies and procedures that address security controls • Identification of individuals within the organization who will have access to electronic protected health information (ePHI) • Procedure that addresses employee access to include authorization, establishment, modification, and termination • Ongoing employee training to address protected health information (PHI) • Third-party (outsourced) verification of compliance to HIPAA standards • Contingency plan for emergencies and disaster management • Internal audits to validate compliance and potential security concerns • Procedures to address security breaches, risks, and vulnerabilities to information
Physical safeguards	Policies and procedures to address physical access and control	• Policies and procedures to specify proper use and access to workstations and electronic media • Access controls to limit use to authorized individuals • Required access controls to include security plans and maintenance records • Management of workstation access in public areas • Policies and procedures regarding transfer, removal, disposal, and reuse of electronic media • Third-party (outsourced) or contractor verification of compliance to physical safeguards

(Continued)

TABLE 10.3 (Continued)

Security Safeguard	Definition	Examples of Safeguard
Technical safeguards	Policies and procedures to address access and transmission of PHI	• Implementation of policies and procedures that allow only authorized persons to access electronic PHI • Use of controls that prevent intrusion from unauthorized individuals • Authentication to validate system entry • Documentation to include access records and technology as well as analysis of risk management programs

Source: Office of the National Coordinator for Health Information Technology (ONC) & DHHS, 2008.

The Nationwide Privacy and Security Framework for Electronic Exchange of Individually Identifiable Health Information was published on December 15, 2008, by the Office of the National Coordinator for Health Information Technology (HIT) of the U.S. Department of Health and Human Services (HHS). This act is part of the American Recovery and Reinvestment Act of 2009, which provided an EHR incentive adoption incentive. The timeline for this program was from 2011 through 2014. Principles of the framework guided actions of all healthcare organizations. These principles were designed to provide privacy and security protections for individual identifiable health information. Principles include the following:

1. Individual access should be provided for individuals in a readable form and format. This is important for self-management of health and wellness.
2. Corrections should be provided with a time-efficient method for resolution of accuracy and integrity disputes. Accurate information is important for the delivery of safe care.
3. Openness and transparency should be maintained regarding policies, procedures and technologies that directly affect individual health information.
4. Individual choice should ensure individuals a reasonable opportunity to make informed decisions about the collection, use, and disclosure of their health information.
5. Collection, use, and disclosure limitation requires that identifiable health information be collected, used, and/or disclosed only to the extent necessary for care delivery.

6. Data quality and integrity should be maintained in order to ensure that individual identifiable information is complete, accurate, and up to date.
7. Safeguards should verify administrative, technical, and physical protection.
8. Accountability should be assured through appropriate methods of monitoring.

Source: Office of the National Coordinator for Health Information Technology, U.S. Department of Health and Human Services, 2008.

Nurses routinely access individual patient identifiable health information during the delivery of care. It is important to remember to access only needed information to assist in patient care delivery based on the need to know. Entry into the system is confidential and should never be shared with another person. Remember to log out of the system to prevent intrusion by unauthorized persons. Violations for breach of organizational policies that address federal guidelines can result in sanctions that include loss of employment.

Nursing Licensure

Licensure is a police power of the state and has evolved over time in the United States and abroad (see Table 10.4). The legislative branch of the U.S. government determines which groups are to be licensed and the limitations of such licenses. Licensure laws may be permissive or mandatory.

In nursing, the permissive license allows nurses to decide whether they will obtain an RN credential after successfully completing an educational program. Permissive law does not protect the title of *nurse*, but it does protect use of the title *registered nurse*. In order for a practitioner to use this title, they must have completed the requirements determined by the state in which they practice. But under permissive law, anyone can practice nursing as long as they do not use the title. They may instead use such terms as *caregiver* or *sitter*. Permissive law allows the public to identify individuals who have met educational and state requirements and serves as a safeguard for identification by the public seeking someone to function as a nurse.

Mandatory law requires licensure by any person who practices as a nurse. No individual can call themselves an RN without completing the required education, successfully passing a licensing examination, and completing state requirements. Initial licensure is the same for all states, but requirements for continued licensure are set by each state and may differ, with some requiring continuing education hours and others not requiring this requirement. All states and territories require that RNs be licensed in order to practice.

TABLE 10.4 History of Nursing Licensure

Year	Event
1867	Henry Wentworth Acland is the first to suggest licensure for nurses in England.
1893	Nursing leaders organize a meeting at the World's Columbian Exposition in Chicago to discuss issues affecting nursing, including education and licensure.
1896	The American Society of Superintendents of Training Schools for Nurses organizes and supports licensure in the United States.
1901	New Zealand is the first country to require licensure of nurses; in the United States, New York, New Jersey, Illinois, and Virginia organize state nurses' associations with a goal of enacting an nurse practice act for their respective states.
1903	North Carolina becomes the first state in the United States to enact permissive licensure for nurses.
1915	ANA drafts its first model nurse practice act.
1919	The first nursing licensure occurs in England.
1923	All 48 states have permissive licensure laws.
1935	New York passes the first mandatory licensure law in the United States (effective in 1947 due to World War II).
1946	Ten states include the definition of nursing in a licensing act.
1947	New York becomes the first state to enact a mandatory licensure law.
1950	This is the first year that the same examination (the State Board Test Pool Examination) is used in all jurisdictions of the United States and its territories.
1965	A total of 21 states have definitions of nursing in the licensing act.
1971	Idaho is the first state to recognize expanded practice in the nursing practice act.
1976	California is the first state to require continuing education for nursing relicensure.
1982	There is a licensure change to process format examination: the National Council Licensure Examination for Registered Nurses (NCLEX-RN).
1986	North Dakota is the only state to require a baccalaureate degree for initial RN licensure and an associate degree for LPN licensure (effective in 1987).
1994	Computerized adapted testing is initiated nationwide for the NCLEX-RN.
1998	The Mutual Recognition Nurse Licensure Compact (multistate licensure) is finalized. Utah is the first state to become part of the compact.
2000	The multistate nurse licensure model called the ***Nurse Licensure Compact (NLC)*** is enacted.
2003	Alternate item formats are operationalized for the NCLEX-RN.
2023	The next-generation NCLEX assesses clinical judgment in innovative ways.
2024	A total of 37 states participate in the compact for multistate licensure.
2025	A total of 43 jurisdictions, 41 states and two territories participate in the NLC. Eight states and the District of Columbia have pending NLC legislation.

Nurse Licensure Compact

The process of nursing licensure began with each state having its own licensing body; after being initially licensed in one state, nurses had to apply to each individual state for work upon relocating. Due to changing economics, nurse work sites have changed, with some nurses living in one neighboring state and working in another state or nurses working in both their state of residence and a neighboring state. Geological changes and other world events resulting in natural disasters have resulted in nurses' mobility to address societal care needs. Alterations have also evolved from changes in care provision, with telehealth (electronic health care) using nurses who live in one state and give care to individuals in another. These evolutionary changes necessitated changes in licensure. The National Council of State Boards of Nursing (NCSBN) developed a mutual recognition model for nurse licensure. This model allows nurses to work physically and electronically outside their state of residence and identifies licensure as long as that state is a member of the compact (Gaines, 2025). Nurses with an active compact state license are not required to apply or pay fees to any state outside the state of residence in order to practice. Licensure in their home state allows nurses the privilege to practice in another compact state. Compact states as of October 2025 included Alabama, Arizona, Arkansas, Colorado, Connecticut, Delaware, Florida, Georgia, Guam, Idaho, Indiana, Iowa, Kansas, Kentucky, Louisiana, Maine, Maryland, Massachusetts, Mississippi, Missouri, Montana, Nebraska, New Hampshire, New Jersey, New Mexico, North Carolina, North Dakota, Ohio, Oklahoma, Pennsylvania, Rhode Island, South Carolina, South Dakota, Tennessee, Texas, Utah, Vermont, Virginia, Virgin Islands, Washington, West Virginia, Wisconsin, and Wyoming. States with pending NLC legislation include Alaska, District of Columbia, Michigan, Oregon, Nevada, Hawaii, Minnesota, Illinois, and New York (Gaines, 2025). In order to have a compact (multistate) license, nurses must:

- Reside in an NLC state and declare this state as their legal place of residence
- Meet the licensure requirements in their home or residence state

Nurses working in a compact state must abide by all the laws and comply with the Nurse Practice Act of the state in which they work. Disciplinary actions may result in the revocation of multistate status, with restriction to the home state mandated.

Nurses residing in a noncompact state are not eligible to practice under the compact multistate license. These nurses are issued a single state-of-residence license. In order to practice in another state, nurses must hold an individual and separate license in each noncompact state where they desire to practice.

Professional Liability Insurance

Nurses are at risk for litigation claims by patients regarding care delivery. **Professional liability insurance**, also called *malpractice insurance*, is a way for nurses to protect themselves against personal payment for these claims that result in judgment. This insurance for nurses is sometimes afforded through their place of employment, but it may only be active while employed at that organization, so any occurrence that is filed after employment may not be covered by the organization. There may also be a limit to the amount of employer coverage, which means that if nurses are named in a malpractice lawsuit and legal costs or the final judgment exceeds employer coverage, they may be legally bound to pay the difference. Carrying one's own insurance affords employment portability, continued protection, and additional financial resources. Personal professional liability insurance can protect nurses while they are at school and work (primary and secondary employment) and during off-duty emergency intervention.

Techniques for Nurse Protection Under the Law

It is important for nurses to practice responsibly. This means that nurses must be knowledgeable about criteria used for care administration and evaluation. Nurses should possess a copy of their nurse practice act for the state in which they practice; the American Nurses Association's (ANA) *Nursing's Social Policy Statement*, which identifies a definition for nursing and the knowledge base for nursing; the ANA's *Nursing: Scope and Standards of Practice*, which defines clinical practice and its safe implementation; and the ANA's *Code of Ethics for Nurses With Interpretative Statements*, which describes the ten ethical provisions that cover all aspects of nursing practice (ANA, 2025; Olsen & Stokes, 2016). Information regarding ANA documents can be accessed at https://www.nursingworld.org. Using the following 12 do's can promote legally responsible care by nurses:

1. **Do:** Know the Nurse Practice Act for their state of practice.
2. **Do:** Adhere to *Nursing's Social Policy Statement*, *Nursing: Scope and Standards of Practice*, and the ANA's Code of Ethics for Nurses.
3. **DO:** Be sure to obtain patient signatures when necessary for procedures. Make sure that patients:
    a. Understand the information given by the physician. If not, notify the physician as further explanation may be needed.

   b. Have had a chance to ask questions and receive answers from the provider.
   c. Understand the risks and benefits of the procedure.
   d. Know that they are free to sign or not sign to have the procedure performed.
4. **DO:** Accurately document care activities and results in a factual manner (e.g., medication administration for pain with subsequent follow-up evaluation for level of pain).
5. **DO:** Effectively and carefully delegate care activities using the five rights of delegation.
6. **DO:** Properly make changes to errors in charting. Follow organizational policy when noting errors and making corrections.
7. **DO:** Maintain privacy for patient records and information by knowing laws and abiding by policies related to protection of identifiable patient health information.
8. **DO:** Report allegations of abuse to the proper authority. These include any allegations of physical, emotional, sexual, or mental abuse toward any member of a vulnerable population (e.g., children, older adults, individuals with mental deficits).
9. **DO:** Use evidence-based research validations for care delivery.
10. **DO:** Use positive interpersonal communications with peers and colleagues to promote communications and interactions that allow for safe patient care delivery.
11. **DO:** Delegate appropriately for the level of the care provider (e.g., peer RN, nursing assistant, care technician) being given the specific task to perform within the organization and that it is based on organizational policies and procedures.
12. **DO:** Carry individual professional liability insurance.

Summary

Nurses are individually responsible and professionally accountable for the nursing care they provide. Nurses must understand the key laws and standards governing their practice, along with core legal responsibilities in patient care, including duty of care, precise documentation, informed consent, and potential liabilities such as malpractice or negligence. Familiarity with common legal terminology such as *liability*, *negligence*, and *malpractice* is also essential, as it helps nurses comprehend the legal implications of their actions. Nurses must be knowledgeable and skilled in delegation, ensuring that they make informed decisions under empowering acts while adhering to scope-of-practice guidelines for safe, effective patient care. Knowledge of HIPAA Security Rule safeguards is crucial for protecting electronic health information (ePHI) and requires administrative, physical, and technical measures to ensure the confidentiality, integrity, and security of patient data.

Knowledge of legal liability is imperative to protect patient safety, health, and rights. Knowledge of organizational policies and procedures and the state nursing practice act can promote safe patient care as they can be used by nurses to administer legally competent care. This knowledge of legal health care components equips nurses with the key information needed to uphold professional accountability and prioritize patient safety.

References

Alder, S. (2024, January 11). *Why is HIPAA important?* HIPAA Journal. https://www.hipaajournal.com/why-is-hipaa-important/

American Nurses Association. (2025). *Code of ethics for nurses with interpretive statements*. Publishing Program of ANA. https://codeofethics.ana.org/provisions

Board of Registration in Nursing. (2000, October 13). *Guideline for compliance with the standard of conduct for a nurse's duty to report to the Board of Registration in Nursing.* https://www.mass.gov/advisory/guideline-for-compliance-with-the-standard-of-conduct-for-a-nurses-duty-to-report-to-the-board-of-registration-in-nursing

Cohen, I. G., & Mello, M. M. (2018). HIPAA and protecting health information in the 21st century. *JAMA, 320*(3), 231–232. https://doi.org/10.1001/jama.2018.5630

Cooper, T. (n.d.). *CPRI toolkit: Managing information security in health care and other HIPAA tools.* https://www.ehcca.com/presentations/HIPAA2/105.PDF

Gaines, K. (2025, June 11). *Compact nursing states list 2025*. Nurse.org. https://nurse.org/articles/enhanced-compact-multi-state-license-eNLC/

International Council of Nurses. (2021). *Code of ethics for nurses*. https://www.icn.ch/sites/default/files/2023-06/ICN_Code-of-Ethics_EN_Web.pdf

Johnson, R. L. (2024, April 23). *Understanding delegation and why it matters.* American Association of Critical Care Nurses. https://www.aacn.org/blog/understanding-delegation-and-why-it-matters

Khalili, H., & Heydari, A. (2022). Poor care: A Walker and Avant concept analysis. *Journal of Caring Sciences, 12*(1), 25–32. https://doi.org/10.34172/jcs.2023.30507

Kim, M. J., Jang, S. G., Kim, S. K., & Lee, W. (2021). A study on the status and contributory factors of adverse events due to negligence in nursing care. *Journal of Patient Safety, 17*(8), e904–e910.

McCoy, A. (2024, January 19). *Understanding the Good Samaritan law as a nurse.* Nursing Education. https://nursingeducation.org/blog/good-samaritan-law/

National Council of State Boards of Nursing & American Nurses Association. (2019, April 29). *National guidelines for nursing delegation.* https://www.ncsbn.org/public-files/NGND-PosPaper_06.pdf

Office of the National Coordinator for Health Information Technology & U.S. Department of Health and Human Services. (2008). *Nationwide privacy and security framework for electronic exchange of individually identifiable health information.* https://www.healthit.gov/sites/default/files/nationwide-ps-framework-5.pdf

Olson, L. L., & Stokes, F. (2016). The ANA code of ethics for nurses with interpretive statements: Resource for nursing regulation. *Journal of Nursing Regulation, 7*(2), 9–20.

Ahrenstedt, O., Westerberg, M., & Rimsten, A. (1985). The assault and battery panorama at a county hospital in Sweden. *Upsala Journal of Medical Science, 90*, 85–90.

Ugoani, J. (2020). Effective delegation and its impact on employee performance. *International Journal of Economics and Business Administration, 6*(3), 78–87. https://ssrn.com/abstract=3666808

USLegal.com. (n.d.). *Good Samaritans law and legal definition.* http://definitions.uslegal.com/g/good-samaritans/

West, B., & Varacallo, M. (2022, September 12). *Good Samaritan laws.* StatPearls Publishing. https://www.ncbi.nlm.nih.gov/books/NBK542176/

CHAPTER 11

Politics and Nursing

Objectives

Upon completion of this chapter, the learner will be able to do the following to:

1. Validate the importance of nursing involvement in politics and policy generation.
2. Explain steps in moving an idea to a law in the political arena.
3. Interpret health equity and its impact on individual patient quality of life and collective societal outcomes.
4. Identify strategies for political action in nursing.

Key Chapter Terms

- Politics
- Affordable Care Act (ACA)
- Policy
- Needlestick Safety and Prevention Act
- Law development
- Nurse activist role
- Nurses as politicians
- National Student Nurses Association (NSNA)
- American Nurses Association (ANA)
- International Council of Nurses (ICN)
- Health equity
- ANA social policy statement
- Political action

Politics and Nursing

Membership in a profession gives one rights and privileges. It also gives them responsibilities that inherently accompany these rights. The focus of nursing is patient-centered, but in order to deliver the best care possible, it is important for nurses to advocate, educate, and serve as models for the public at large. Often nurses focus on tasks only and fail to put time and effort into visualizing future directions. Targeting efforts in this one direction does not promote all components of the profession that are required in order for nursing to have the impact it should on societal management. It is important for nursing to promote leadership among its members in order to promote professional credibility and political impact.

Politics and Policy

Politics

Politics can be defined as "the process by which a community's decisions are made, rules for group behavior are established, competition for positions of leadership is regulated, and the disruptive effects of disputes are minimized" (Bakwesegha, 2013). This political approach is presented as a system of activity and is concerned with understanding the authoritative allocation of public values and decisions about societal resources (Easton, 1965). A graphic descriptive systems analysis of political life proposed by Easton is seen in Figure 11.1.

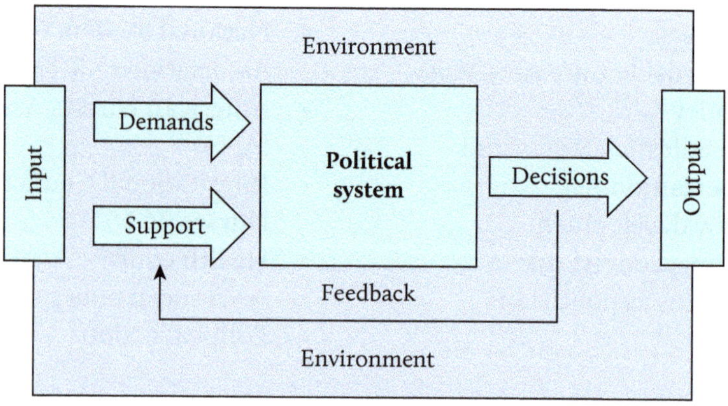

FIGURE 11.1 A Systems Analysis of Political Life

Easton's (1965) approach represents an approach to politics that proposes that a political system has designated boundaries that are fluid or changing. Following are the steps to this approach:

- Step 1: Alterations in the environment that surrounds the political system will create demands and supports for individual actions, which result in a system input of political behavior.
- Step 2: Demands and supports for action cause political system competition, which leads to decisional outputs.
- Step 3: Outputs (e.g., policies) interact with the environment and cause a change.
- Step 4: Environmental output interactions further create group demands or supports for or against the new policy or policy change (feedback).
- This returns the cycle to Step 1 and reinitiates the cycle.

This directly relates to how decisions are made regarding resource allocation. Let's look at this system related to health care. No country or community has enough healthcare resources for 100% of the individuals who reside in that country or community. These resources must be efficiently allocated among individual residents. Demands and support for action related to healthcare changes caused political system competition for resources based on specific state, county, and/or congressional district. The output in this system occurred in the form of an initiative. One example of an initiative was the **Affordable Care Act (ACA)** (Kenton et al., 2025), passed by Congress and signed into law by the president. This law stated that (a) health insurance companies were to remove out-of-pocket charges for preventive services and give consumers an opportunity to appeal coverage decisions as well as a choice for the selection of a primary care provider, (b) healthcare costs for consumers and companies must be reduced through implementation of specific actions, and (c) a new competitive insurance marketplace was to be established for individuals and companies. This law was an output that caused a significant change in the U.S. environment. As a result of this change, more group demands were created, and support for and against this law resulted, which then returned the system to Step 1.

Incorporated into this system are events and activities that significantly affect whether an initiative gets through the political system. These may be at the national or state level, with individuals who are proponents for or against an initiative. They lobby and rally to support their cause and garner support of individuals who have power, influence, or a vote in a certain political arena (e.g., city counselors, state representatives, senators, members of the House of Representatives) that could affect the outcome of their supported

Box 11.1

Case Demonstrating Use of Lawmaker Influence

Examine this case that demonstrates an example of influence and why it is important as a nurse to be involved in what happens in the nursing profession. The Board of Nursing in each state regulates the profession. In one southern U.S. state, this ability is under investigation. This is on the heels of a formal suspension of the licenses of three advanced practice nurses due to accusations of overprescribing narcotics. During this period of suspension, the Board of Nursing's right to exist as a regulatory board was up for reauthorization or renewal by the state legislature. At least two lawmakers (state representatives) used their influence to delay the reauthorization vote. These lawmakers used their position and vote—which equaled power—to influence the Board of Nursing to rescind or reverse the three suspensions, which occurred prior to the vote for renewal. Following the board rescinding the suspensions, the two state representatives voted in favor of the reauthorization. These lawmakers openly admitted to the press their involvement in using the threat of legislative action to push the state Board of Nursing into reversing revocation of the three nurses' licenses. Following this incident, the state bureau of investigation explored the possibility of official misconduct by these legislators.

initiative. Individual placement in an elected or appointed position in these situations give government officials the right to exercise power and influence. Occasionally, this power is not exercised as it should be in the best interest of constituents (see Box 11.1). This demonstrates the importance for nurses to be involved both directly (i.e., running for elected positions) and indirectly (i.e., voting to elect individuals) in the political arena.

Policy

Policy is defined as "a plan or course of action, as of a government, political party, or business, intended to influence and determine decisions, actions, and other matters" (Farlex, n.d.). These plans reflect the values of those involved. Resource allocation is then based on these values. Government policy represents a strategic plan or course of action designed to address and resolve specific societal issues or problems.

At the federal level, government policies are reflected through (a) constitutions, (b) the chief executive's (i.e., the president's) agenda, and (c) legislative policies. These can emerge as policies or mandates that are then translated into services that reflect a strategic plan or policy memoranda. The plan or policy can be translated into workable components such as rules and regulations, requests for proposals, and contractual agreements. Budgets can reflect service decisions based on these items.

Policies are generated from the ideas of elected individuals, citizens, or special interest groups. Decision-maker values and beliefs also go into this decision equation. Some take into consideration constituent values and beliefs. Ideas that generate policy can result from constituent influences. These ideas result from life events, such as the parental loss of a child who committed suicide due to being bullied, personal experiences such as a debilitating personal trauma from being hit by a drunk driver, and high-visibility issues such as health care. These triggers can cause momentum for change and push these issues to the forefront of social concern.

Policies can evolve from philosophies that stem from the personal and political values of individuals along party lines. Personal philosophies can be developed in the early years. People learn from exposure to situations and through their education what might, can, and will work along policy lines. Personal philosophies also encourage individuals to identify with specific political parties and organized constituencies. Politicians work to identify and support the will of those they represent. This influences their policy decisions.

Policies may result in laws, regulations, or guidelines that govern behavior in public or private areas. They can evolve from a single constituent idea. Sometimes these constituents are nurses. This was the case with needlestick legislation. Karen Daley, RN, MPH, helped pass the **Needlestick Safety and Prevention Act** *(Public Law 106-430, 106th Congress, H.R. 5178)* of 2000. This requires that healthcare facilities provide safe-engineered needles/sharps devices for employees providing direct patient care. In 1998, Daley sustained a needlestick injury despite using all the necessary safety precautions. She was stuck while disposing of a second needle in a sharps container. She found out later that she had become infected with both hepatitis C and HIV due to this injury. This life-changing event led Daley to work toward preventing other healthcare workers from experiencing the trauma that she experienced. This demonstrates the importance of putting vision into reality in an effort to make work safer for those in the healthcare profession.

Law Development

There are numerous steps in moving an idea to the development of a specific law. Initial thoughts are generated and written as an idea for a law or rule comes from an individual or group. The following list of steps takes you through this process:

1. *Idea formation:* The process starts with identifying a need or problem that requires a legislative solution. The idea can come from concerned citizens, advocacy groups, business leaders, government agencies, and/or lawmakers.

2. *Drafting the bill:* The idea needs to be clearly defined in a proposal. The proposal is then drafted into a bill, which is a formal document. A bill is often written with the assistance of legal experts, interest groups, or government attorneys in order to ensure precise language that follows legislative rules.
3. *Introduction of the bill:* The bill is introduced in either the House of Representatives or the Senate by a legislator in that body. The bill is sent to the clerk of their house, and it is given a specific reference number and labeled with a sponsor's name (bills may be co-sponsored). The bill is then read in its entirety (first reading) and referred to the proper committee.
4. *Committee review:* The bill is examined by a committee that aligns with its subject matter (e.g., a healthcare bill would go to the Health Committee). The committee may hold public meetings to gather input from experts, industry representatives, public officials, or citizens. The committee has the power to determine that the idea is not in the best interest of others or unnecessary, which immediately kills the bill. If the bill is identified as credible, it is debated, and amendments are made if they are found to be necessary. Following a favorable vote, the bill is sent back to the floor of the house.
5. *Subcommittee review:* Many committees have subcommittees. These committees focus on more specialized topics within the bill and may address information from the initial review or conduct further hearings in close analysis of the bill. If there is subcommittee approval, the bill is then sent back to the full committee for consideration.
6. *Markup and committee voting:* Necessary edits, amendments, or bill adjustments occur in the markup phase. There can be minor adjustments or major structural adjustments to the bill at this point. Members debate the bill vote on whether it should advance. If there is a favorable committee vote, the bill moves to the full legislative chamber (House or Senate). If the bill doesn't pass the committee stage, it is typically "tabled" or "killed," ending its progress.
7. *Debate and vote in the House/Senate:* Legislators have the opportunity to debate the bill in the full chamber. During this stage, lawmakers present arguments for or against the bill, and additional amendments may be proposed. Each chamber follows its own rules for debate. Steps for discussion differ between the Senate and the House of Representatives. In the latter, the time for debating is limited. There is no such standing rule in the Senate, and individuals can filibuster (i.e., talk a bill to death) to defeat it. If successful in the appropriate house, the bill

goes forward. After debate concludes, the chamber votes. A majority vote allows the bill to advance to the other chamber of Congress.

8. *Process in the second chamber:* A vote is now taken, and, if favorable, the bill is sent to the other house of Congress (transmitted from the House of Representatives to the Senate or from the Senate to the House of Representatives). Here it undergoes a similar review process: committee assignment, hearings, possible subcommittee review, markup, and a final vote. The second chamber often makes changes or amendments to the bill. If the bill passes the second chamber with identical language, it can move directly to the president. However, if differences arise between the House and Senate versions, further steps are needed.
9. *Conference committee:* This step is needed if the House and Senate pass different versions of the bill. This committee works to reconcile the differences. It has members from both chambers who work to reach a compromise for the two versions. Once there is committee agreement, a final version is sent back to both chambers for approval.
10. *Final approval in both chambers:* The reconciled bill requires approval from both the House and the Senate. No further amendments can be made at this stage, and the bill must be either passed or rejected. If there is approval from both chambers, the bill proceeds to the president.
11. *Presidential action:* The president has several options. They may sign the bill into law or refuse to sign the bill (veto) and return it to Congress with an explanation. Congress can override a veto with a two-thirds majority vote in both chambers. The president can take no action on the bill. If no action is taken within 10 days (excluding Sundays) while Congress is in session, the bill will become law without presidential signature. If Congress adjourns at any time prior to the end of the 10-day waiting period, the bill is automatically killed. This action is called a *pocket veto.*

The process uses vigorous debate and careful consideration by both the House and the Senate. This complex process assures everyone that sufficient time and effort is placed on issues that will become laws for U.S. citizens. This demonstrates why it is important to vote for individuals who represent personal values and beliefs. This is a significant way for citizens to have sufficient influence in politics and on policies.

Getting Involved

Knowledge of government processes is the first step to involvement. Increasing communication and leadership skills also facilitate involvement by adding to one's scientific knowledge and skill foundation. Involvement can take many forms, from an individual who desires to directly affect the political scene by running for a political office to an organizational member who promotes changes in a collective fashion.

Individual Involvement

Nurses as Citizens

Knowledge of issues, laws, and health policy is a starting place for individual nurses as citizens. It is important to get involved and stay involved at this level by maintaining momentum to move forward and vote for individuals at every election—from local to national. This is a significant way to influence the political outcome on key issues that affect nurses and the health care of those whom they serve. Political awareness requires continuous monitoring of political stances by elected officials. This can be done through their individual websites, which identify a politician's involvement in issues that relate to the community or country at large. Online access to political information allows any citizen the ability to review activities of the politician, including their accomplishments and votes cast on issues before their legislative body of membership.

Nurses as Activists

This step moves nurses from bedside patient advocacy to active involvement in political processes. This is a key method to be visible and vocal about healthcare issues and those that affect the nursing profession. The ideas and issues from citizen nurses are captured and moved forward to the politician through this mechanism. This level of activity involves lobbying for these ideas and issues in order to let politicians know whether nurses do or do not support these issues and the rationale for their decision. The **nurse activist role** works within the political system to positively affect issue outcomes. This was never more apparent than the support that nurses provided for federal legislation, namely the Nurse Staffing Standards for Hospital Patient Safety and Quality Care Act (H.R. 2530 and S. 1113), which addressed the nurse-patient ratio. This was supported in order to guarantee a single standard for quality of care. These bills were introduced to Congress on March 30, 2023. This legislation was endorsed by the **American Nurses Association (ANA)**. Nurses expressed strong approval that they aimed to establish a minimum nurse-to-patient ratio in hospitals. These bills did not become law as they failed to pass and were referred to committees but did not advance further. This is just one of many illustrations of nurse activism activities that occur in this country (Chinn & Kennedy, 2023; Svetvilas & Morris, 2023). This example reflects the persistent engagement of nurses in policy advocacy and highlights the necessity of sustaining these efforts through diversified strategies to advance legislative and systemic change in healthcare.

Nurses as Politicians

The policy process of idea generation, action to identify potential solutions, and initiation of solution activities is inherent in solving issues relative to the nursing profession. **Nurses as politicians** are in a unique place to make a direct impact in this process outcome (Wilson et al., 2022). There is no doubt that the political arena can be intimidating. But nurses have a skill set that makes them effective in political office. Nurses are educated to solve problems using a process that can be adapted to any situation. They learn astute communication skills in managing all types of patient communications that require different approaches for success, they must multitask on a daily basis to address issues as they prioritize them for intervention, and they think holistically in managing patient situations. Additionally, on a foundational level, people trust nurses. Putting in the time and effort can be rewarding and beneficial for nurses and citizens alike.

Collective Involvement

Involvement in a collective fashion can start in a nursing program. Many schools have student nurse associations, which are part of the **National Student Nurses Association (NSNA)**, with online information located at https://www.nsna.org. This gives you the opportunity to start in a manner that promotes peer support and assistance in developing leadership skills to influence policies at various levels. The organization mentors professional development and serves as a nursing education and career resource. Following graduation and licensure, nurses can join the ANA (https://www.nursingworld.org). This organization is a broad-purpose professional organization as it is open to all nurses regardless of area of specialization. The ANA represents all nursing interests and advances the profession of nursing by "fostering high standards of nursing practice, promoting a safe and ethical work environment, bolstering the health and wellness of nurses, and advocating on healthcare issues that affect nurses and the public" (ANA, n.d.).

Often nurses work in a certain area of patient care and identify specifically with that type of nursing personally and professionally. As they advance their education, they select a specialized area and focus their career along that path.

As a result, many will join specialty organizations that allow involvement with this group. These may be focused on such nursing areas as acute care, emergency, oncology, geriatric, pediatric, neonatal, and many more (see a more complete listing at https://www.nurse.org/orgs.shtml). Individual nurses can belong to a specialty nursing organization and the ANA simultaneously. This allows individuals to promote nursing initiatives for the profession as a whole as well as stay focused on an area of specialization. As members of both the broad-purpose ANA organization and a specialty organization, nurses can help effect standards of nursing practice on both levels.

Health care is a global issue, and nurses can connect internationally through the **International Council of Nurses (ICN)**, founded in 1899. The organization has three key programs, called the *ICN's Pillars*. These are professional practice, nursing regulation, and socioeconomic welfare for nurses (Farrah, 2014). This organization is a federation of more than 140 national nurses' associations and represents over 30 million nurses worldwide (International Council of Nurses, n.d.). This organization is nurse-driven and works

Box 11.2

Benefits to Professional Organizational Membership

- **Networking** with peers and professional role models who have similar interests
- **Job opportunities** through awareness of available positions of interest from networking opportunities and information received through membership
- **Organizational power** through the numbers of individuals who can effect change in policy and issues of importance identified by the organization
- **Education and research** opportunities, including exposure to journal and electronic updates with area-of-interest highlights
- **Leadership opportunities** within and outside the organization based on the level of involvement desired
- **Career development** opportunities, which can involve committee work and potential positions within the organization (e.g., board member, officer, committee chairperson)
- **Certification** in a specialty field, which can be promoted and facilitated through a professional organization, which may be used to climb an organizational job ladder
- **Personal growth** through the development of communication and leadership skills
- **Travel** to meetings in various parts of the country, which promotes personal and professional networking

to ensure quality nursing care for all individuals, promote comprehensive global health policies, advance nursing knowledge, and promote the professional respect and satisfaction of working nurses (International Council of Nurses, 2024). There is no individual membership for this organization. Nurses who are members of their national nurses association are automatically part of the ICN. The nursing organization that represents U.S. nurses in the ICN is the ANA.

Working through local, national, and international nursing organizations can provide a collective vehicle for change. This level of involvement demonstrates a commitment to the profession and society. It allows for unity in the development of public policy. Members allow associations to accomplish their goals and objectives. It is only through the collective work of the members that nursing can protect, promote, and optimize health care for individuals, families, and populations. Some benefits to belonging to a professional organization are presented in Box 11.2.

Health Equity

Health equity is a global concern. *Health inequities* have been defined as "differences in health that are not only unnecessary and avoidable but, in addition, are considered unfair and unjust" (Whitehead, 1992, p. 430). *Health inequities* and *health disparities* are terms often used interchangeably to identify differences among population groups that are defined by specific characteristics. Not only is there inequity in the distribution of health care from country to country, but this inequity also exists within countries. The United States is not alone in working to address this concern (Avanceña et al., 2021). In order to ensure that this issue is addressed from multiple directions, it is important for nurses to be present at the discussion table (National Academies of Sciences, Engineering, and Medicine; National Academy of Medicine; Committee on the Future of Nursing 2020–2030, 2021; Reutter & Kushner, 2010). The foundation of this inequity lies in social, economic, environmental, and structural determinants of health that perpetuate disparities in health outcomes among individuals, families, and communities (Arcaya et al., 2015; Brannon et al., 2010; National Academies of Sciences, Engineering, and Medicine; Health and Medicine Division; Board on Population Health and Public Health Practice; Committee on Community-Based Solutions to Promote Health Equity in the United States, 2017). Recognizing and addressing these underlying determinants is essential to advancing health equity and guiding nursing practice toward more just and inclusive care systems (LaVeist et al., 2023). These inequities may be reflected in public policy.

Health care outcomes are based on four broad categories: personal attributes (biological and genetic), access to health care, health behaviors, and social determinants of health (social, economic, cultural, and environmental) (Braveman et al., 2010; Tiase et al., 2022). These categories incorporate areas that can and cannot be changed. It is the areas that can be changed that are the ones that affect overall health care and the outcomes for disease interventions, with which nurses can get involved. These areas include access to health care through collaborative work with organizations to promote this concept and working with consumers to improve health behaviors (Hewitt et al., 2024).

The next section will address how the United States is addressing this issue through healthcare reform. Nurses are prime candidates to work in the area of healthcare reform due to their background in the sciences and patient management.

Social Policy Statement: Nursing's Link to Society

Social policy statements guide decision-making. They serve three main purposes: "(1) to operationalize the public's mandate; (2) to establish the professional's scope of practice; and (3) to formulate a framework for influencing health policy" (Gorenberg et al., 1991, p. 11). It is the responsibility of the nursing profession to provide written clarification of its mission, purpose, goals, responsibility, and accountability to the public. Social policy statements serve as the platform for disseminating this information. Nursing is but one part of a larger healthcare system that is involved with patient care. The social policy statement serves to delineate what part of this system expressly belongs to nursing. The **ANA social policy statement** serves to define nursing and address issues related to knowledge, standards, and professional regulations. According to this policy, nurses are a critical part of the healthcare profession and are highly respected and valued for their knowledge, skills, and care delivery (Fowler, 2015). Using their value as a foundation, nurses must identify barriers and overcome them to become politically active (Han & Kim, 2024)

The ANA stresses the social contract the profession of nursing has with society. The contract is directed toward nurses' work with all individuals in society, which includes individuals, families, groups, communities, and populations. Elements of the social contract are as follows:

- Humans manifest an essential unity of mind, body, and spirit.
- Human experience is contextually and culturally defined.

- Health and illness are human experiences. The presence of illness does not preclude health, nor does optimal health preclude illness.
- The relationship between the nurse and patient occurs within the context of the values and belief of the patient and nurse.
- Public policy and the healthcare delivery system influence the health and well-being of society and professional nursing.
- Individual responsibility and interprofessional involvement are essential (ANA, 2010).

As the collective voice for nurses in the United States, the ANA links nursing to society through a social policy statement that addresses key issues inherent in an evolving society. The social policy statement is foundational to establishing the context of nursing, both within and outside of the profession. It serves as a unifying framework for nurses to influence health policy.

Strategies for Political Action

Effecting a change means getting involved in strategies for **political action** (Boswell et al., 2005). There are many strategies that can be used to promote participation in political activities, including the following:

- Become a registered voter and cast your vote in elections. Investigate the candidates and vote for the one who is reportedly the closest to your values and philosophy for healthcare management.
- Incorporate political science courses in an educational foundation. This is an excellent way to keep abreast of how political activities are being managed, along with the potential to expand expertise in policy and politics specifically related to an area of interest.
- Strategically use the communication mechanisms to keep current of the issues that are of importance in the government. This can be done through print media, news releases on television, or online through news and political websites.
- Get involved in organizational committees that form the foundation for effective patient management and nursing practice. Take the initiative to get started. Work closely with an area of interest in order to maintain momentum for a specific political policy.
- Get involved in nursing organizations that promote the welfare of all nurses. Join organizations that are aligned with you as a professional nurse in addition to an area of specialization if that is your desire. There is power in numbers, and increasing numbers in a broad-purpose organization can increase the political potential of the organization and profession.

Nurses can also get involved in specific activities in order to promote individual and professional initiatives. Be proactive in politics and not *reactive* after an issue has been made into law. Many activities can be accomplished without a significant outlay of effort or time. Specific activities can include those in Box 11.3.

Ways to Get Politically Involved in Nursing

1. **Apply for the White House Fellows program.** This program is a prestigious, nonpartisan leadership development program that offers exceptional professionals first-hand experience working at the highest levels of the federal government.
2. **Become a Washington nurse intern.** The Nurse in Washington Internship program is a professional development program that prepares nurses to engage in health policy by providing hands-on experience in advocacy, legislative processes, and effective communication with policymakers.
3. **Join the ANA.** This professional organization represents registered nurses in the United States, setting standards of practice, advocating for the nursing profession, and advancing health policy.
4. **Stay informed.** Research and stay up to date on current bills and resolutions that affect healthcare and the nursing profession. Visit https://www.govtrack.us/congress/bills/subjects/nursing/6180 to browse nursing bills.
5. **Engage in legislative advocacy.** Contact legislators, submit written testimony, or participate in legislative days to share nursing expertise on healthcare issues. Directly communicate with policymakers to ensure that frontline perspectives are represented in decisions that shape healthcare delivery and funding.
6. **Participate in grassroots campaigns.** Support local and national initiatives such as petition drives, letter-writing campaigns, or community forums to improve chances to amplify nursing voices and mobilize action around key issues such as staffing ratios, access to care, or public health policy.
7. **Serve on boards or committees.** Contribute to policy development by serving on hospital committees, advisory boards, or governmental health councils. Through this level of involvement nurses can influence organizational and public health decisions while highlighting nursing's essential role in leadership.
8. **Ethically use media and social platforms.** Engaging in social media advocacy or participating in professional blogs allows nurses to raise public awareness about healthcare issues. This visibility helps shape public opinion and can place pressure on policymakers to act.
9. **Educate others as a political pathway.** Educating others is a powerful strategy for nurses to create change. Sharing legislative issues or advocacy resources with colleagues, friends, and family can spark greater awareness and encourage collective action.

Source: Adapted from Bethany Derricott, "Political Activities for Nurses – Get Involved," BellaOnline: The Voice of Women. Copyright © 2023 by BellaOnline.

Summary

Learning is a lifelong process that involves active engagement. Nurses are responsible for shaping their practice and effecting policies that are important to promoting the best outcome for patients, families, communities, and populations. Developing professional agendas that incorporate active involvement will move the profession forward and promote nursing control over the profession's destiny. Involvement can give individuals a competitive edge because it keeps them informed and engaged. It will also serve to promote personal success and may initiate lasting networking relationships. It is through these relationships that important issues can be addressed in unison and outcomes focused on delivery of evidence-based care at the local, state, and federal levels.

References

American Nurses Association. (n.d.). *About ANA*. https://www.nursingworld.org/ana/about-ana

American Nurses Association. (2010). *Nursing's social policy statement: The essence of the profession.*

Arcaya, M. C., Arcaya, A. L., & Subramanian, S. V. (2015). Inequalities in health: Definitions, concepts, and theories. *Global Health Action*, *8*, 27106. https://doi.org/10.3402/gha.v8.27106

Avanceña, A. L. V., DeLuca, E. K., Iott, B., Mauri, A., Miller, N., Eisenberg, D., & David W. Hutton, D. W. (2021). Income and income inequality are a matter of life and death. What can policymakers do about it? *American Journal of Public Health, 111*, 1404–1408. https://doi.org/10.2105/AJPH.2021.306301

Bakwesegha, C. J. (2013, March 7). *Politics, democracy and governance in Africa: A bird's eye view.* Human Services Today. https://www.uwosh.edu/hst/politics-democracy-and-governance-in-africa-a-birds-eye-view/

BellaOnline. (n.d.). *Political activities for nurses—get involved.* http://www.bellaonline.com/articles/art60390.asp

Boswell, C., Cannon, S., & Miller, J. (2005). Nurses' political involvement: Responsibility versus privilege. *Journal of Professional Nursing*, *21*(1), 5–8. https://doi.org/10.1016/j.profnurs.2004.11.005

Brannon, K. (2023, May 16). *Study: Rising cost of racial and ethnic health inequities in US surpasses $450 billion.* Tulane University. https://sph.tulane.edu/study-rising-cost-racial-and-ethnic-health-inequities-us-surpasses-450-billion

Braveman, P. A., Cubbin, C., Egerter, S., Williams, D. R., Pamuk, E. (2010). Socioeconomic disparities in health in the United States: What the patterns tell us. *American Journal of Public Health,* 100(Suppl 1), S186–S196. https://doi.org/10.2105/AJPH.2009.166082

Chinn, P. L., & Kennedy, M. S. (2023). Activism is an essential nursing role. *American Journal of Nursing, 123*(10), 52–58. https://doi.org/10.1097/01.NAJ.0000979100.16233.cc

Easton, D. (1965). *A Systems Analysis of Political Life*. Wiley.

Farlex. (n.d.). *Policy*. The Free Dictionary. https://www.thefreedictionary.com/policies

Farrah, M. (2013, May 10). *The Internatinal Council of Nursing and you; learning, legislation and networking*. https://www.nurses.co.uk/blog/opinion/international-council-nursing-and-you-learning-legislating-and-networking

Fowler, M. (2015). *Guide to nursing's social policy statement: From social contract to social covenant* (1st ed.). American Nurses Association.

Gorenberg. B. D., Alderman, M. C., & Cruise, M. J. (1991). Social policy statements: Guidelines for decisionmaking. *International Nursing Review, 38*(1), 11–13.

Han, N. K., & Kim, G. S. (2024). The barriers and facilitators influencing nurses' political participation or healthcare policy intervention: A systematic review and qualitative meta-analysis. *Journal of Nursing Management*, 606855. https://doi.org/10.1155/2024/2606855

Hewitt, S., & Padya, S. (2024, January 18). *ANA on Capital Hill—federal legislative update*. Capitol Beat. https://anacapitolbeat.org/2024/01/18/ana-on-capitol-hill-federal-legislative-update/

International Council of Nurses. (n.d.). *Who we are*. https://www.icn.ch/who-we-are

International Council of Nurses. (2024). *Strategic plan 2024–2028*. https://www.icn.ch/sites/default/files/2024-05/ICN_Strategic-Plan_2024-2028_EN.pdf

Kenton, W., Boyle, M. J., & Kvilhaug, S. (2025, January 27). *Affordable Care Act (ACA): What it is, key features, and updates*. Investopedia. https://www.investopedia.com/terms/a/affordable-care-act.asp

LaVeist, T. A., Pérez-Stable, E. J., Richard, P., Anderson, A., Isaac, L. A., Santiago, R., Okoh, C., Breen, N., Farhat, T., Assenov, A., & Gaskin, D. J. (2023). The economic burden of racial, ethnic, and educational health inequities in the US. *JAMA, 329*(19), 1682–1692. https://doi.org/10.1001/jama.2023.5965

National Academies of Sciences, Engineering, and Medicine; Health and Medicine Division; Board on Population Health and Public Health Practice; Committee on Community-Based Solutions to Promote Health Equity in the United States. (2017, January 11). The root causes of health inequity. In A. Baciu, Y. Negussie, A. Geller, & J. N. Weinstein (Eds.), *Communities in action: Pathways to health equity*. National Academies Press (U.S.). https://www.ncbi.nlm.nih.gov/books/NBK425845/

National Academies of Sciences, Engineering, and Medicine; National Academy of Medicine; Committee on the Future of Nursing 2020–2030. (2021, May 11). The future of nursing 2020–2030: Charting a path to achieve health equity. In M. K. Wakefield, D. R. Williams, S. L. Menestrel, & J. L. Flaubert (Eds)., *The role of nurses in improving health care access and quality*. National Academies Press (U.S.). https://www.ncbi.nlm.nih.gov/books/NBK573910/

Needlestick Safety and Prevention Act of 2000, Public Law 106-430, 106th Congress, H.R. 5178.

Reutter, L., & Kushner, K. E. (2010). Health equity through action on the social determinants of health: Taking up the challenge in nursing. *Nursing Inquiry, 17*(3), 269–280. https://doi.org/10.1111/j.1440-1800.2010.00500.x

Svetvilas, C., & Morris, M. (2023). *Federal safe staffing bill introduced in House and Senate*. https://www.nationalnursesunited.org/article/federal-safe-staffing-bill-introduced-in-house-and-senate

Tiase, V., Crookston, C. D., Schoenbaum, A., & Valu, M. (2022). Nurses' role in addressing social determinants of health. *Nursing, 52*(4), 32–37. https://doi.org/10.1097/01.NURSE.0000823284.16666.96

Whitehead, M. 1992. The concepts and principles of equity in health. International *Journal of Health Services* 22(3):429–445. https://doi.org/10.2190/986L-LHQ6-2VTE-YRRN

Wilson, D. M., Underwood, L., Kim, S., Olukotun, M., & Errasti-Ibarrondo, B. (2022). How and why nurses became involved in politics or political action, and the outcomes or impacts of this involvement. *Nursing Outlook, 70*(1), 55–63. https://doi.org/10.1016/j.outlook.2021.07.008

Image Credits

Fig. 11.1: Adapted from David Easton, "A Systems Analysis of Political Life: ," https://en.wikipedia.org/wiki/File:Easton-System_of_political-life.PNG. Copyright © 1965 by John Wiley & Sons, Inc..

CHAPTER 12

Technology and Nursing Practice

Charles W. Revell, MCP, MCAD, MCSD, MCT

Objectives

Upon completion of this chapter, the learner will be able to do the following:

1. Discuss informatics nursing and its role in supporting safe patient activities.
2. Identify how technology has changed the role of nursing.
3. Explain the impact of technology on patient care outcomes.
4. Understand the role of artificial intelligence (AI) in health care.
5. Describe how robotics are being used to promote healthy patient outcomes.

Key Chapter Terms

- Nursing informatics
- Data
- Information
- Knowledge
- Data gatherer
- Information user
- Knowledge user
- Knowledge producer
- Electronic health records (EHRs)
- Health Insurance Portability and Accountability Act (HIPAA)
- Medical errors
- Informatics competencies
- Technology Informatics Guiding Education Reform (TIGER) international project
- American Association of Colleges of Nursing (AACN) essentials
- Beginning nurse
- Experienced nurse
- Informatics nurse specialist
- Informatics innovator
- Artificial intelligence (AI)
- Robotics

Technology and Nursing: An Effective Combination

Effective utilization of technology is imperative to patient safety in nursing practice. Technological changes are foundational in order to provide continuous quality care, which is at the forefront of nursing practice in today's healthcare environment. Despite the numerous technological changes made to the healthcare environment, nurses continue to play a critical role in the delivery of care. They serve as conduits to safety through which technological changes play out their role in care delivery.

The American Nurses Association (ANA) defines ***nursing informatics*** as a specialty that:

> integrates nursing science, computer science, and information science to manage and communicate data, information, knowledge, and wisdom into nursing practice ... facilitates the integration of data, information, knowledge and wisdom to support patients, nurses, and other providers in their decision-making in all roles and settings. This support is accomplished through the use of information structures, information processes, and information technology. (ANA, 2007, p. 1)

Technological innovations are transforming the culture of care in many organizations. The use of information technologies is one of the five core competencies required of nurses, according to a 2003 Institute of Medicine (IOM) document. This impetus gives the nursing profession a fundamental requirement to educationally prepare individuals to deliver care in the technologically based healthcare organization of the present and future.

Nursing Informatics

Technology is inherent in patient management, from entry into the healthcare system until discharge. In this realm of healthcare information technology (IT), a need has evolved for nurses who not only are clinical experts but also have technological know-how. Technologically savvy individuals have the expertise to develop systems but are not knowledgeable in the language or patient care aspects for which they are developing these systems. It requires a blend of education and skills that include technology and nursing. Nursing informatics is a form of health informatics that applies IT to the skills and work of nurses in health care. It integrates nursing science, computer technology, and information science to effectively enhance the quality of nursing practice. This blending promotes improved communication, documentation, and efficiency in healthcare delivery by nurses.

Technology supplies fingertip access to information needed to develop individualized plans for patient care management. Integration of technology into nursing allows for an appropriate flow of data collected by nurses in the course of patient management.

From Data to Knowledge

In technology, ***data*** consists of characters, numbers, and/or facts gathered for analyses. This analysis can occur at the time of data collection or be deferred to a later time when additional data are gathered for comparative analyses. Data that are interpreted are further moved to the category of information as they are now usable for patient management. One blood pressure measurement alone gives you only part of the patient's picture. Correlation of these blood pressure data with prior and current readings allows you to put together ***information*** for interpretation and use for effective patient management. From these data to information retrieval, ***knowledge*** results in a decision regarding the best course of action for patient management (see Figure 12.1).

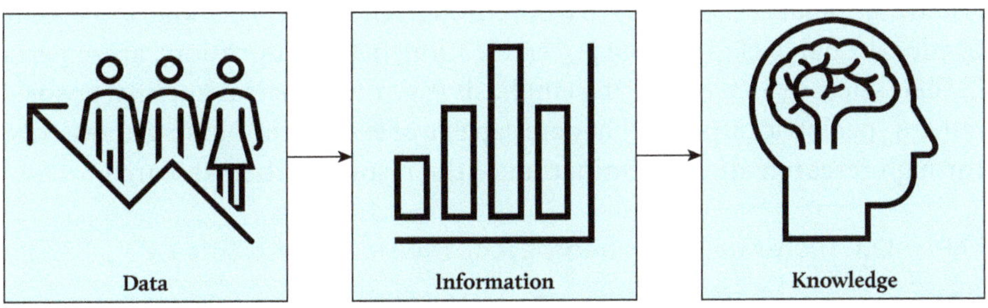

FIGURE 12.1 Data to Knowledge Transition

Each level increases in complexity and requires greater application of expertise and intellect to follow through to safe patient care practice and efficient care delivery.

Healthcare settings are knowledge-intensive. Nurses need to exponentially grow in order to effectively use this information. Technology supports knowledge acquisition by allowing just-in-time access to evidence-based information. Nurses have access to this information through handheld devices, stationary and mobile computer setups, and bedside computer systems, which allow for retrieval of information that promotes decisions made on the most current research-based information.

Nurses function in several roles in moving data to decision. These roles can extend from foundational to expert. These roles include (a) data gatherer, (b) information user, (c) knowledge user, and (d) knowledge producer (see Table 12.1). *Data gatherers* are individuals whose task is to collect data from patients in various situations. These individuals can either use the information themselves if they are the care nurse or move this information to another care provider who has the primary responsibility to function in other roles of the technological movement. Nurse preceptees are new to the healthcare environment and are just learning to critically think and use information gathered or delivered to them by other care providers. As new nurses, these individuals are in transition from studying at an educational facility to becoming full-time care providers who use the knowledge acquired over prior years of learning. Through the process of orientation and preceptorship, nurses learn to coordinate care and organize information for effective and safe care delivery. After several years of nursing and countless hours of experience, nurses are proficient at delivery of care. This level of expertise allows for development of foundational information that can be integrated into a format that promotes individualized care delivery. Information is collectively retrieved and quickly organized into a usable format that allows for on-the-spot retrieval, enhancing decision-making skills. *Knowledge producers* are nurses who, through their years of experience and/or educational background (e.g., certification, higher education), are experts in their selected area of nursing emphasis (e.g., neurological nursing, hospice nursing, pediatric nursing). They are capable of expanding nursing knowledge through research and dissemination of the results of their research.

TABLE 12.1 Potential Roles and Descriptive Healthcare Titles

Role	Healthcare Title
Data gatherer	**Nursing assistant/novice nurse:** An individual who gathers and collects data for delivery to the appropriate care provider, which can include self, in order to promote health care decisions.
Information user	**Nurse preceptee:** An individual who is new to the nursing profession and in the initial stages of using information for healthcare decisions for patient management.
Knowledge user	**Proficient nurse:** An individual who has been in nursing for several years and is capable of quickly moving data through the information stage to knowledge use for decisions that promote safe and efficient care delivery.
Knowledge producer	**Expert nurse:** An individual who has been in nursing and has acquired an educational base in a specific area of nursing that allows for correlational analyses and differentiation of data to produce evidence that is research-based to promote delivery of care, which is shared with the nursing profession.

These roles are not mutually exclusive. Individuals may move from role to role based on their care delivery position, such as to another area of nursing (e.g., an experienced home health nurse moving to an acute care surgical setting), and their need to obtain information. For example, expert nurses may function in all roles when delivering care to a critically ill patient.

In order to make healthcare decisions, nurses must be able to access important information when needed. Moving from data to knowledge requires that nurses have access to critical information at a moment's notice. It is important that the system in place affords nurses the ability to retrieve and manage information. With nursing involvement, this integration of critical information and system usability will be promoted. It is nurses' responsibility to learn how to effectively access this information for the best possible outcome for patient management.

Electronic Records and Care Delivery

Healthcare organizations have computerized systems for some part or all of care documentation. This can range from such services as laboratory and radiological information to total documentation of care by nurses at the bedside or point-of-care delivery. The end result can be a totally paperless system that requires awareness of information flow and management by nurses.

Electronic patient-based records are also known as electronic medical records, ***electronic health records*** **(EHRs)**, *electronic patient records*, or *computerized patient records*. All these terms refer to a systematic collection of patient-based information. The Health Information Management Systems Society defines an EHR as "a secure real-time, point-of-care, patient-centric information resource for clinicians" (Handler et al., 2003). This digitalized record can include current and past health encounter information. Some of the information included can include patient demographics, past medical history, immunizations, chief complaints with interventions and progress notes, vital signs, medications, laboratory results, and radiology reports, among others. EHRs can generate a total record of a health care visit. Nurses and other providers have immediate access to information and can generate trend reports and algorithms that support care decisions and delivery. This allows for interdisciplinary interventions specifically designed for individualized patient interventions to promote evidence-based decisions for quality health care outcomes.

Electronic patient-based information may be static or dynamic. Static records include information placed in a record at a designated time, such as during a wellness physician visit and not updated hourly or daily. These records remain in a database state until acted upon at a specific time. Some examples of these include patient demographic data and prior health historical information. Dynamic records are those that accept constant input of information from seconds to minutes to hours. These are used in care facilities that require continuous input of information. Some examples of these include incremental information entered in acute care settings through electronic devices, such as intravenous medication delivery machines and continuous blood pressure devices. Regardless of the type of record, EHRs can be shared across various healthcare settings and provide instant access to critical information needed for care decisions by nurses and other healthcare providers. Dynamic records allow for actionable opportunities to close healthcare risks and quality gaps.

Each patient encounter results in the capture of data. The EHR network integrates data from all participating systems (e.g., administration, nursing, laboratory, radiology, pharmacy) and organizes them to create EHRs for specific patients. This information can then be retrieved for coordination of care (see Figure 12.2).

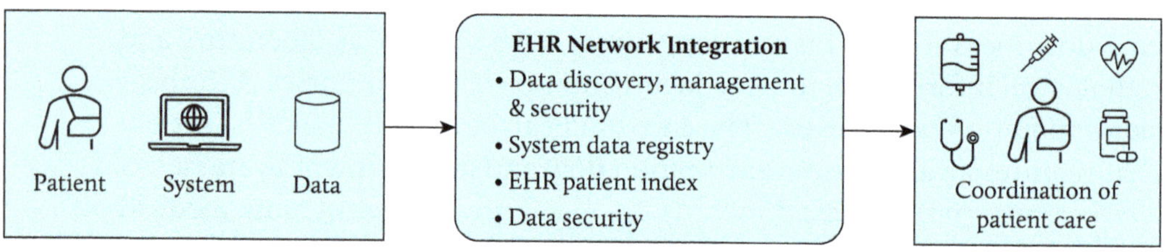

FIGURE 12.2 EHR: Nursing Concept Overview

EHRs now have the ability to allow nurses to retrieve patient data from a multitude of sources inside and outside their organization. All incorporate supporting security measures that allow for access across organizational, state, and country-of-origin boundaries. These systems can be nationwide and worldwide, integrating language (e.g., French to English) and results (e.g., meters to inches) translational components to allow for enhanced operation across nationalities and cultures. EHR capability can also translate information into analytics and generate algorithms that promote diagnosis and treatment options for better patient diagnosis and management. EHR integration allows for care continuity and collaboration, employee efficiency, patient engagement, and scalable insights into future patient needs.

Information Security

Security in the IT world is a significant issue. Security must ensure that the **Health Insurance Portability and Accountability Act (HIPAA)** is addressed in an effort to provide continuity of care without risk to health information for patients. Information about health care crosses many areas within acute and extended care facilities, physician offices, outpatient settings, as well as others. It is important that security be addressed in an effort to assure access in an effort to improve quality of care, prevent medical errors, reduce paperwork, and expand access for individuals seeking care. Nurses should access only the records of those for whom they have direct care or about whom they have a need to know regarding information in an effort to render safe care. HIPAA violations carry stiff penalties, up to and including immediate employment termination.

Measures to control threats and vulnerabilities in information systems can be organized into three categories of safeguards. These include administrative, physical, and technical. HIPAA security standards fall in the administrative category. These administrative safeguard actions, policies, and procedures manage the selection, development, implementation, and maintenance of measures that manage patient information (U.S. Department of Health and Human Services, 2007). Physical safeguard actions include policies, procedures, and measures that control physical access to information devices that house information such as computers, servers, networks, and buildings in which devices that house information are stored. Technical controls include devices associated with security of information, including passwords, firewalls, and encryptions that ensure integrity of patient health information (Alder, 2024).

Security is imperative in health care in order to protect the rights of individuals regarding their health information. Organizations must ensure that security addresses confidentiality, integrity, and availability of information. A patient data system must be secure in that it does not allow information to undisclosed individuals. Access must be restricted to individuals who have a right to know. Systems must be password-restricted and partitioned in segments that give specific individuals access to designated information. The system must have data integrity. Information must be correct and unalterable by persons without specific access and privileges. This ensures that information is correct as entered and does not allow misrepresentation of information within the system. *Availability* is the property that data or information is accessible and usable on demand. In health care, it is imperative to be able to access specific information when necessary to ensure continuity of patient care.

Nursing's responsibility for security encompasses user awareness. Nurses gain entry to patient healthcare information systems through passwords, specific system keys, badges, or other security components. When logging in or accessing the system for input, alteration, or review of patient information, it is imperative to log out or return the system to a user-ready state. This prevents access by unauthorized individuals under another's specific user information. Consistent awareness of the general extent of security measures, practices, and procedures for security of the system is a must. It is the ethical and legal responsibility of all healthcare professionals to protect patient information from unauthorized access.

Patient Safety

Patient safety is of utmost concern in health care. Keeping patients safe through the reduction of accidental injury is part of nurses' responsibility. Errors can be costly in terms of quality of life for patients and families and fiscal recovery from an organization for such errors (e.g., judgment against an organization by a court system or federal/state fines for not adhering to safe practice standards). Patient safety is not only a responsibility of nurses but has been championed by other organizations in an effort to reduce the number of errors and subsequent negative outcomes. In 2000, the Institute of Medicine (IOM) published a landmark report that heightened public awareness of healthcare errors. According to this report, as many as 98,000 Americans die in any given year in hospitals from **medical errors**. Even today, error rates are difficult to validate and are reported as varying units of measure, but approximately 210,000 to 400,000 deaths are identified as being associated with medical errors in U.S. hospitals (Aryankhesal et al., 2023). Medical errors continue to be a significant issue. Many occurrences are due to human error, and in an industry in which service from people is a standard, it is important to address these errors. Technology is a foundational strategy that can be used to address medical errors and promote patient safety. Technology can be used to promote safe care activities through the following:

- Use of prompts to identify inconsistencies or alerts in a computerized system (e.g., an alert for a medication that is ordered that is on a patient's allergy list, inappropriate medication dose alert, retrieval of blood pressure or heart rate prior to administration of a specific medication)
- Use of constraints or forcing functions, which require that the individual act on a presented situation before being allowed to progress to the next action
- A plan-for-recovery system that would allow for reversal of an operation with validation, such as deletion or moving information within the system
- Standardization of actions that would require the use of preset protocols in order to complete an action

Patient safety is the underlying premise for technological use. This can be promoted through a safe infrastructure, technologies and medical devices, and education for staff and patients regarding the use of technology in patient safety programs. Usage of technological innovations can reduce unsafe patient situations and occurrences of what are called *sentinel events* in patient care. A sentinel event is one in which an unexpected situation occurs that places a patient at risk of death or actually results in death or serious physical or psychological injury. An example of serious physical injury might include the discharge of an infant to the wrong family, a medication error that results in death or major permanent loss of function, or a patient fall that results in death or major permanent loss of function. A psychological injury might include a stress-related emotional condition resulting from real or imagined threats, such as an event that might cause substantial and lasting psychological damage, including depression or significant anxiety. These events are termed *sentinel* because they identify an immediate need for investigation and response by the organization. Nurses should be proactive in embracing a technology that promotes patient safety through early identification and alert systems. These systems serve to identify needs that require immediate action.

Informatics Competencies

Technology Informatics Guiding Education Reform

Nurses must be competent users of technology and possess foundational competencies. Nurse **informatics competencies** have a significant effect on patient outcomes and organizational success (Hübner et al., 2019). The **Technology Informatics Guiding Education Reform (TIGER)** (2020) international project identified core competencies by role. The role that specifically related to direct patient care for nurses included core competencies of communication, documentation and information, and knowledge management in patient care as the top three of 10 competencies.

It is important that nurses know not only how to enter information into an electronic system but also how to use it in planning care. They must be able to identify needed information and analyze it to make informed decisions regarding care delivery (Khezri & Abdekhoda, 2019). The TIGER (2020) international project further identified roles correlated to competencies, which included clinical nursing (direct patient care); coordination of interprofessional care (see Table 12.2); and four data, information, and knowledge (DIK) domains of core competency areas, including an information exchange and sharing (IEIS) domain and an ethics and legal issues (EL) domain (see Table 12.3), which are applicable to the new nurse graduate.

TABLE 12.2 TIGER-Applicable Roles and Competencies for New Nurses

Role	Core Competency
Clinical nursing (direct patient care)	• Nursing documentation (including terminologies) • Information and knowledge management • Principles of nursing informatics • Data protection and security • Ethics and IT • Information and communication
Coordination of interprofessional care	• Data protection and security • Information and knowledge management • Nursing documentation (including terminologies) • Ethics and IT

Source: Adapted from TIGER, 2020.

TABLE 12.3 Four TIGER-Applicable DIK Domains of Core Competency Areas

DIK Domain	Domain Component	Associated Core Competency Areas
Information exchange and sharing (IEIS) domain	• Continuity of care	• Information and communication systems; eHealth, telematics, and telehealth
	• The sharing of information with the patient, working in partnerships, learning to listen	• eHealth, telematics, and telehealth; assistive technology for ageing people
	• Health information exchange (HIE)	• Information and communication systems; eHealth, telematics, and telehealth
Ethics and legal issues (EL) domain	• Ethics	• Ethics and IT
	• Security and privacy	• Data protection and security
	• Use of social media and ethical use of data	• Ethics and IT; data protection and security

Source: Adapted from TIGER, 2020.

American Association of Colleges of Nursing

The AACN has identified critical components for nursing education. The association has presented these in ***essentials*** for nursing education specific to the level of competency. The AACN document identifies domains that are considered essential to nursing education. The domain specific to Informatics and Healthcare Technologies is Domain 8, which states that graduates must be able to "[describe] the various information and communication technology tools used in the care of patients, communities, and populations" (AACN, 2021).

Education is important to ensure that nurses have the skills and knowledge to interact with technologies and communicate effectively with patients and colleagues. Knowledge to promote correct and effective interactions with team members, patients, and consumers can serve to promote safe, effective care management and improve overall health. Domains are divided into subdomains for entry and advanced levels (see Table 12.4).

TABLE 12.4 AACN Domain 8 Subdomains and Taxonomy Descriptive Level Outcomes

Entry-Level Professional Nursing Education	Advanced-Level Nursing Education
8.1 Describe the various information and communication technology tools used in the care of patients, communities, and populations.	
8.1a Identify the variety of information and communication technologies used in care settings.	8.1g Identify best evidence and practices for the application of information and communication technologies to support care.
8.1b Identify the basic concepts of electronic health, mobile health, and telehealth systems for enabling patient care.	8.1h Evaluate the unintended consequences of information and communication technologies on care processes, communications, and information flow across care settings.
8.1c Effectively use electronic communication tools.	8.1i Propose a plan to influence the selection and implementation of new information and communication technologies.
8.1d Describe the appropriate use of multimedia applications in health care.	8.1j Explore the fiscal impact of information and communication technologies on health care.
8.1e Demonstrate best-practice use of social networking applications.	8.1k Identify the impact of information and communication technologies on workflow processes and healthcare outcomes.
8.1f Explain the importance of nursing engagement in the planning and selection of healthcare technologies.	
8.2 Use information and communication technology to gather data, create information, and generate knowledge.	
8.2a Enter accurate data when chronicling care.	8.2f Generate information and knowledge from health IT databases.

(Continued)

TABLE 12.4 (Continued)

Entry-Level Professional Nursing Education	Advanced-Level Nursing Education
8.2b Explain how data entered on one patient impact public and population health data.	8.2g Evaluate the use of communication technology to improve consumer health information literacy.
8.2c Use appropriate data when planning care.	8.2 Use standardized data to evaluate decisionmaking and outcomes across all systems levels.
8.2d Demonstrate the appropriate use of health information literacy assessments and improvement strategies.	8.2i Clarify how the collection of standardized data advances the practice, understanding, and value of nursing and supports care.
8.2e Describe the importance of standardized nursing data to reflect the unique contribution of nursing practice.	8.2j Interpret primary and secondary data and other information to support care
8.3 Use information and communication technologies and informatics processes to deliver safe nursing care to diverse populations in a variety of settings.	
8.3a Demonstrate appropriate use of information and communication technologies.	8.3g Evaluate the use of information and communication technology to address needs, gaps, and inefficiencies in care.
8.3b Evaluate how decision support tools impact clinical judgment and safe patient care.	8.3h Formulate a plan to influence decision-making processes for selecting, implementing, and evaluating support tools.
8.3c Use information and communication technology in a manner that supports the nurse-patient relationship.	8.3i Appraise the role of information and communication technologies in engaging the patient and supporting the nurse-patient relationship.
8.3d Examine how emerging technologies influence healthcare delivery and clinical decision-making.	8.3j Evaluate the potential uses and impact of emerging technologies in health care.
8.3e Identify impact of information and communication technology on quality and safety of care.	8.3k Pose strategies to reduce inequities in digital access to data and information.
8.3f Identify the importance of reporting system processes and functional issues (e.g., error messages, misdirections, device malfunctions) according to organizational policies and procedures.	

Entry-Level Professional Nursing Education	Advanced-Level Nursing Education
8.4 Use information and communication technology to support documentation of care and communication among providers, patients, and all system levels.	
8.4a Explain the role of communication technology in enhancing clinical information flows.	8.4e Assess best practices for the use of advanced information and communication technologies to support patient and team communications.
8.4b Describe how information and communication technology tools support patient and team communications.	8.4f Employ electronic health, mobile health, and telehealth systems to enable quality, ethical, and efficient patient care.
8.4c Identify the basic concepts of electronic health, mobile health, and telehealth systems in enabling patient care.	8.4g Evaluate the impact of HIE, interoperability, and integration to support patient-centered care.
8.4d Explain the impact of HIE, interoperability, and integration on health care.	
8.5 Use information and communication technologies in accordance with ethical, legal, professional, and regulatory standards and workplace policies in the delivery of care.	
8.5a Identify common risks associated with using information and communication technology.	8.5g Apply risk mitigation and security strategies to reduce misuse of information and communication technology.
8.5b Demonstrate ethical use of social networking applications.	8.5h Assess potential ethical and legal issues associated with the use of information and communication technology.
8.5c Comply with legal and regulatory requirements while using communication and information technologies.	8.5i Recommend strategies to protect health information when using communication and IT.
8.5d Educate patients on their rights to access, review, and correct personal data and medical records.	8.5j Promote patient engagement with their personal health data.
8.5e Discuss how clinical judgment and critical thinking must prevail in the presence of information and communication technologies.	8.5k Advocate for policies and regulations that support the appropriate use of technologies impacting health care.
8.5f Deliver care using remote technology.	8.5l Analyze the impact of federal and state policies and regulation on health data and technology in care settings.

Source: American Association of Colleges of Nursing, "AACN Domain 8 Sub-domains and Taxonomy Descriptive Level Outcomes," The Essentials: Core Competencies for Professional Nursing Education, pp. 46-48. Copyright © 2021 by American Association of Colleges of Nursing (AACN). Reprinted with permission..

Skill Levels of Informatics Competencies

Nurses must have a positive attitude toward the use of computers and technology in general in order to address any skill level and promote the best outcomes for themselves and others. There are four skill levels commonly recognized in nursing informatics: (a) **beginning nurse**, (b) experienced nurse, (c) informatics nurse specialist, and (d) informatics innovator (Staggers et al., 2001). These levels promote a format that allows nurses to identify where they are on the knowledge scale of IT. This knowledge encourages further acquisition in order to understand the intricate skill set required for the use of technology in health care.

Beginning Nurse

Skills include those basic to computer use such as demonstrating keyboard skills, using the internet, and conducting searches. These skills extend to electronic communication in the form of email skills, including generating messages, using an appropriate tone for communication, and securely forwarding information from one individual to another. In relationship with health care, these categories go much further. Basic computer skills include administration, communication, data access, decision support, documentation, education, monitoring, and desktop software and systems. Word-processing skills are elementary to communication, as they include the ability to generate, edit, and save information in various formats, allowing for later retrieval. This information is then used for developing care plans and promoting decision-making for care delivery. Informatics knowledge for this level includes data, impact, privacy, and security and systems. Data are important to decisions that are made for implementation of care and in relaying patient information to peers and interdisciplinary care providers throughout the course of patient management. The impact of these data on management and future potential health problem developments can be assessed with proper data entry through algorithm generation and comparison with national datasets. Privacy and security are required at all levels and begin as one enters the nursing profession.

Experienced Nurse

Experienced nurses expand on the skills of beginning nurses. In addition to possessing entry-level skills, these nurses support their specific specialty area with quality improvement activities and other activities to promote safe and skilled patient care using technology. This level of informatics nurses use evidence-based databases to promote high-level nursing care activities for patients. These nurses use research to identify gaps in practice for appropriate interventions. Through the promotion of technology applications, nurses can improve patient outcomes. Experienced nurses work with the organization's IT department to promote system improvements. These improvements allow for nurses to deliver quality, safe care to patients in all environments.

Informatics Nurse Specialist

Informatics nurse specialists possess beginning and experienced nurse skills. They also possess all the skills required to be proficient with technological applications that are used to support all areas of nursing practice. They are engaged in analysis of systems inclusive of fiscal management for hardware and software integration within the organization. They are skilled in data management, programming, system development and testing, and use of computer applications. Their involvement in data management may include data design or the way data are structured in the organization's system, *data storage*, which refers to the many ways data can be stored (e.g., primary, secondary or tertiary storage; magnetic disk; futuristic five-dimensional optical storage) and/or data security that involves management of firewalls or other security encryptions that may exist to maintain data and system integrity.

Informatics Innovator

Informatics innovators possess all prior skills and have an in-depth understanding of the various levels of technology. This extends from the user interface to security technology. They are proficient in data structures, conduct research, and generate theoretical foundations for informatics nursing. These nurses are pivotal to evidence-based validation of technology-based solutions that improve nursing communication and increase the efficiency of patient care. These individuals are often members of the multidisciplinary team for an organization that promotes the integration of beginning nurses with computer technology to improve patient care. Informatics innovators often promote strategic planning and determination of system solutions that support patient care through research activities. They work to develop standards for technology use in clinical applications while conforming to organizational accreditation standards and regulatory requirements.

The Impact of Technology on Patient Care Outcomes

Technology has changed the nursing role. It has streamlined communication between healthcare providers with tools such as secure messaging apps, telehealth platforms, and shared EHRs, which enable nurses to effectively collaborate with multidisciplinary team members. Nurses can now monitor patients remotely, provide education, and follow up with patients without the need for physical visits, especially during pandemics and disasters and regarding managing chronic conditions.

The introduction of sophisticated health technologies has expanded nursing roles. Nurses are now responsible for more than just direct patient care; they are tasked with managing healthcare technologies. This involves training in the use of EHR system capabilities, participating in technology policy development, and contributing to the implementation of new health IT systems. Nurses also need to stay current with technological advancements to provide optimal patient care and act as intermediaries between patients and technologies (Brennan & Bakken, 2019).

The impact of technology on health care is profound and will continue to expand as innovative technologies are developed. These impacts include a reduction in errors and improved information accuracy, increased efficiency and workflow optimization, enhanced patient engagement in their health through online portals, and increased communication and collaboration.

Reduced Errors and Improved Information Accuracy

One of the most significant technological impacts in healthcare is the reduction of medical errors. EHRs and automated systems reduce errors that result from manual paper-based documentation, which include legibility issues, decimal place errors in medication orders, missed treatments, and duplication of laboratory or radiological tests. Barcoding systems in medication administration ensure that the right patient receives the correct medication at the right dose and time, which reduces adverse drug events (Poon et al., 2010).

Increased Efficiency and Workflow Optimization

The adoption of automated tools and electronic records has optimized nursing workflows. Routine tasks, such as documentation of treatments and care activities and medication administration, have become faster and more accurate. This significantly reduces charting, data input time, and administrative tasks, which allow nurses to spend more time with patients. Telehealth solutions, wearable patient monitors, and real-time data analytics also enable more proactive care management, especially for patients with chronic diseases.

Enhanced Patient Engagement

Technology has empowered patients to take an active role in managing their health. Patient portals allow individuals to access their health records. This gives them an opportunity to see their historical data for vital signs, diagnoses, medications, healthcare provider notes, and radiological and laboratory findings. They can even schedule appointments and securely communicate directly with their healthcare providers. These portals also have the ability to send alerts for future medical interventions needed. By fostering better communication and increasing patient involvement, technology improves adherence to treatment plans and overall patient satisfaction, which ultimately leads to better health outcomes (Adeniyi et al., 2024).

Communication and Collaboration

Technology has streamlined communication between healthcare providers. Tools such as secure messaging apps, telehealth platforms, and shared EHRs enable nurses to efficiently collaborate with multidisciplinary team members in order to deliver holistic care. Nurses now have the capability to remotely monitor patients, deliver education, and conduct follow-up care without requiring in-person visits, a practice that has proven particularly valuable during pandemics and public health emergencies. This capability also extends to patients who require chronic illness management.

The Role of Artificial Intelligence in Health Care

AI is increasingly becoming a key component in health care, particularly in areas such as diagnostics, predictive analytics, and personalized care. AI algorithms can quickly analyze vast amounts of data, promoting the identification of trends that would be difficult for humans to detect in a short period of time. For instance, AI tools can analyze patient histories and diagnostic images to support early detection of diseases, such as cancer, enhancing the likelihood of successful treatment outcomes. AI technology is not one technology but a collection of various technologies that have a variety of processes and tasks. Some of these technologies include machine learning, which uses a statistical technique to fit models to data and learn, and natural language processing, in which applications recognize speech and analyze text and then analyze and classify this language information (Davenport & Kalakota, 2019).

Various AI programs are being used for nurse and physician education focused on clinical simulation, communication skills, and administrative task automation. These AI programs offer AI-driven case-based scenarios with adaptive guidance for clinical reasoning and decision-making skill development, have real-time AI guidance to help clinicians with cardiac ultrasound imaging experience, and AI-enhanced virtual reality (VR) for immersive training in procedures like intubation or emergency medication administration.

AI-driven chatbots are emerging as versatile tools across health care settings, providing services such as patient education, symptom triage, appointment scheduling, chronic disease self-management, and mental-health support (Böhm et al., 2024). These conversational agents, powered by natural-language processing and machine learning, can engage patients 24/7, automate routine interactions, and help reduce provider workload while improving access and efficiency (Xu et al., 2024). However, despite promising findings, limitations remain which include concerns about accuracy, user trust, integration into clinical workflows, and safeguarding patient data privacy and ethical standards (Hindelang et al., 2022). As such, nurse leaders and healthcare organizations should consider chatbots as supplementary supports rather than replacements for clinician-led care, with careful attention to implementation, oversight, and continuous evaluation.

The adoption of AI in health care raises ethical concerns, especially around data privacy, consent, and potential biases in AI algorithms. It is essential for nurses to work closely with other healthcare providers, technology engineers, and policymakers to ensure that AI applications are used ethically and equitably, with a focus on an ultimate outcome of patient-centered care.

Robotics in Promoting Healthy Patient Outcomes

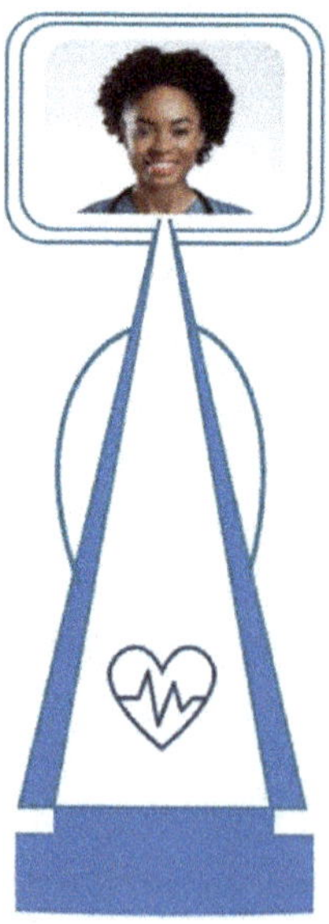

FIGURE 12.3 Example of a Telepresence Robot

Robotics has been significant in health care, particularly in enhancing patient care and outcomes (Maibaum et al., 2022). Surgical robots, such as the da Vinci Surgical System, have enabled minimally invasive surgeries, reducing recovery times, decreasing pain, and minimizing the risk of infections. In nursing, robots may assist in routine tasks, such as lifting patients for care activities and transferring patients from their bed to other modes of transportation. These robot-assisted activities can reduce the physical strain on nurses and reduce nurse injuries. Using robots for routine tasks assistance can also minimize patient injuries during these procedures (Sharkey & Sharkey, 2012).

Telepresence robots (see Figure 12.1) can promote interpersonal communication. Robots equipped with telepresence capabilities allow nurses to provide care remotely. For example, telepresence robots in a clinic can enable real-time interactions between patients and healthcare providers, facilitating monitoring, consultations, and patient education. This technology is particularly beneficial in rural and outlying areas where access to healthcare services is limited, ensuring that patients receive timely and high-quality care.

In addition to physical care, robots are being used to provide emotional support to patients, particularly the elderly, individuals with disabilities, and those with cognitive impairments (Goda et al., 2020). These service robotic companions which are specifically designed to be interactive and therapeutic in their interactions to reduce stress and anxiety in patients thereby promoting a better sense of well-being. These robots can provide companionship and cognitive stimulation, especially in long-term care settings, improving patients' overall mental health outcomes (Sawik et al., 2023; Wada et al., 2005).

Summary

Technology unfolds over time, allowing for improved access to patient information at the point of care and enhancing nurses' ability to benchmark, monitor, and audit quality measures. Effective implementation of technology in nursing care requires behavioral adaptations regarding patient care management. These adaptations allow the nursing profession to promote technological use in building a strong base of support for administering high-quality, safe, effective, patient-centered care. As technology continues to advance, nurses will further develop their proficiency in utilizing innovative tools to enhance the delivery of high-quality, safe, effective, and patient-centered care. With nursing informatics, a passion for nursing, and technological knowledge and skills, nurse can build a strong base of support to improve patient outcomes and experience high-quality patient-nurse interactions.

References

Adeniyi, A. O., Arowoogun, J. O., Chidi, R., Okolo, C. A., & Babawarun, O. (2024). The impact of electronic health records on patient care outcomes: A comprehensive review. *World Journal of Advanced Research and Reviews*, *21*(02), 1446–1455. https://doi.org/10.30574/wjarr.2024.21.2.0592

Alder, S. (2024, January 2). *HIPAA administrative safeguards*. HIPAA Journal. https://www.hipaajournal.com/hipaa-safeguards/

American Association of Colleges of Nursing. (2021, April 6). *The essentials: Core competencies for professional nursing education*. https://www.aacnnursing.org/Portals/0/PDFs/Publications/Essentials-2021.pdf

Aryankhesal, A., Aghighi, N., Raeissi, P., & Najafpour, Z. (2023). Recurrence of medical errors despite years of preventive measures: A grounded theory study. *Journal of Education and Health Promotion*, *12*, 329. https://doi.org/10.4103/jehp.jehp_17_23

Böhm, J., Smith, L., & Nguyen, T. (2024). Roles, users, benefits, and limitations of chatbots in health care. *Journal of Medical Internet Research, 26*, e56930. https://doi.org/10.2196/56930

Brennan, P. F., & Bakken, S. (2019). Nursing needs big data and big data needs nursing. *Journal of Nursing Scholarship, 47*(5), 477–484.

Davenport, T., & Kalakota, R. (2019). The potential for artificial intelligence in healthcare. *Future Healthcare Journal*, *6*(2), 94–98. https://doi.org/10.7861/futurehosp.6-2-94

Goda, A., Shimura, T., Murata, S., Kodama, T., Nakano, H., & Ohsugi, H. (2020). Psychological and neurophysiological effects of robot assisted activity in elderly people with cognitive decline. *Gerontology & Geriatric Medicine*, *6*. https://doi.org/10.1177/2333721420969601

Handler (2003, July 7). HIMSS Electronic Health Record definition model version 1.0. HIMSS The Source for Healthcare Information. https://www.researchgate.net/publication/247151484_HIMSS_electronic_health_record_definitional_model_version_10

Hindelang, M., Sitaru, S., & Zink, A. (2024). Transforming health care through Chatbots for medical history-taking and future directions: Comprehensive systematic review. *JMIR Medical Informatics*, *12*, e56628. https://doi.org/10.2196/56628

Hübner, U., Thye, J., Shaw, T., Elias, B., Egbert, N., Saranto, K., Babitsch, B., Procter, P., & Ball, M. J. (2019). Towards the TIGER International Framework for Recommendations of Core Competencies in Health Informatics 2.0: Extending the scope and the soles. *Studies in Health Technology and Informatics*, *264*, 1218–1222. https://doi.org/10.3233/SHTI190420

Institute of Medicine (U.S.) Committee on Quality of Health Care in America; Kohn, L. T., Corrigan, J. M., & Donaldson, M. S. (Eds.). (2000). *To err is human: Building a safer health system*. National Academies Press (U.S.).

Khezri, H., & Abdekhoda, M. (2019). Assessing nurses' informatics competency and identifying its related factors. *Journal of Research in Nursing*, *24*(7), 529–538. https://doi.org/10.1177/1744987119839453

Maibaum, A., Bischof, A., Hergesell, J., & Lipp, B. (2022). A critique of robotics in health care. *AI & Society*, *37*, 467–477. https://doi.org/10.1007/s00146-021-01206-z

Poon, E. G., Keohane, C. A., Yoon, C. S., Ditmore, M., Bane, A., Levtzion-Korach, O., & Gandhi, T. K. (2010). Effect of bar-code technology on the safety of medication administration. *New England Journal of Medicine*, *362*(18), 1698–1707. https://doi.org/10.1056/NEJMsa0907115

Sawik, B., Tobis, S., Baum, E., Suwalska, A., Kropińska, S., Stachnik, K., Pérez-Bernabeu, E., Cildoz, M., Agustin, A., & Wieczorowska-Tobis, K. (2023). Robots for elderly care: Review, multi-criteria optimization model and qualitative case study. *Healthcare (Basel, Switzerland)*, *11*(9), 1286. https://doi.org/10.3390/healthcare11091286

Sharkey, A., & Sharkey, N. (2012). Granny and the robots: Ethical issues in robot care for the elderly. *Ethics and Information Technology*, *14*(1), 27–40. https://doi.org/10.1007/s10676-010-9234-6

Staggers, N., Gassert, C. A., & Curran, C. (2001). Informatics competencies for nurses at four levels of practice. *Journal of Nursing Education*, *40*(7), 303–316. https://doi.org/10.3928/0148-4834-20011001-05

Technology Informatics Guiding Education Reform. (2020, April). *TIGER international competency synthesis project.* Health Information and Management Systems Society. https://gkc.himss.org/sites/hde/files/media/file/2021/01/29/tiger-icsp-recommendations.pdf

U.S. Department of Health and Human Services. (2007, March). *Security safeguards: Administrative safeguards*. https://www.hhs.gov/sites/default/files/ocr/privacy/hipaa/administrative/securityrule/adminsafeguards.pdf

Wada, K., Shibata, T., Musha, T., & Kimura, S. (2005). Effects of robot therapy for demented patients evaluated by EEG. *IEEE/RSJ International Conference on Intelligent Robots and Systems*, 1552–1557. https://doi.org/10.1109/IROS.2005.1545304

Image Credtis

Fig. 12.1a: Copyright © by Microsoft.
Fig. 12.1b: Copyright © by Microsoft.
Fig. 12.1c: Copyright © by Microsoft.
Fig. 12.2a: Copyright © by Microsoft.
Fig. 12.2b: Copyright © by Microsoft.
Fig. 12.2c: Copyright © by Microsoft.
Fig. 12.2d: Copyright © by Microsoft.
Fig. 12.2e: Copyright © by Microsoft.
Fig. 12.2f: Copyright © by Microsoft.
Fig. 12.2g: Copyright © by Microsoft.
Fig. 12.2h: Copyright © by Microsoft.
Fig. 12.3a: Generated using Adobe Firefly.

CHAPTER 13

Advocacy and Leadership

Martina Suttle Harris, EdD, RN, CNE, ANEF

Objectives

Upon completion of this chapter, the learner will be able to do the following:

1. Understand the role of advocacy in protecting patient rights, health, and safety.
2. Identify the role of nurses as formal and informal leaders who advocate for others, share knowledge, and promote quality care.
3. Recognize the need for resilience in leadership roles.
4. Explain critical skills needed for effective nursing leadership.

Key Chapter Terms

- Advocacy
- Leadership
- Resilience
- Culturally competent care
- Safe patient care environments
- Unsafe practices or policies
- Advocacy framework
- Formal leader
- Informal leader
- Leadership skills
- Effective communication
- Teamwork and collaboration
- Adaptability
- Professional growth
- Mentorship

Advocacy in Nursing and Its Significance

Advocacy is a fundamental aspect of nursing practice. Concepts related to advocacy include patient support, compassionate care, and empathy (Sanford, 2012).

Advocacy involves acting in the best interests of patients, ensuring that their voices are heard, and safeguarding their rights, health, and safety (Abbasinia et al., 2020). The nurse advocacy responsibility extends beyond direct patient care and includes influencing healthcare policies, addressing inequities, and fostering environments conducive to optimal health outcomes (Walker et al., 2015, Water et al., 2016). Advocacy is rooted in ethical principles such as autonomy, beneficence, and justice, reflecting nurses' commitment to upholding patient dignity and promoting well-being. Historically, individuals such as Florence Nightingale demonstrated the transformative power of nursing advocacy. She and others challenged systemic barriers, which served to advance public health initiatives and improve patient care.

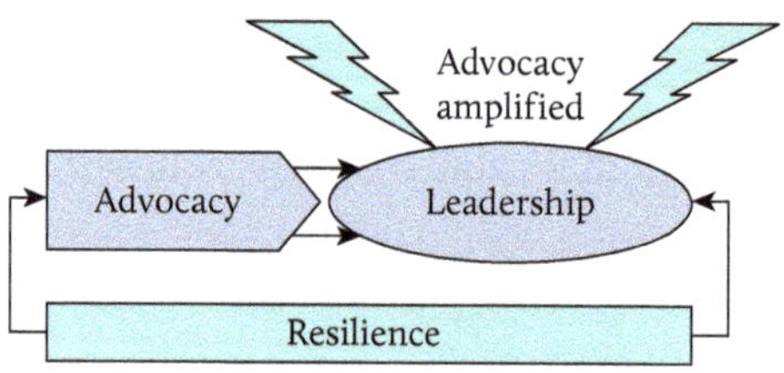

FIGURE 13.1 Interconnectedness of Advocacy, Leadership, and Resilience

Advocacy, **leadership**, and **resilience** are interconnected elements of nursing (see Figure 13.1). Advocacy drives leadership by compelling nurses to take initiative, guide teams, and influence systems to address patient and community needs. Leadership amplifies advocacy efforts, equipping nurses with the authority and skills to effect change. Resilience underpins both advocacy and leadership as it enables nurses to navigate emotional and physical challenges of their multiple roles. Combined, these components empower nurses to champion patient care, lead transformative initiatives, and sustain their professional growth amid healthcare complexities.

In today's healthcare environment, advocacy and leadership are even more critical. Nurses face complex challenges, which include health disparities and technological advances that necessitate ethical decisions while maintaining resilience in the face of these highly stressful situations. By maintaining a strong foundation of advocacy and leadership skills, nurses can improve patient outcomes while shaping the future of health care.

Advocacy and Its Historical Perspective in Nursing

According to the American Nurses Association (ANA, n.d.), advocacy is a pillar of nursing. "Advocacy means leveraging one's position to support, protect, or speak out for the rights and interests of others" (Haebler & Fitting, 2018). Advocacy in nursing is the active pursuit of ensuring that patients' rights, needs, and preferences are respected and prioritized within the healthcare system. This means that nurses represent patients who may be vulnerable, voiceless, or unable to navigate the complex medical environment without assistance. Advocacy also extends beyond patients to systemic issues, which include inequities in access to care or inadequate policies that affect patient outcomes. Central to this concept is nurses' role as a liaison, educator, and protector. These roles ensure that care decisions align with the best interests and informed choices of patients or representatives who know patients' wishes. Advocacy reflects the ethical principles of beneficence, autonomy, and justice. It is foundational to the delivery of compassionate and patient-centered care.

Nursing Advocacy: Historical Perspective

The roots of nursing advocacy can be traced back to the profession's earliest foundations, with Nightingale serving as its pioneer. While Nightingale never used the word *advocacy*, her actions demonstrated this concept. During the 19th century, Nightingale championed public health reforms that improved sanitation and reduced mortality rates. Her actions redefined patient care practices. During the Crimean War, she tirelessly advocated for better conditions for wounded soldiers, demonstrating how nursing could influence broader societal change. Nightingale's legacy set the standard for nurses as advocates. This laid the foundation for the nursing profession to embrace a commitment to safeguarding patients' health and rights.

The rise in advocacy occurred in Western society and culture in the 1960s to 1970s. These changes mirrored the women's and civil rights movements. The critical review of the power relations that suppressed women and minority groups had a significant impact on nursing as a profession since nursing was—and still is—a predominantly female profession. At this time, the rise in consumerism placed emphasis on consumer choice, including those related to health care. These cultural shifts, which occurred in the second half of the 20th century, placed an increased emphasis on individual autonomy and self-determination.

Healthcare system evolution expanded the scope of advocacy in the nursing profession. In the mid-20th century, advocacy expanded to include addressing disparities in healthcare access, especially for marginalized populations. Nurses have become instrumental in civil rights and public health movements, advocating for policies to reduce inequities and improve overall community health outcomes. The first formal code of ethics for nurses was formalized in 1950 through the ANA. This validated advocacy as an obligation of all nurses to incorporate as part of their patient management. The code continues to require the nurse to use advocacy efforts to improve patient safety, influence health policy, and promote health equity (Epstein & Turner, 2015).

Nursing Advocacy: Today

Advocacy is a vital aspect of the nursing profession. It is secure in the trust that patients have for nurses. In this way, nurses can influence not only individual patient care but also care delivered in their communities, states, and the nation overall. Nurses are a powerful profession due to their numbers. According to the National Center for Health Workforce Analysis (2024), as of 2022, there were more than 4 million registered nurses, licensed practical nurses, and advanced practice nurses. There is strength in these numbers that can be used for advocacy efforts at all levels (Hewitt & Champlin, 2024).

Advocacy requires the nurse to ever-changing technology components in health care. This is required in order to address not only current challenges such as technological advancements but also those related to complex healthcare delivery models and population health issues. Nurses today advocate for not only individual patients but also for communities and the profession itself, striving to ensure that healthcare systems are equitable and sustainable. The advocacy role intersects with leadership, as nurses increasingly take on influential management roles that promote the shaping of policies and practices that enhance patient care. By drawing on its rich historical foundations, nursing advocacy continues to be a powerful force for improving health outcomes and advancing the profession.

The Role of Advocacy in Ensuring Culturally Competent Care

Advocacy is vital in promoting **culturally competent care** which is essential for providing care for individuals from different cultural backgrounds (Červený et al., 2022). According to Cross et al. (1989), "cultural and linguistic competence is a set of congruent behaviors, attitudes, and policies that come together in a system, agency, or among professionals that enables effective work in cross-cultural situations." Culture involves the integration of human behavior patterns that include "language, thoughts, communications, actions, customs, beliefs, values, and institutions of racial, ethnic, religious, or social groups" (Cross et al., 1989). Competence involves the ability to understand and effectively function in the context of others regardless of their cultural beliefs, behaviors, or needs. Cultural competence requires nurses to respect the diverse cultural, religious, and social backgrounds of patients (Breier-Mackie, 2007).

Nurses act as advocates by addressing cultural barriers that may hinder effective communication or treatment. This might involve seeking an interpreter for a patient with limited or no English proficiency, facilitating accommodations for a patient's dietary restrictions due to religious practices, or tailoring health education activities to align with cultural norms. Advocacy also includes challenging biases within the healthcare system and advocating for policies that promote inclusivity and equity in care delivery.

Ensuring culturally competent care extends beyond individual patient interactions. It encompasses systemic change. Systemic changes require addressing the root in an overall system, as the U.S. healthcare system is made up of several layers. These layers include healthcare providers, insurance companies, pharmaceutical companies, technology companies, and many others that collaborate to provide quality patient care. For the nursing profession to effectively change the landscape of culturally competent care, it will take interprofessional collaboration to design and implement solutions.

Nurses advocate for the inclusion of cultural competence training in healthcare education and the development of policies that address disparities in patient access and outcomes. By fostering an inclusive environment that respects diverse needs, nurses contribute to a healthcare system that is equitable and responsive to the populations whom it serves. Advocacy for culturally competent care is not only an ethical obligation but also a practical strategy to enhance the quality of care and build trust within diverse communities.

Advocacy Promotes Safe Patient Care Environments

Advocacy plays a crucial role in promoting **safe patient care environments** for patients, where they can receive quality care that is free from harm. Nurses are patient advocates. In this advocacy role, they are uniquely positioned to identify potential risks, implement preventive measures, and raise concerns about unsafe practices. This includes advocating for (a) access to the necessary resources to ensure quality delivery of patient care, (b) adherence to evidence-based safety protocols, and (c) adequate staffing levels based on patient numbers and the degree of care requirements. Creating a safe care environment also extends to care providers. It involves fostering a culture of transparency and accountability for healthcare provider team members in which they feel empowered to report errors or near-misses without fear of retribution or retaliation. By advocating for patient safety, nurses uphold the ethical principle of nonmaleficence, ensuring that care processes prioritize patient well-being.

Addressing Unsafe Practices or Policies

A key aspect of nursing advocacy is addressing **unsafe practices or policies**. As nurses are front-line providers, they are in a strategic position to identify and address real and potential error situations. For instance, a nurse might notice the improper use of a specific piece of medical equipment or an outdated infection control policy and procedure based on current evidence. It is important that they report concerns to the appropriate authorities for them to be addressed. Another example could involve advocating for policies that promote proper staffing ratios in order to prevent comprising patient safety and reduce the likelihood of errors. Nurses may also participate in initiatives to reduce medication errors, such as implementing barcode scanning systems, revising protocols for high-alert medications, promoting proper medication reconciliation, or using a system to reduce distractions and interruptions during medication administration. By actively identifying and correcting such issues, nurses contribute to safer healthcare environments and, ultimately, better patient outcomes.

The Impact of Healthcare Policies on Advocacy Efforts

Even though there are policies that affect advocacy implementation, nurse leaders play a crucial role in advocating for patients by ensuring their safety, autonomy, and access to quality care. A structured **advocacy framework** includes several key components (see Figure 13.2). First, nurse leaders prioritize patient safety by implementing evidence-based practices, reducing risks, and fostering a culture of accountability in healthcare settings. They also uphold patient autonomy, ensuring that individuals have the right to make informed decisions about their care while respecting their values and preferences. Additionally, nurse leaders promote care policies that enhance healthcare delivery, advocating for ethical and effective standards that benefit both patients and healthcare providers. Finally, they act on patients' behalf, speaking up for those who may be vulnerable or unable to advocate for themselves. Through this comprehensive approach, nurse leaders strengthen patient-centered care and contribute to a more ethical, safer, and more effective healthcare system while working within policy structures. Nurses work within these structures to ensure advocacy for patients.

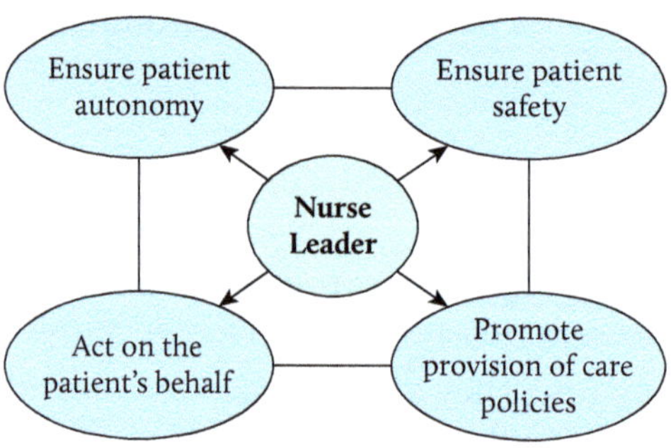

FIGURE 13.2 An Advocacy Framework for Nursing

Policies that prioritize patient safety play a crucial role in enabling nurses to advocate effectively for their patients. Regulations such as mandated safe staffing ratios and the promotion of electronic health records help create safer environments, improve communication, and enhance patient outcomes. When nurses have policies that support safe work environments and adequate resources, they can focus on providing high-quality care, reducing errors, and ensuring patient-centered decision-making. However, when policies fail to address critical issues such as workload management or patient safety protocols, nurses may struggle to uphold advocacy efforts. Ensuring that healthcare policies align with best practices is essential for empowering nurses to fulfill their professional and ethical responsibilities.

On the other hand, restrictive policies can hinder advocacy efforts by creating barriers that limit nurses' ability to provide optimal care. Policies that reduce funding for healthcare organizations at the state or federal level may lead to outdated medical equipment, inadequate training opportunities, or a lack of continuing education for nurses. Excessive administrative burdens, such as extensive documentation requirements or bureaucratic hurdles, can distract nurses and move their attention away from direct patient care. These challenges force nurses to balance competing priorities, potentially compromising patient safety and quality of care. Therefore, advocacy in nursing extends beyond implementing policies. It also involves actively influencing policy changes to address systemic challenges, secure necessary resources, and improve working conditions. By engaging in policy reform and speaking out on behalf of their patients and profession, nurses can drive meaningful improvements in healthcare delivery.

Formal and Informal Nurse Leaders

In leadership, nurses can be **formal leaders** or **informal leaders**. Both roles are essential components that shape healthcare teams and influence patient outcomes. *Formal nursing leadership* refers to roles specifically designated within the organizational hierarchy, such as nurse managers, charge nurses, or directors of nursing. These leaders have specific responsibilities, such as staffing, policy implementation, budget management, and ensuring compliance with healthcare regulations. Formal leaders are accountable for maintaining organizational standards and fostering a work environment that supports professional development and high-quality patient care. Their authority is derived from their position. They are expected to provide guidance, resolve conflicts, advocate for others, and move the team toward achieving strategic organizational goals.

In contrast, informal nursing leadership emerges organically. The position of these leaders does not come from an organizational title or formal authority given by the organization but rather from the respect and influence they command within a team. Informal leaders are often experienced, highly skilled nurses who inspire confidence, model professional behavior, and provide mentorship and advocacy. They can play a critical role in shaping the culture of a nursing team by promoting collaboration, offering emotional support, and fostering a positive work environment. Informal leaders often act as intermediaries, bridging communication gaps between peers and formal leaders. Their ability to influence without official authority makes them key people in driving change, improving morale, and encouraging adherence to best practices.

Both formal and informal nursing leadership roles are vital for the effective functioning of a healthcare team and the promotion of advocacy. Formal leaders set the framework for policies, accountability, and resource allocation, while informal leaders reinforce these efforts through interpersonal influence and peer support. Both roles work together to enhance team effectiveness and ensure that objectives are met to improve patient care.

Resilience in Nursing Leadership

Resilience in nursing is the ability to cope despite adverse circumstances. In this way, nurses can adapt and recover from difficult challenges, stress, and adversity while maintaining a high standard of care and professionalism (Henshall et al., 2020). Resilience is applicable to all nurses but specifically needed by nurse leaders. Characteristics of resilience include physiological as well as psychological aspects, such as emotional regulation, self-awareness, adaptability, problem-solving skills, and a strong sense of purpose. Resilient nurses demonstrate the capacity to maintain a sense of calmness under pressure, keep the focus on patient needs, and find constructive solutions to problems and adverse situations. In leadership roles, resilience is particularly important because leaders often face complex demands, such as managing team conflicts, navigating organizational changes, and addressing critical situations. Resilience enables nurse leaders to effectively manage stress, inspire their teams, and create a supportive work environment. By modeling resilience, leaders can foster a culture of strength and adaptability, encouraging their teams to thrive despite challenges, maintain optimal performance, and deliver high-quality care.

Critical Skills for Effective Nursing Leadership

Critical **leadership skills** include communication, decision-making, teamwork, adaptability, and emotional intelligence. These form the foundation of effective nursing leadership. These skills affect the overall work environment for an organization. A leader who excels in these areas can inspire confidence, drive innovation, and create a supportive work environment that prioritizes both patient safety and staff well-being.

Communication Skills

Effective communication is at the heart of successful nursing leadership. Nurse leaders must clearly convey treatment plans to staff, patients, and families as well as medical information to interdisciplinary healthcare team members. Leaders must be able to deliver clear information clearly displaying empathy and assertiveness in order to promote understanding and trust team members, patients, and families. This communication is important for team efficiency. The use of active listening by leaders ensures that all voices are heard and valued. It also allows for any necessary information clarification that might be needed to address diverse audiences of individuals.

Leaders need strong written communication skills as well. This is necessary to ensure accuracy in written documents, policies, and reports. Miscommunication can lead to errors or conflicts. Clear and consistent communication provides proper team guidance to maintain patient safety.

Decision-Making and Critical Thinking

Nurses in leadership roles are frequently faced with complex situations that demand sound decision-making. This decision-making must use critical thinking and be supported with evidence. Leaders must assess multiple situational components, which can include patient needs, resource availability, and organizational goals, to make informed decisions. Nurse leaders can use the nursing process and evidence-based practice models to help them analyze situations, identify options, decide on a solution among these options, and implement the effective solution. By using decision-making and critical thinking, nurse leaders can effectively address organization-based challenges and ethical dilemmas that are aligned with evidence and best practices.

Teamwork and Collaboration

It is important that nurse leaders be able to build and lead a cohesive team. In order to enhance **teamwork and collaboration**, leaders must foster an environment of mutual respect, trust, and shared accountability. They must be able to recognize individual team member strengths, mediate conflicts and know when to elevate them to another level, and promote interdisciplinary cooperation to achieve the best patient outcome. Collaborative leadership is important in healthcare settings, where diverse professionals must work together to deliver comprehensive patient care. By supporting inclusiveness and shared decision-making, leaders can strengthen working teams and improve patient outcomes.

Adaptability and Emotional Intelligence

Adaptability enables nursing leaders to navigate the rapid healthcare changes occurring at record speed. Whether responding to technological advancements; policy updates; or unforeseen local, national, or worldwide crises; leaders must remain flexible and open to change. Leaders who display emotional intelligence (EI) have the ability to monitor the feelings of themselves and others, discriminate among them, and use this information to guide their thinking and actions (Prezerakos, 2018). This enhances leaders' ability to be self-aware. This self-awareness allows leaders to manage their feelings in a way that benefits themselves and others while supporting their team through current challenges. Adaptability and EI allow leaders to build resilience, maintain morale, and ensure organizational advancement through challenging times.

Promoting Professional Growth for Self and Others

Professional growth through lifelong learning is key to the success of all, but especially nurse leaders. Leaders promote self-growth through continued education, self-reflection, networking, EI work (self-awareness, empathy, and stress management), and time management. Leaders not only focus on self-growth but also promote elevating the skills and knowledge levels of others. They achieve this by encouraging professional development, providing constructive feedback, fostering a learning environment, empowering team member decision-making, recognizing and rewarding growth, promoting work-life balance, and creating leadership opportunities for team members. Promoting the professional development of others can be accomplished through mentorship. This allows leaders to transfer knowledge and enhance others' leadership skills in preparation for this role in the future (Rosser et al., 2023).

Mentorship

Mentorship is a vital component of effective nursing leadership. It fosters professional development and creates a supportive environment for both novice and experienced nurses. Leaders who serve as mentors guide others by sharing their knowledge, skills, and experiences. This helps mentees navigate challenges and develop confidence. Mentorship promotes the transfer of institutional knowledge, enhances clinical competence, and strengthens

TABLE 13.1 Benefits of Mentoring

Benefits of mentoring for the mentee	• Improves job effectiveness and career satisfaction • Receives support from a designated role model • Promotes ongoing support, direction, and advice while moving into a role • Facilitates refinement of problem-solving skills • Expands one's professional network • Facilitates identification of career opportunities • Reduces role-related anxiety and stress
Benefits of mentoring for the mentor	• Promotes career development of self • Allows one to learn and understand potential generational differences • Encourages retrieval of current research evidence in order to teach up-to-date practices and policies • Contributes to a positive work environment • Improved leadership, empathy, and active-listening skills • Promotes the expansion of effective communication skills in various teaching/learning situations

leadership pipelines. There is value in mentorship and often gains for both the mentor and mentee (see Table 13.1).

Through maintaining open communication, offering constructive feedback, fostering accountability, and celebrating achievements, mentors inspire growth and empower mentees. This allows mentees to increase their skill level and accept more complex patient care responsibilities while building their confidence. This improves their ability to deliver high-quality patient care.

Professional Growth

Professional growth is a continuous process that nurse leaders must prioritize for self-growth and the growth of their team members. Leaders encourage growth and promote lifelong learning by encouraging the retrieval and use of online evidence-based information as well as organization-based educational programs. This promotes skill development, improves knowledge, and supports nurses who may be pursuing advanced certifications or degrees. Cultivating leadership qualities in others, such as strategic thinking, advocacy, and innovation, is also part of professional leader growth. Fostering education-based activities enhances self-improvement of others, which strengthens the overall team's capacity to provide high-quality, patient-centered care. Through professional growth, nurses are prepared to meet evolving healthcare demands and take future leadership roles.

Summary

Advocacy and leadership are vital to the nursing profession. By protecting patient rights, sharing knowledge, and demonstrating resilience, nurses drive meaningful change. Advocacy and leadership are cornerstones of nursing practice. Nurses serve as their patients' voice, ensuring that their rights, health, and safety are prioritized in all care aspects. Nurses embody leadership, whether formally as managers or informally through everyday actions that inspire and guide others. Resilience plays a crucial role in navigating the challenges of leadership, while critical skills such as communication, teamwork, and decision-making are indispensable. Through the continual development of leadership competencies, nurses can rise to the challenges of modern healthcare, fostering an organizational culture that values excellence, collaboration, and continuous improvement. Embracing leadership roles enables nurses to influence healthcare systems and improve patient outcomes. As the healthcare landscape continues to evolve, the need for strong nursing leaders will continue to increase.

References

Abbasinia, M., Ahmadi, F., & Kazemnejad, A. (2020). Patient advocacy in nursing: A concept analysis. *Nursing Ethics, 27*(1), 141–151. https://doi.org/10.1177/0969733019832950

American Nurses Association (ANA). (n.d.). Federal advocacy. https://www.nursingworld.org/practice-policy/advocacy/

Breier-Mackie, S. (2007). Cultural competence and patient advocacy: The new challenge for nurses. *Gastroenterology Nursing, 30*(2), 120–122. https://doi.org/10.1097/01.SGA.0000267933.36748.e4

Cross, T., Bazron, B., Dennis, K., & Isaacs, M., (1989). *Towards A Culturally Competent System of Care, Volume I.* Washington, DC: Georgetown University Child Development Center, CASSP Technical Assistance Center.

Červený, M., Kratochvílová, I., Hellerová, V., & Tóthová, V. (2022). Methods of increasing cultural competence in nurses working in clinical practice: A scoping review of literature 2011-2021. *Frontiers in Psychology, 13*, 936181. https://doi.org/10.3389/fpsyg.2022.936181

Epstein, B., & Turner, M. (2015). The nursing code of ethics: Its value, its history. *Online Journal of Issues in Nursing, 20*(4), 4. https://doi.org/10.3912/OJIN.Vol20No02Man04

Haebler, J., & Fitting, M. (2018, January 11). *Advocacy at the bedside and beyond.* American Nurses Association. https://www.myamericannurse.com/advocacy-bedside-beyond/

Henshall, C., Davey, Z., & Jackson, D. (2020). Nursing resilience interventions—A way forward in challenging healthcare territories. *Journal of Clinical Nursing, 29*(19–20), 3597–3599. https://doi.org/10.1111/jocn.15276

Hewitt, S., & Champlin, E. (2024). *Elevating the voice of nurses through advocacy.* American Nurse. https://www.myamericannurse.com/elevating-the-voice-of-nurses-through-advocacy/

National Center for Health Workforce Analysis. (2024, May). *State of the U.S. health care workforce, 2023.* https://bhw.hrsa.gov/sites/default/files/bureau-health-workforce/data-research/state-of-the-health-workforce-report-2023.pdf

Prezerakos, P. E. (2018). Nurse managers' emotional intelligence and effective leadership: A review of the current evidence. *Open Nursing Journal, 12*, 86–92. https://doi.org/10.2174/1874434601812010086

Rosser, E. A., Edwards, S., Kwan, R. Y. C., Ito, M., Potter, D. R., Hodges, K. T., & Buckner, E. (2023). The Global Leadership Mentoring Community: An evaluation of its impact on nursing leadership. *International Nursing Review, 70*(3), 279–285. https://doi.org/10.1111/inr.12860

Sanford, K. (2012, January 31). Overview and summary: Nurse advocates: Past, present, and future. *Online Journal of Issues in Nursing, 17*(1). https://doi.org/10.3912/OJIN.Vol17No01ManOS

Walker, D. K., Barton-Burke, M., Saria, M. G., Gosselin, T., Ireland, A., Norton, V., & Newton, S. (2015). Everyday advocates: Nursing advocacy is a full-time job. *The American Journal of Nursing, 115*(8), 66–70. https://doi.org/10.1097/01.NAJ.0000470409.04919.of

Water, T., Ford, K., Spence, D., & Rasmussen, S. (2016). Patient advocacy by nurses—past, present and future. *Contemporary Nurse, 52*(6), 696–709. https://doi.org/10.1080/10376178.2016.1235981

CHAPTER 14

Nursing Education

The Path to a Nursing Career

Objectives

Upon completion of this chapter, the learner will be able to do the following:

1. Identify various educational programs that lead to entry into the nursing profession.
2. Differentiate between various nursing-level competencies.
3. Explain the intent and overall goal of the Quality and Safety Education for Nurses (QSEN) project in addressing nurse knowledge, skills, and attitudes (KSAs) necessary to improve patient care quality and safety.
4. Explain the three landmark reports that influence nursing's past and future.

Key Chapter Terms

- *Assessing Progress on the Institute of Medicine Report* The Future of Nursing (2016)
- Prelicensure education
- Licensed Practical Nurse (LPN)
- Registered nurse (RN)
- Diploma nursing
- Associate degree program
- Baccalaureate degree program
- Graduate programs
- Advanced practice nurse (APN)
- Master of Science in Nursing (MSN)
- Doctor of Philosophy (PhD)
- Doctor of Nursing Practice (DNP)
- Quality and Safety Education for Nurses (QSEN)
- Patient-centered care
- Teamwork and collaboration
- Evidence-based practice
- Quality improvement (QI)
- Safety

- Informatics
- The Institute of Medicine's (IOM) *The Future of Nursing: Leading Change, Advancing Health* (2011)
- The National Academy of Medicine (NAM) et al.'s *The Future of Nursing 2020–2030: Charting a Path to Achieve Health Equity* (2021)

Nursing Education: The Path to a Nursing Career

In order to achieve the goal of becoming a nurse, one must select a route and educational delivery that supports their ability to learn information and fit within their overall personal life situation. The educational process of nurses can take many routes. Even after successfully completing a basic education, nurses must be licensed in order to administer care. This two-step process—education and licensure—are an introduction to the lifelong process of learning that nurses undertake.

Nursing's Educational Pathways

One may enter the nursing profession in one of four ways. These include a **licensed practical nurse** program, diploma program, an **associate degree program**, or a baccalaureate degree program. All programs offer theoretical and clinical components. These programs are different in their basic educational preparation, which includes length of the program and number and type of courses offered, affecting the cost of each program type. Upon successful completion of a basic education, new graduates are eligible to take the National Council Licensure Examination for Practical Nurses (NCLEX-PN) or the National Council Licensure Examination for Registered Nurses (NCLEX-RN) in their state of choice, as all states have the ability to offer these examinations. When successful, graduates can legally use the credential LPN or RN and practice as nurses in the healthcare setting of their choice.

The route for **prelicensure education** from student to nurse can be achieved by one of three different routes (see Figure 14.1). It is not uncommon that nurses prepared through all educational routes work within an organization to deliver care. This can be confusing for many individuals receiving health care from these nurses as they may work side by side in the healthcare delivery system.

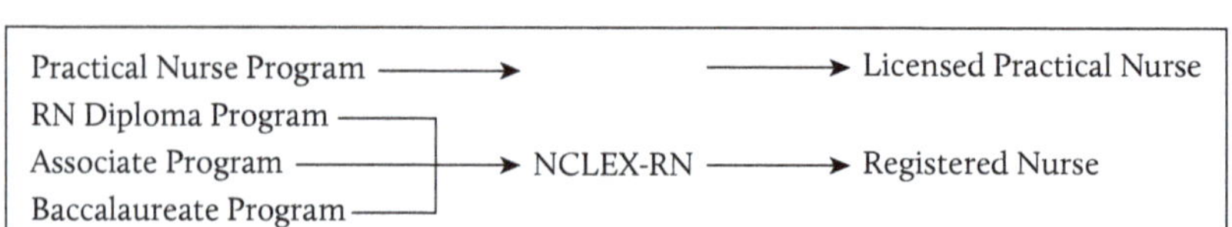

FIGURE 14.1 Educational Route for Nurses

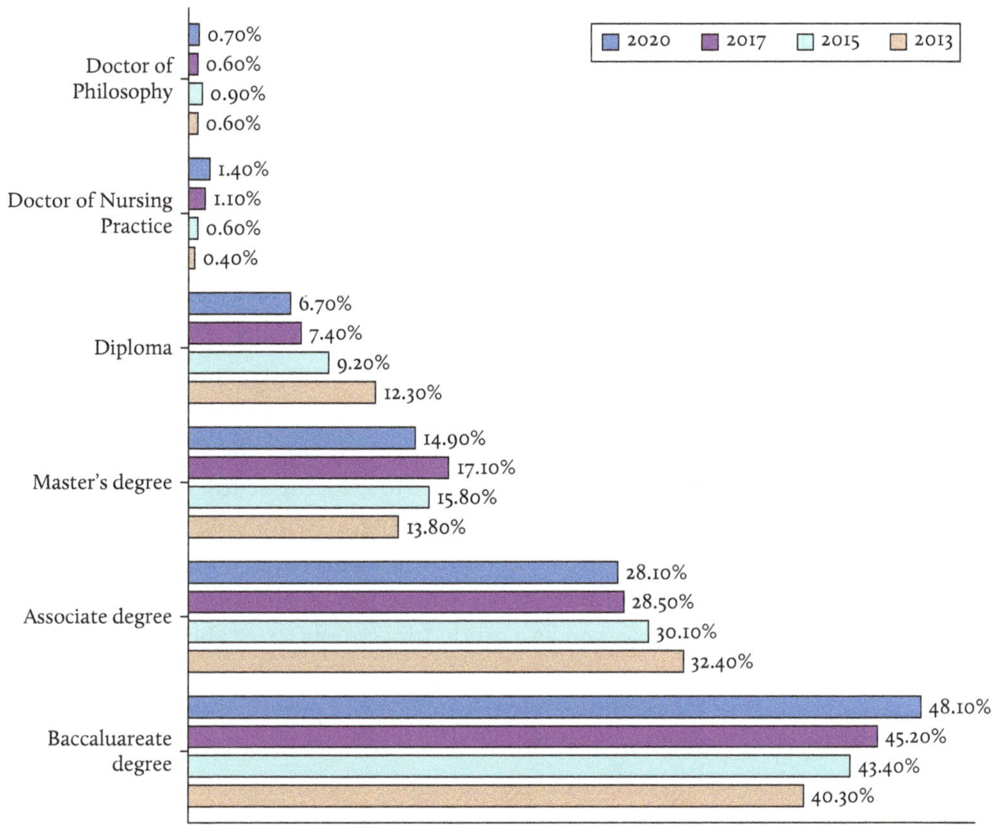

FIGURE 14.2 Nursing Education Statistics

The most common route for entering the nursing profession reported in 2022 was the bachelor's degree, with nearly 2.0 million RNs (45.4% of the workforce) indicating that they entered the workforce with this degree. More nurses reported having this degree as their highest obtained degree in the profession as of 2022 (see Figure 14.2).

From 2015 to 2022, the number of nurses with both baccalaureate and master's degrees increased. Nurses reporting a baccalaureate degree increased 7.7%, and those reporting a master's degree increased 2.1% between 2015 and 2022. The number of graduates prepared at the diploma level has declined since 2015.

Some educational programs have evolved that prepare nurses at higher levels. These programs promote completion of education with educational termination at the master's or doctoral level (e.g., Associate Degree in Nursing [ADN] to MSN or Bachelor of Science in Nursing to DNP). Some MSN programs cater to individuals with non-nursing bachelor's degrees. They allow individuals with a background outside of nursing to transition into the nursing field and obtain a master's degree. These programs may be promoted for individuals with some previous educational experience or degree. They allow entry at an advanced level into the academic process, and upon completion of a designated program of study, the individual can exit the higher educational institution with a master's or doctoral degree in nursing.

Licensed Practical Nurse Programs

The concept of practical nursing began in the late 19th century in the United States. In 1892, the Young Women's Christian Association (YWCA) in New York City established the Ballard School, which was the first formal training for practical nurses. The school offered a three-month training program. This program emphasized home care and focused on essential skills such as personal hygiene, nutrition, and sanitation. By 1917, the National League of Nursing Education (NLNE; now the National League for Nursing) began emphasizing a structured role for nurse training, although the focus remained on RNs. The NLNE published *Standard Curriculum for Schools of Nursing.* It was written by the Committee on Education, which was chaired by M. Adelaide Nutting. This served as a guide for schools to establish training for the nursing profession.

The name of the first school of training for the practical nurse was established in 1892 in Brooklyn, New York. It was the Bellevue Hospital School of Nursing and was founded as a training center for nurses to provide practical care for patients. The school played a crucial role in the development of nursing education and the professionalization of nursing in the United States.

The Great Depression of the 1930s placed a significant strain on the healthcare system. This need soared during World War II, which led to the establishment of wartime training programs for nurses. The U.S. army and other organizations created training programs for nurses and quickly developed the Cadet Nurse Corps in 1943. This provided training for both **LPN** graduates and RNs to meet wartime nursing needs.

Many LPN programs can be found at vocational and community colleges and may be 12 to 18 months in length. These programs can be accredited by the Accreditation Commission for Education in Nursing (ACEN). As of 2024, on the ACEN website, there were 256 accredited practical nursing programs in the United States. It is important to attend an accredited program in order to sit for the NCLEX-PN examination.

LPNs' role has evolved over the years due to the aging U.S. population and has required more long-term and chronic care services. The role may vary by state, with some allowing activities and others restricting them (e.g., drawing blood from a vein). It is important for LPNs to know their scope of practice laws in the state where they practice. LPN work settings include hospitals (acute, psychiatric, and substance abuse), rehabilitation centers, extended

TABLE 14.1 Projected Supply and Demand for LPNs

Projections	2027	2032	2037
Supply	592, 960	570,780	545, 870
Demand	739,670	795,750	848,310
Percentage adequacy	80%	72%	64%

Source: HRSA, 2024

care facilities or nursing homes, home care agencies, medical offices or urgent care clinics, and school settings. According to U.S. Bureau of Labor Statistics (2024), 12.42% of LPNs are employed in nursing care facilities, with the second highest percentage (4.88%) working in home care agencies. According to the Health Resources and Services Administration (2022), the demand for LPNs is projected to increase between 2020 and 2035. This projection identifies that the number educated will not meet 100% of the workforce demands.

LPNs have a long and evolving history in the United States, which, through their adaptability, has served to assist in meeting the demands of an ever-changing healthcare system throughout economic shifts, wars, and a changing population. They remain a significant component in the workforce in long-term care, home care, and outpatient care settings.

RN Diploma Programs

Diploma nursing or hospital-based programs in nursing were the first U.S. programs for nurses. These appeared in the late 1800s and transitioned from the Nightingale School in 1860 in England. These schools spread quickly and grew to approximately 2,000 by 1930. Programs used the fundamental hospital as a training laboratory, and this allowed these organizations to reduce labor costs for nursing staff. These programs had some classroom learning activities, but most were delivered in an apprenticeship format. Classroom and clinical activities were often combined in a 24-hour day, with minimal time for rest and relaxation. Courses were offered in areas of nursing currently used, as these correlated to the medical model that was familiar to many hospitals. Obstetrics, pediatrics, and surgery were among courses offered over the three-year study period. This allowed the hospital to have students deliver care throughout the 24-hour period, seven days a week. Nurse graduates were awarded a diploma upon successful completion of the program, since these schools could not grant academic credit for a degree.

Following transition from a hospital-based program to an academic setting, the numbers of diploma programs significantly declined in the mid-1960s. These numbers continued to decrease through 2024 (ACEN, 2024). This decline was in part due to the growth of associate and baccalaureate programs, and some diploma programs were actually phased into these programs. Changes in healthcare financing and fiscal reductions for organizational education also caused the closure of some programs. Program requirements also changed with the transition to academia. State requirements for operating schools of nursing were required to be met in order to prepare students for success on the state licensure examination.

Nurses who graduated from these one- to two-year **RN diploma programs** were at a disadvantage when they desired to continue their nursing education. Hospital-based courses were not offered by an organization that was part of the higher education system. In an effort to expand opportunities for diploma graduates, some programs developed articulation agreements with universities and colleges. Alignment with these programs of higher education promoted transition to associate or baccalaureate degree programs, with some academic credit toward degree completion upon successful completion of the diploma program.

Many diploma programs are now accredited by the ACEN. As of 2024, on the ACEN website, there were 27 accredited diploma nursing programs, mainly in the Northeastern United States. It is important to attend an accredited program in order to sit for the NCLEX-RN examination. Accreditation validates that programs meet standards for the following:

1. **Administrative capacity and resources:** The nursing program mission and/or philosophy reflects the mission, goals, and/or values of the governing organization, and there is administrative capacity and sufficient resources to support program delivery and achievement of student end-of-program learning outcomes.
2. **Faculty:** Staff are educationally qualified and experienced for their assigned roles and responsibilities and maintain expertise, which is annually evaluated to verify their ability to support student end-of-program learning outcomes.
3. **Students:** Policies and services for students support the achievement of end-of-program learning outcomes.
4. **Curriculum:** The curriculum used supports students' achievement of end-of-program learning outcomes and is consistent with safe practice in healthcare environments.
5. **Outcomes:** Assessment demonstrates the extent of student learning at or near the end of their program of study as well as outcome achievement using a systematic plan for evaluation.

Diploma nursing evolved from an apprenticeship-based program to a profession with rigorous educational standards. These programs laid the groundwork for nursing as both a science and an art. Nursing has moved more towards degree-based programs, but the clinical skills and work ethics fostered by diploma programs remain central to nursing's identity.

Associate Degree Programs

ADNs arose out of a need to produce nurses faster than over a four-year time span. This increased need resulted from healthcare innovations in surgery, the discovery of antibiotics, and the Hill-Burton Act of 1946, which funded construction of new hospitals in communities nationwide. Four-year nursing programs could not meet the need for nurses, so in the early 1950s, a two-year ADN was developed to provide technically skilled nurses and address the immediate nurse need. Enrollment in ADN educational programs was accelerated in 1964 with the Nurse Training Act.

The educational development of ADN programs was a direct result of a model for education developed by Mildred Montag (Harker, 2017). The Montag model identified bedside nurses who were dedicated to performing nursing functions without administrative responsibilities. The functions of these nurses focused on:

1. Assisting with planning nursing care activities
2. Giving supervised general nursing
3. Assisting in evaluation of nursing care activities

ADN graduates have instruction with prerequisites and co-requisites inclusive of clinical requirements. The initial education model proposed by Montag focused on such topics as fundamentals, maternal care, pediatrics, physical and mental illness, and medical-surgical nursing. As expectations for ADN graduates increased in the work setting, educational programs modified their curriculum to include such components as management and team leader roles. These courses are outside the original model proposed by Montag. As a result of educational curriculum changes and modifications, some programs of study expanded beyond two years. These changes added up to a year of additional education to some programs. These programs now graduate nurses who are difficult to differentiate within an organizational structure from baccalaureate graduates in function and employment setting. Many ADN nurses work alongside baccalaureate degree nurses as peers. Some even assume charge or head nurse positions in healthcare organizations.

The Health Resources and Services Administration's National Sample Survey of Registered Nurses (2022) identified that the number of nurses educated at the ADN level (1,921,377; 44%) dropped below the number of nurses educated at the BSN degree (1,976,426; 45%). Some rationales for this increase in BSN degree graduates are as a result of nurses moving into organizations that seek to obtain or maintain Magnet status, where nurses educated at the BSN level are preferred; a desire for individuals to move into higher-level organizational administrative positions; and individuals seeking to move into graduate education. A comparison of ADN curriculum outcomes with the *AACN Baccalaureate Essentials* revealed that 38.5% (42 of 109) of the *Baccalaureate Essentials for Professional Nursing Practice* outcomes were met within ACEN-accredited ADN programs in a single-state study This might explain why some individuals also seek to attend BSN programs versus ADN programs for nursing (Kumm et al., 2014).

ADN graduates may often transition seamlessly into the baccalaureate program of study. As a result of ADN courses being in academic settings, unlike diploma graduates, some of the courses taken by ADN graduates may be recognized in the baccalaureate program of study. Articulation agreements with baccalaureate programs facilitate this transition.

The ADN pathway has made a lasting impact on nursing by increasing access to the profession and quickly supplying qualified nurses to the healthcare system (Mahaffey, 2002). Although some nursing organizations advocate for a BSN as the minimum standard, ADN programs remain essential in meeting healthcare demands, particularly in community and rural settings (Orsolini-Hain & Waters, 2009). They continue to evolve with articulation agreements that highlight their adaptability and ongoing importance in nursing.

Baccalaureate Degree Programs

The first **baccalaureate degree program** was established in 1909 at the University of Minnesota. This program resulted from research that promoted a move for nursing education to shift from a hospital-based educational component to colleges and universities. Nursing leaders identified that this educational foundation was needed to promote nursing as a profession. It was believed that a BSN degree would prepare nurses to assume leadership positions.

Since the initial program inception, BSN programs have continued to develop at universities and allow individuals the opportunity to obtain a degree and prepare for nursing licensure simultaneously. Courses in a BSN program of study include liberal arts, science, and nursing. Many programs are structured to allow for electives in these areas. This permits individuals to select courses that work to complete a minor study area, if desired. Nursing courses focus on various settings that include public or community health. Extending skills in this area promotes independence while managing patients in the public or community health setting. This area is unique to the baccalaureate degree curriculum.

Nurses may enter BSN programs as extensions of their program of study as the basis of their initial RN licensure. In some programs, RNs receive credit for prior education and/or experience. This may be achieved through validation of prior education on a transcript from an educational institution or by successfully challenging knowledge in an area by examination. Programs are often flexible to permit part-time education as nurses continue to work. Some programs offer courses outside of typical on-ground classroom settings, with many offering them in a full or partial (hybrid) computer-based or online format.

In 1965, the American Nurses Association (ANA) published a position paper that addressed educational preparation. This document was foundational in defining nurse graduate knowledge, skills and values. The ANA's first position paper, entitled *Educational Preparation for Nurse Practitioners and Assistants to Nurses, a Position Paper,* made the following four major recommendations:

1. Education for all who are licensed to practice nursing should take place in institutions of higher education.
2. Minimum preparation for beginning professional practice should be baccalaureate degree education in nursing.
3. Minimum preparation for beginning technical practice for nursing should be the associate degree education in nursing.
4. Education for assistants in the health service occupation should be a short, intensive preservice program in vocational education institutions rather than on-the-job training programs (ANA, 1965).

The 1965 position document was not widely accepted by those inside or outside of the nursing profession. Many nurses were educated at the diploma level, and there was no recognition of these nurses in the document. The document would require a new way of thinking and have unique regulatory and licensure implications. This brainstorm of responses spanned the continuum of acceptance to rejection. It segmented nurses into those who could use the terms *professional* and *RN* from those who could not. The term *technical* was interpreted to mean a level below the one currently occupied by ADNs. It was also interpreted to mean that these nurses would have limited responsibilities related to patient care. Many organizations devoted much time and energy to address both ends of the acceptance continuum.

In 1970, a document entitled *An Abstract for Action* was published by the National Commission for the Study of Nursing and Nursing Education (Lysaught, 1970). This document presented the outcome of a study that addressed nursing practices and patterns and assessed future needs. Four key recommendations from this study centered on (a) the need for resources to study nursing's practice impact on health care, (b) the establishment of state master plans to ensure that nursing education is positioned in education's mainstream, (c) the formation of a National Joint Practice Commission and state counterparts, and (d) the adoption of governmental measures to support research in nursing. This document did not defuse all controversy related to nursing's educational foundation. Comments included criticism about the research process, which made results less than credible and shared perspectives that the study offered no new information for the nursing profession.

In 1979, the ANA placed a timeline on the preparation and differentiation of nursing. They proposed that changes to the entry level of nursing practice be the baccalaureate degree by 1985. Nursing should be identified by two levels (professional and technical) by 1980, with competencies identified for each level. Accessibility was also identified as a component to be addressed that would allow for career mobility, with flexibility in approaches to addressing this issue. The 1980s saw these dates come and go with no action by the profession.

Baccalaureate degree programs were challenged by the American Association of Colleges of Nursing (AACN) with its 1987 document written to ensure the abilities of its graduates. The document, entitled *Essentials of College and University Education for Professional Practice: Report to the Membership of AACN, October 1986*, discussed nursing's context and its effect on student education and socialization. It identified abilities that baccalaureate degree programs should ensure in their graduates. These included the following:

1. Read, write, and speak English clearly and effectively to acquire knowledge, convey and discuss ideas, evaluate information, and think critically.
2. Think analytically and reason logically using verifiable information and past experience.
3. Understand a second language at a minimum of an elementary level to widen access to diversity.
4. Understand other cultural traditions to gain perspective on personal values and similarities and differences among individuals and groups.
5. Use mathematical concepts, interpret quantitative data, and [use] computers and other information technology to analyze problems.
6. Use concepts from the behavioral and biological sciences to understand oneself and one's relationship with other people and to comprehend the nature and function of communities.
7. Understand the physical world and interrelationship with human activity to make decisions based on scientific evidence and be responsive to individual and community values and interests.

8. Comprehend life and time from historical and contemporary perspectives and draw from past experiences to influence the present and future.
9. Gain a perspective on social, political, and economic issues for resolving societal and professional problems.
10. Comprehend the meaning of human spirituality to recognize the relationship of beliefs to culture, behavior, health, and healing.
11. Appreciate the role of the fine and performing arts in stimulating individual creativity, expressing personal feelings and emotions, and building a sense of the commonality of human experience.
12. Understand the nature of human values and develop a personal philosophy to make ethical judgments in both a personal and professional life (AACN, 1987).

This document also addressed critical components for faculty of nursing programs. It identified nursing faculty as being responsible for integrating liberal arts and science knowledge into professional nursing education and practice. This "essentials" document has been revised in response to changes in health care over the years. The last document published to date was in 2021 and entitled *The Essentials: Core Competencies for Professional Nursing Education*. This document provides a framework for the preparation of individuals in the nursing profession at various educational levels. Ten domains expected of graduates from baccalaureate programs as a generalist are identified as follows:

- Domain 1: Knowledge for Nursing Practice
- Domain 2: Person-Centered Care
- Domain 3: Population Health
- Domain 4: Scholarship for Nursing Discipline
- Domain 5: Quality and Safety
- Domain 6: Interprofessional Partnerships
- Domain 7: Systems-Based Practice
- Domain 8: Informatics and Healthcare Technologies
- Domain 9: Professionalism
- Domain 10: Personal, Professional, and Leadership Development (AACN, 2021)

As a result of a generalist four-year education, baccalaureate-prepared nurses have a variety of healthcare settings in which they can practice at various levels, from the bedside or home care to administration. These nurses can serve as advocates to ensure quality healthcare practices and promote nursing as a profession.

Graduate Education

Graduate education can be an individual's initial degree into the nursing profession, but this is not common. Many nurses enter graduate programs following completion of a BSN and work experience that allows them to specialize in an area of special interest. This prepares individuals for advanced practice in their area of interest.

Due to the limited number of **graduate programs** in nursing prior to 1960, many nurses desiring to obtain graduate degrees were forced to select other disciplines of interest. Most nurses in the 10-year span between 1950 and 1960 viewed the master's degree as a terminal degree for nurses' educational experience. This view of the master's degree as the final educational experience was soon overshadowed by the recognition that doctoral degrees were needed in order to place nurses on a par with other disciplines. As a result, there has been a substantial growth of graduate nursing programs.

Entry into graduate nursing programs vary, with most requiring a baccalaureate degree in nursing from an accredited program, an unencumbered nursing license (a license free of any restrictions by the state for potential sanctions), a designated grade point average on undergraduate study, and letters of recommendation and/or professional references. Some programs require some work experience, but in response to encouragement to increase the numbers of **APNs**, some programs permit continuation from the baccalaureate degree directly into MSN graduate study.

Many graduate programs can be completed in 12 to 18 months of full-time study and 24 months of part-time study. Students have an option to select an area of advanced practice to focus on, such as adult health, pediatrics, critical care, administration, education, informatics, nurse anesthesia, nurse practitioner, and other areas of clinical specialization. The curriculum will generally include a core of courses taken by all students regardless of the specific area of study, which might include theory, research, advanced health assessment, advanced pharmacology, advanced pathophysiology, and/or other courses that are identified by the specific nursing program. Completion of graduate programs may include a research study or thesis, successful completion of a comprehensive examination, and/or completion of a clinically based project.

Nurses graduating from master's degree programs usually earn a Master of Science or a **Master of Science in Nursing (MSN)** degree. Some graduate programs offer combination degrees for nurses with a non-nursing degree being earned simultaneously with one in nursing. These can include Master of Science in Nursing/Master of Business Administration (MSN/MBA), and Master of Science in Nursing /Master of Health Administration (MSN/MHA), etc. These degrees are not offered by all programs. Many continue to offer a nursing degree with a single focal area.

Doctoral education in nursing began in 1910 at Teachers College, Columbia University. The degree offered was a **Doctor of Philosophy**, or **PhD**. This degree was and is still considered to not be specific to nursing but rather a research degree. Graduates from these programs are expected to expand theory and conduct research. Some nurses, in an effort to focus their doctoral study in an area directed toward education, obtain the Doctor of Education (EdD) degree. Graduates from this program are expected to work in academia or administration or specialized educational positions. There are still individual nurses who are enrolled in doctoral study outside of nursing, but the preference for employment in nursing education and other areas that are nursing-focused is a degree that is in the discipline.

The **DNP** is a degree focused on moving the current level of advanced nursing practice from master's preparation to doctoral level. This degree grew out of the AACN, 2004's *Position Statement on the Practice Doctorate in Nursing*. This nursing doctorate (ND) was first offered at Case Western Reserve University in 1979. Prior to this time, nursing focused on research-based doctoral degrees or professional doctorates. Professional doctorates at most universities included the Doctor of Nursing Science (DNS or DNSc). These degrees were closely aligned to the PhD in preparation of graduates, and many have since been converted to PhD degrees. A doctoral degree that resulted from a practice-focused curriculum in nursing was offered by some programs under varying programs of study, which included nurse doctorate (ND) or DNP.

In 2005, the National Research Council Committee for Monitoring the Nation's Changing Needs for Biomedical, Behavioral, and Clinical Personnel called for nursing to develop a nonresearch clinical doctorate to address the need for expert practitioners to serve to fill the need for clinical faculty. The AACN's work advanced this call to action for a doctoral degree. This was one of many factors that set the foundation for promoting a change in nursing education to the graduate level. These included the rapid increase in knowledge required to move health care forward, the increased complexity of patient care, national concerns about the need to offer and maintain high-quality care to promote patient safety, the need for nurses with higher education to serve in leader roles who can design and implement care that meets assessment criteria, the need for nursing faculty to be prepared at the doctoral level, and increasing educational expectations by society regarding the preparation of members of the healthcare team, including nurses.

Doctoral education as the terminal degree has been recognized and promoted by all in the nursing profession. Some organizations have even gone as far as to make it the entry-level degree for practice. The Council on Accreditation of Nurse Anesthesia Educational Programs established a requirement that, by 2025, all entry-level nurse anesthesia programs confer a doctoral degree. The entry level for new certified nurse anesthetists can be either a DNP or Doctor of Nurse Anesthesia Practice (DNAP). This mandate applies to new graduates entering the profession, while currently certified nurse anesthetists are exempt from returning to school to meet this standard.

In 2022, the AACN released a report titled *The State of Doctor of Nursing Practice Education in 2022*. This updated information from the initial 2004 AACN position statement in support of the DNP as the graduate degree for advanced nursing practice preparation. This document, along with then-current data, identified that doctoral programs had increased over the past several years and were now available in all 50 states, with a reported 433 programs currently enrolling students as of 2023 (AACN, 2024). This number represented a 69% increase in programs since 2013. These programs also now include alternate routes of entry, such as post-baccalaureate to DNP and post-master's to DNP. This education option has grown in popularity among nurses.

Quality and Safety Education for Nurses

Nursing is a profession that requires knowledge and skills in order to safely manage patient health care in various settings. In an effort to address this challenge to nursing education, the **QSEN** was funded by the Robert Wood Johnson Foundation (RWJF) in 2005. The basis of this project is to educate nursing students on patient safety issues and mechanisms to improve healthcare quality. This project addresses not only the knowledge and skills but also the attitudes necessary for individuals who desire to become a nurse. The (KSA) combination is designed to promote continuous improvement in the healthcare setting by future nurses who will work there. The QSEN promotes the use of patient-centered care, teamwork and collaboration, evidence-based practice in care delivery, quality improvement, safety, and informatics in nurses' learning environments (Cronenwett et al., 2007). These aspects will be reviewed in the following sections.

Patient-Centered Care

Patient-centered care promotes patient or designee as the source of control and by allowing them to be a full partner in their care. They have ultimate control of care activities and decisions regarding their health care activities. It is important for nurses to be aware of the many dimensions of patient-centered care. These dimensions include knowledge of preferences and values in care based on interactions of the patient, family, and community in which they live; coordination and integration of care among all providers; the need for information, communication, and education regarding care activities and health status updates; the need for physical comfort and emotional support during their illness episodes; involvement of family as well as friends; and patients' transition from nurse-given care to self-care and continuity of care. Skills include the ability to elicit patient values, preferences, and expressed patient needs during the clinical interview as well as care implementation, communication with other healthcare team members, and the ability to provide patient-centered care with sensitivity and respect. Attitudes are important and affect care components. It is imperative that patients be viewed with respect and their knowledge base be recognized regarding their individual illness or disease process. It is important for nurses to be self-aware and willingly support individuals whose values differ from their own.

Patient-centered care extends to comprehensive understanding of the many disease processes that result in pain and suffering, an awareness of patient empowerment aspects in health care, ethical and legal issues in patient-centered care, and collaboration and communication in promoting care. Nurses need to be astute in their assessment skills and implementation of techniques to address pain and suffering as well as removing barriers to the promotion of empowerment. Valuing active partnerships can assist in increasing patient respect and increasing active engagement of both patients and their family. The use of shared decision-making can promote success in patient outcomes.

Teamwork and Collaboration

Nurses are just one member of an interdisciplinary team that interacts with patients in the delivery of care. **Teamwork and collaboration** require that nurses know their own strengths, limitations, and values in order to function effectively in intercollaborative teams with other healthcare professionals in health promotion and disease prevention activities. Successful patient outcomes can depend on the attainment of this collaboration. It is important for nurses to be knowledgeable of the roles of individuals on the team. Often, roles overlap in their responsibilities in patient care management. It is important for all care providers to be able to work through clearly identifying roles and accountabilities that demonstrate recognition of the value, expertise, and perspective of each team member. This is imperative in order for the team to function cohesively in the delivery of safe care. This allows team members to initiate request for assistance that acknowledges the expertise of each team member and promotes team success in care activities and patient management.

Nurses must learn skills that promote cohesive team functioning inclusive of conflict resolution. Conflict resolution strategies include such things as listening with respect and responding with care while using breathing techniques to convey calmness and confidence. It is important to know when to assert one's own position versus support that of another team member. It is important to effectively use communication styles based on the situation and personality of individuals involved. There are basically three communication styles: aggressive, passive, and assertive. Becoming more self-aware and understanding one's own personal style of communication can assist in creating a good working care delivery team.

It is important for nurses to assess their own communication strengths and weaknesses in an effort to promote the improvement of this skill. Use of communication practices promoted to reduce patient risks when engaging in hand-off activities (e.g., giving a patient condition report to a nurse or another care provider who will assume care from a designated point in time for continued care or administration of specific interventions) should be followed. These improve patient outcomes and promote quality and safe care.

Evidence-Based Practice

Current **evidence-based practice (EBP)** knowledge is foundational to quality care delivery. Nursing has its history in borrowed knowledge from other disciplines. The profession is continuously working to develop a research or EBP environment that validates nursing activities. It is important that quality care be based on research and not opinion. Research plays a critical role in determining the best patient care practices. Nurses have a responsibility to validate the strength of the evidence used for choices made regarding nursing interventions. Nurses should be able to evaluate the quality of research studies and select those that best demonstrate research processes and outcomes toward success. This is important in initial selection, continued use, or modification of best-practice decisions.

Research is used in the clinical and/or classroom preparation of nurses. An appreciation of this information is important. Validation of care activities through the use of research is integral. New-graduate nurses are consumers of research, using it to promote understanding and verification of care. This allows nurses to effectively validate care activities and outcomes. Nurses at all levels must learn to value research as well as appreciate the strengths and weaknesses of this process in the delivery of care. Knowledge of how to evaluate research is an important skill, from its ethical underpinnings to its quality in methodology and results. Knowledge of the research process and how it is integral to validation of patient outcomes is foundational to the learning process. This is necessary in order to continue to improve care through use and involvement in the research process at all levels of nursing. Identifying self-limitations and acquiring increased knowledge regarding research and its use allows nurses to increase their knowledge base in this area. The ultimate outcome is increased quality and safety in patient care.

Quality Improvement

Data are used to monitor outcomes and continuously improve quality and safety in healthcare systems. Knowledge regarding **quality improvement (QI)** and outcomes is important to include in the educational process. This is a continuous process in organizations, and QI affects patient safety. Students are part of the healthcare system and affect the overall quality of patient care. It is important for them to be familiar with tools that are used for care and evaluation of sentinel events (events that occur due to failure to adhere to preidentified policies and procedures, such as a patient fall). Health care is constantly changing in an effort to give safe, economical care. Effective changes need a collaborative team approach for success. Changes should be initiated based on evidence, and proper change strategies are important to use in an effort to promote the change in an organization.

Safety

System effectiveness and individual performance can be used to minimize the risk of harm to patients and providers. **Safety** initiatives include human and safety-enhancing technologies (e.g., barcodes, medication pumps, automatic bed alarms). Knowledge and effective use of strategies are important factors in patient safety. All nurses need to know and value their role in preventing errors in promoting safe patient care. Strategies such as effective open communication can promote safety for patients and providers. Communication strategies reduce the probability of error in receiving orders and delegation of care activities. Promoting vigilance and monitoring performance of self and others can facilitate safe patient outcomes.

Informatics

Technology is the basis of many healthcare organizations. **Informatics** applications include electronic charting to requisitions for laboratory or radiological information. Patient personal information databases in the computerized system can be readily accessed for update or verification of care activities. Knowing the legal and ethical mechanisms for management of this information is a must. There are technological benefits and limitations. Many systems are designed to initiate alerts and monitor activities related to care activities (e.g., medication removal from a computerized system will be logged into a computer database). Knowledge of technology and information management tools that support safe care initiatives are imperative. It is important to recognize the need for nurse involvement in designing, selecting, implementing, and evaluating technology-based systems in healthcare organizations.

Landmark Nursing Reports

Three landmark nursing reports have had a significant impact on the profession. These are the ***IOM's The Future of Nursing: Leading Change, Advancing Health*** (IOM Committee on the RWJF Initiative on the Future of Nursing, 2011); ***Assessing Progress on the Institute of Medicine Report* The Future of Nursing** (Committee for Assessing Progress on Implementing the Recommendations of the Institute of Medicine Report, IOM, National Academies of Science, Engineering, and Medicine et al., 2016), and the **NAM's *The Future of Nursing 2020–2030: Charting a Path to Achieve Health Equity*** (NAM et al., 2021).

The IOM's *The Future of Nursing: Leading Change, Advancing Health* (2011)

The IOM Committee on the RWJF Initiative on the Future of Nursing published a landmark document in 2011 that explored nurses' roles, responsibilities, and education that needed to change to meet the increased care demands of society. These changes would be fueled by impending healthcare reforms. The changes promoted for nurses would also advance improvements in society's increasingly complex healthcare system. The committee engaged in several deliberations and concluded that outdated regulations, attitudes, policies, and habits related to the nursing profession restricted innovations needed to promote the transformation needed in education. Its recommendations for transforming the nursing profession were as follows:

1. Nurses should practice to the full extent of their education and training.
2. Nurses should achieve higher levels of education and training through an improved education system that promotes seamless academic progression.
3. Nurses should be full partners, with physicians and other health professionals, in redesigning health care in the United States.
4. Effective workforce planning and [policymaking] require better data collection and an improved information infrastructure. (IOM Committee on the RWJF Initiative on the Future of Nursing, 2011)

This landmark, 620-page document served as a framework for changes needed in the nursing profession to address an ever-changing healthcare system.

Assessing Progress on the Institute of Medicine Report The Future of Nursing (2016)

The second report, entitled *Assessing Progress on the Institute of Medicine Report* The Future of Nursing (2016), highlighted promising progress made since the 2011 report but also identified that much more work needed to be done relative to the nursing profession. It outlined three themes that were identified as central to the future success of the RWJF/AARP Future of Nursing Campaign for Action, which was developed as a result of the initial report. These included:

> the need to build a broader coalition to increase awareness of nurses' ability to play a full role in health professions practice, education, collaboration, and leadership; the need to continue to make promoting diversity in the nursing workforce a priority; and the need for better data with which to assess and drive progress. (NAM et al., 2021, p. x)

Nursing continues to work toward the development of these recommendations in the profession.

The IOM's *The Future of Nursing 2020–2030: Charting a Path to Achieve Health Equity* (2021)

The third report, *The Future of Nursing 2020–2030: Charting a Path to Achieve Health Equity* (2021), focused recommendations for charting a 10-year path forward for the nursing profession to support society's health and well-being initiatives not only for today but in the future (National Academies of Sciences, Engineering, and Medicine et al., 2021). These recommendations focused on the Social Determinants of Health (SDOH) and the elimination of inequities in health as well as health care. Specific recommendations addressed the following:

1. The initiation of work to develop a shared agenda for addressing SDOHs of health and equity in 2021 by all national nursing organizations
2. The initiation of substantive changes to enable nurses to comprehensively address SDOHs by state and federal agencies, healthcare organizations, public health organizations, payers, and foundations, by 2023
3. The implementation of structures, systems, and evidence-based interventions to promote the health and well-being of nurses as they take on new roles to advance health equity by nursing education programs, employers, nursing leaders, licensing boards, and nursing organizations, by 2021

4. The removal of state, federal, and organizational barriers that prevent nurses from practicing to the full extent of their education and training, in order to fully address social needs and SDOHs to improve health access, quality, and value, by 2022
5. The establishment of sustainable and flexible payment mechanisms to support nurses in health care and public health to address SDOHs and health equity by federal, tribal, state, local, private payers, and public health agencies
6. The recommendation that nursing expertise should be included in designing, generating, analyzing, and applying data to support SDOH initiatives and health equity using all platforms, artificial intelligence, and other innovative technologies in all public and private healthcare systems
7. The need to ensure that nurses are prepared to address SDOH achievement of health equity through inclusion of core concepts and competencies in didactic and clinical courses, and experiential learning activities in nursing education academic and continuing education programs, and by accreditors and the National Council of State Boards of Nursing
8. The recommendation to convene representatives from nursing, public health, and health care to develop and support a research agenda and evidence-based foundation for nursing to identify and describe the nursing intervention impact on SDOHs by the National Institutes of Health, the Centers for Medicare & Medicaid Services, the Centers for Disease Control and Prevention, the Health Resources and Services Administration, the Agency for Healthcare Research and Quality, the Administration for Children and Families, the Administration for Community Living, and private associations and foundations

These recommendations provide a comprehensive path forward for all, including nurse educators, policymakers, practicing nurses in all areas, leaders, and researchers and payers alike, to support nursing's current path and future initiatives in promoting societal well-being. Through nursing collaboration and partnerships with key stakeholders, policies and initiatives can be developed and implemented to promote nursing's positive impact on the SDOHs and health equity for society at large.

Summary

The nursing profession's history has demonstrated a slow but deliberate move from hospital to higher education. There are several educational routes to the nursing profession. There is no consensus on the entry level for nursing, although one was proposed more than 40 years ago. Graduate education is on the rise, with education moving toward a practice doctorate for advanced practice entry. The doctorate is now considered the terminal degree for nursing practice. The two reports by the IOM and the NAM are key components to nurses' current path and future initiatives as the profession continues to evolve. The educational pathway for nurses continues to respond to societal challenges as needs change and care becomes more complex.

References

American Association of Colleges of Nursing. (1987). Essentials of college and university education for professional nursing: Report to the membership of AACN, October 1986. *Journal of Professional Nursing, 3*(1), 54–69. https://doi.org/10.1016/S8755-7223(87)80028-5

American Association of Colleges of Nursing. (2004, October). *AACN Position Statement on the Practice Doctorate in Nursing.* https://www.aacnnursing.org/portals/42/news/position-statements/dnp.pdf

American Association of Colleges of Nursing. (2021). *The essentials: Core competencies for professional nursing education.* https://www.aacnnursing.org/Portals/0/PDFs/Publications/Essentials-2021.pdf

American Association of Colleges of Nursing. (2024, May). *Associate degree in nursing programs and AACN's support for articulation.* https://www.aacnnursing.org/news-data/fact-sheets/adn-programs-and-aacns-support-for-articulation

Accreditation Commission for Education in Nursing. (2024). *Search programs: Diploma programs.* https://www.acenursing.org/search-programs?program-type=Diploma

American Nurses Association. (1965, December). *Educational preparation for nurse practitioners and assistants to nurses, a position paper.* ERIC, Institute of Education Sciences. https://files.eric.ed.gov/fulltext/ED021059.pdf

Committee for Assessing Progress on Implementing the Recommendations of the Institute of Medicine Report, Institute of Medicine, National Academies of Science, Engineering, and Medicine; Altman, S. H., Butler, A. S., & Shern, L. (Eds.). (2016). *Assessing progress on the Institute of Medicine report* The future of nursing. National Academies Press (U.S.).

Cronenwett, L., Sherwood, G., Barnsteiner, J., Disch, J., Johnson, J., Mitchell, P., Sullivan, D. T., & Warren, J. (2007). Quality and Safety Education for Nurses. *Nursing outlook, 55*(3), 122–131. https://doi.org/10.1016/j.outlook.2007.02.006

Harker, M. (2017). History of nursing education evolution Mildred Montag. *Teaching and Learning in Nursing, 12*(4), 295–297. https://doi.org/10.1016/j.teln.2017.05.006

Health Resources and Services Administration. (2022). *NCHWA nursing workforce dashboard*. https://data.hrsa.gov/topics/health-workforce/nursing-workforce-dashboards

Health Resources and Services Administration. (2024, November). *Nurse workforce projections, 2022–2037*. https://bhw.hrsa.gov/sites/default/files/bureau-health-workforce/data-research/nursing-projections-factsheet.pdf

Institute of Medicine (U.S.) Committee on the Robert Wood Johnson Foundation Initiative on the Future of Nursing. (2011). Key messages of the report. In *The future of nursing: Leading change, advancing health*. National Academies Press. https://www.ncbi.nlm.nih.gov/books/NBK209880/pdf/Bookshelf_NBK209880.pdf

Kumm, S., Godfrey, N., Martin, D., Tucci, M., Muenks, M., & Spaeth, T. (2014). Baccalaureate outcomes met by associate degree nursing programs. *Nurse Educator, 39*(5), 216–220. https://doi.org/10.1097/NNE.0000000000000060

Lysaught, J. (1970). *An abstract for action*. McGraw-Hill.

Mahaffey, E. H. (2002). The relevance of associate degree nursing education: Past, present, future. *Online Journal of Issues in Nursing, 7*(2), 3. https://doi.org/10.3912/OJIN.Vol7No02Man02

National Academy of Medicine; National Academies of Sciences, Engineering, and Medicine; Committee on the Future of Nursing 2020–2030; Wakefield, M. K., Williams, D. R., Le Menestrel, S., & Flaubert, J. L. (Eds.). (2021). *The future of nursing 2020–2030: Charting a path to achieve health equity*. National Academies Press (U.S.). https://doi.org/10.17226/25982

National Research Council (U.S.) Committee for Monitoring the Nation's Changing Needs for Biomedical, Behavioral, and Clinical Personnel. (2005). *Advancing the nation's health needs: NIH research training Programs*. National Academies Press (U.S.). https://doi.org/10.17226/11275

Orsolini-Hain, L., & Waters, V. (2009). Education evolution: A historical perspective of associate degree nursing. *Journal of Nursing Education, 48*(5), 266–271. https://doi.org/10.3928/01484834-20090416-05

U.S. Bureau of Labor Statistics. (2024, April 3). *Occupational employment and wage statistics: 29-2061 licensed practical and vocational nurses*. https://www.bls.gov/oes/current/oes292061.htm#top

Image Credits

Fig. 14.2: Richard A. Smiley et al, "Nursing Education Statistics from 'The 2020 National Nursing Workforce Survey,'" Journal of Nursing Regulation, vol. 12, no. 1. Copyright © 2021 by Elsevier B.V.

CHAPTER 15

Evidence-Based Nursing Practice

Objectives

Upon completion of this chapter, the learner will be able to do the following:

1. Define evidence-based practice (EBP) as it relates to the nursing profession.
2. Explain some of the basic steps used in EBP to develop solutions for healthcare problems.
3. Understand various types of research and their application to scientific inquiry for a phenomenon of concern in nursing.
4. Summarize the research process inclusive of its steps in research design.

Key Chapter Terms

- EBP
- PICO (patient/problem [P], intervention [I], comparison [C], and outcome [O])
- Focus question
- Nursing research
- Quantitative research
- Qualitative research
- Research process
- National Institute of Nursing Research
- Council for the Advancement of Nursing Science
- Midwest Nursing Research Society
- Western Institute of Nursing Research
- Southern Nursing Research Society
- Eastern Nursing Research Society

Evidence-Based Nursing Practice

EBP is nursing care with a foundation in research validation for implementation. As with some other components of nursing, nursing research dates back to Florence Nightingale and her validation of observations made related to issues that significantly affected patient care and outcomes. Nursing's research history began slowly and was mainly used for education rather than validation of patient care outcomes. This was in part due to the fact that nursing was only beginning to have nurses with educational expertise to conduct research studies. Nursing research was also not highly financially subsidized for intense research or longitudinal studies over time. But times have changed. Research has evolved to be a critical foundation for nursing practice (Alay-odao et al., 2024), and this chapter will explore EBP and its link to nursing research.

Evidence-Based Nursing Practice

EBP is a problem-solving method for healthcare delivery that integrates the best evidence from research studies to develop solutions for a healthcare problem. This information is further integrated with relevant patient care data, preferences, and values and then merged with nurse expertise to develop a strategy that promotes the best healthcare outcome possible for a patient (Chien, 2019; Cardoso et al., 2021).

There are some basic steps to EBP, which are as follows:

1. **ASK:** Convert information needed into an answerable question.
2. **ACQUIRE:** Find the best evidence.
3. **APPRAISE:** Critically appraise results of the literature search for validity and usefulness.
4. **APPLY:** Apply findings to clinical practice.
5. **ASSESS:** Evaluate professional performance.

Sources: Adapted from Straus et al., 2011, & Flemming, 1998.

These steps will be briefly reviewed in the following sections.

Step 1: ASK: Convert information needed into an answerable question. This involves formulation of a clinical question. Here, nurses need to ask questions in a format that can be answered with specific information. It is important to define the question and structure it for the appropriate setting, as this technique is applicable to not only the clinical environment but also management. The question may be directed to a management issue relevant to nursing. There are usually four parts to question construction: the patient/

problem (P), intervention (I), comparison (C), and outcome (O). The acronym for this is ***PICO*** (Gray & Grove, 2021, p. 560). Using this framework for question development allows for structured follow-through for the following steps.

The four PICO elements should be evident in a well-structured question. This way you can develop a focused question that will allow for retrieval of specific research results in the next evidence-based step. If your question is too broad, you may end up with thousands of results; if it is too narrow, you may not have any results of your search. A well-formed question also allows for identification of key words to use in Step 2 of the EBP process. This can save a lot of valuable time during research study retrieval. Let's use a situation to develop a question using PICO.

Suppose that you work in a busy labor and delivery unit. Patients are admitted for a brief period for delivery of their newborn. All patients admitted who report "smoking during pregnancy" in history retrieval are given a brochure about quitting smoking. The nurse interacts with the mother for a very brief period of time, addressing this brochure. This information is reviewed only once during the admission. You and other coworkers are concerned that these mothers will resume smoking with the new infant in the home and that the one-time brochure review is not adequate to cause cessation of smoking in the mother after discharge. You and several other nurses working on the unit decide to identify if this minimal contact and brochure review is adequate based on the available research to affect smoking. See Table 15.1 for how to use PICO to develop the question.

TABLE 15.1 Using PICO in the ASK Step of EBP

P	I	C	O
Hospitalized maternal smokers	A short, one-time educational nursing intervention	No treatment	Smoking cessation (patient-reported)

Focus question result: In hospitalized maternal patients, does a short, one-time educational nursing intervention, compared with no intervention, lead to smoking cessation? This allows for identification of key words such as *smoking cessation* and *education* for information retrieval. This would lead to more specific studies being returned in the search results database.

Step 2: ACQUIRE: Find the best evidence. This is a critical step. It is important to make sure you locate information that both supports and negates interventions. These are best located in peer-reviewed journals, which is where published articles are reviewed by other nurse researchers for quality and relevance before they are published in the journal. Many times, the perfect article is located, but there is a cost associated with retrieval. The local hospital librarian may be able to assist with retrieval at no cost. There may also be information located online, but this information must be critically reviewed for quality. Literature searches through well-known search engines may also retrieve thousands of hits, but their relevance and quality must be reviewed individually. This can be a time-consuming endeavor.

Step 3: APPRAISE: Critically appraise results of the literature search for validity and usefulness. Critical analysis of the article type is where to begin for this step. It is important to identify only research studies or systematic analyses of the research for inclusion in the list of articles for use. Use only articles that fit the format for quantitative research, qualitative research, or a systematic review of the literature. Systematic reviews of research are articles where authors have collected numerous research studies and based on criteria for inclusion or exclusion, compared and contrasted these studies to determine their findings. They appraise these articles and arrive at conclusions from all the included studies. They can be very beneficial in validating a thorough review of key research studies for certain topics of interest.

Step 4: APPLY: Apply findings to clinical practice. In this step, you integrate the evidence into practice decisions and activities. This information is combined with the unique needs and values of patients to achieve the best outcome.

Step 5: ASSESS: Evaluate professional performance. This allows for critical appraisal of the outcome following implementation of the EBP-validated activity. Assessment should take into account the perspective of other healthcare providers, which can give varying perspectives and credibility to the assessment. After identifying the fiscal efficacy and clinical effectiveness of the intervention, changes can be made to policies and procedures.

It is important to bridge the gap between the evidence and the bedside use of it. Nursing students should take any research course seriously, knowing that this information will be foundational to their future practice. Nursing is ever evolving, and information is increasingly available. This can present an overwhelming task for review and critique related to research relevance and use. There is also a current nursing shortage, which adds to the demand of nurses working with patients in various settings. These things make it difficult for nurses to engage in activities that require time and effort that some may feel distract from the importance of patient care. A balance is imperative to continually address nursing research topics of interest in the delivery of care that promotes the best patient outcome.

What Is Nursing Research?

Nursing research is applying scientific inquiry to a phenomenon of concern for nursing. It is to search and search again for an answer to this phenomenon

TABLE 15.2 Comparison of Steps in the EBP Problem-Solving Process and the Research Process

EBP Problem-Solving Process	Research Process
1. ASK: Convert information need into an answerable question.	1. Identify a research topic.
2. ACQUIRE: Find the best evidence.	2. Review the literature to identify what is already known.
3. APPRAISE: Critically appraise results of the literature search for validity and usefulness.	3. Define the research purpose and formulate questions or hypotheses.
No comparative step	4. Select the research design.
No comparative step	5. Select the sample or population.
No comparative step	6. Collect study data.
4. APPLY: Apply findings to clinical practice. 5. ASSESS: valuate professional performance.	7. Analyze study data to generate conclusions and implications.
No comparative step	8. Communicate study results.

of interest. It is specifically defined by Gray and Grove (2021) as "the diligent, systematic inquiry or investigation to generate new knowledge, validate existing knowledge, and refine knowledge by incorporating new research findings" (p. 1). Nurses conduct research in an effort to build a body of knowledge that is unique to nursing, validate improvements that are proposed for nursing interventions, and promote cost management in health care. Nursing research is a more formalized process than that used for EBP problem-solving (see Table 15.2).

There are two broad categories of research: **quantitative research** and **qualitative research.** *Quantitative research* uses methods that are more objective and uses techniques that allow replication or duplication of the research study. This type of research is based more on the retrieval of numbers or data that can be counted or measured with standardized instruments or questionnaires. Statistical techniques are used that allow quantification and numerical differentiation or similarity identification (Rivera et al., 2020). Quantitative research is deductive in its approach. Deductive approaches move from a general case—which, in research, is identifying a research question or hypothesis—to a specific instance or precise measurements and analyses. *Qualitative research* uses methods that are more subjective in their approach. This approach uses methods of inquiry that emphasize retrieval of the meaning of the experience for a given individual (Li et al., 2022). Researchers are an integral part of this process. They may conduct or work with others to conduct interviews or methods of verbal interaction, which are often used to obtain data from subjects involved in the study. Researchers reduce these words to themes (single words or phrases) that evolve from critical analyses of words retrieved through the data collection process. Qualitative research is inductive in its approach. Inductive approaches move from specific situations, which are the interviews of individuals who address the common topic of the research, to broader generalizations or themes (specific topics) derived from the numerous interviews. See Box 15.1 for examples of the two general types of research.

Box 15.1

Example of Types of Research

Quantitative Research Abstract

Rivera, J., Donohoe, E., Deady-Rooney, M., Douglas, M., & Samaniego, N. (2020). Implementing a pressure injury prevention bundle to decrease hospital-acquired pressure injuries in an adult critical care unit: An evidence-based, pilot initiative. *Wound Management & Prevention, 66*(10), 20–28.

Abstract

Title: Implementing a pressure injury prevention bundle to decrease hospital-acquired pressure injuries in an adult critical care unit: An evidence-based, pilot initiative

Aim: This article is a report of a study of the implementation of a pressure injury prevention bundle to reduce hospital-acquired pressure injuries (HAPIs) in an 11-bed adult critical care unit in a tertiary, acute care hospital in New York City. An underlying purpose was to standardize interdisciplinary care for prevention of HAPIs.

Background: Patients in critical care units are at high risk for pressure injuries due to their clinical instability and comorbidities. Additional factors include immobility, sedation, and mechanical ventilation. A research-based question was generated. An initial literature review was done to validate bundle components and implementation processes for the study. Education was used as a critical implementation component. Special wound, ostomy, and continence (WOC) nurses provided education for morning and night shift staff inclusive of patient care associates on the bundle. The bundle consisted of use of the Braden scale to promote early identification of patient risks, a repositioning system, nutrition consultations, audits, WOC nurse consultations, establishment of an interdisciplinary team, WOC rounds to maintain motivation, and educational tips on how to correctly document for accuracy.

Methods: A pilot study design was used. Data were collected throughout February 2018. Educational sessions were held by the WOC nurses during morning briefs for staff. Meetings included all nurses as well as patient care associates. Audits were used to validate compliance and areas needing further review and revision. Feedback was obtained from resources nurses and staff regarding perceived concerns, which included additional time for implementation. Assistant nurse managers worked with nurses at the bedside to ensure bundle implementation, when needed.

Results: The bundle audit tool provided valuable information for this study. Implementation of the pressure injury prevention bundle resulted in a considerable decrease in HAPIs. The preintervention HAPI score was 3.4, and the postintervention score decreased to 0.48 over a 13-month time frame. Preintervention pressure injuries were three stage 2 pressure injuries, five deep-tissue pressure injuries, and one unstageable. Postintervention pressure injuries consisted of one stage 2 injury.

Conclusion: Initiation of a pressure injury prevention bundle significantly reduced HAPIs in the studied critical care unit. Staff involvement and leadership support were integral to the study's success.

Qualitative Research Study

Li, Z., Marshall, A. P., Lin, F., Ding, Y., & Chaboyer, W. (2022). Registered nurses' approach to pressure injury prevention: A descriptive qualitative study. Journal *of Advanced Nursing, 78*(8), 2575–2585. https://doi.org/10.1111/jan.15218

Abstract

Title: Registered nurses' approach to pressure injury prevention: A descriptive qualitative study

Aim: This article is a report of a study aimed at exploring registered nurses approaches to pressure injury prevention.

Background: Nurses are the largest healthcare provider group. They are responsible for delivering quality patient pressure injury prevention care. Key pressure injury prevention includes repositioning, use of skin protection, and selection of appropriate support surfaces. Research has shown that internationally, there are varying degrees of compliance with the use of pressure injury strategies for patients. The purpose of this study was to gain an understanding of how medical and surgical nurses approached pressure injury prevention.

Methods: A descriptive qualitative approach was used in this research study. Audiotaped face-to-face interviews were conducted in a large tertiary hospital in China from August to December 2020. Thirty-seven female nurses were interviewed. Semistructured interviews were used to collect data regarding the nurses' understanding of pressure injury prevention and their practices. Data were transcribed and verified.

Results: Analysis identified four themes. Theme 1 identified "Nurses lead and coordinate pressure injury prevention," which further expanded to state that pressure injury prevention is led by nurses, patients, and carers' participation in prevention; nurses desire better physician engagement with pressure injury prevention; and a variety of tools, equipment, and devise are used by nurses to support pressure injury prevention. Theme 2 identified "Individualized pressure injury prevention is founded on comprehensive patient assessment," which further expanded to state that risk assessment goes beyond completing a risk assessment tool and that high-risk patients need care supplemented with other components. Theme 3 identified "Collaborating ensures patients receive appropriate pressure injury prevention," which further expanded to state that nurses support each other in delivery of pressure injury prevention, wound care experts provide care advice for these patients, and a wound care team supports nurses in delivery of pressure injury prevention strategies. Lastly, Theme 4 identified "Competing factors influence the delivery of appropriate pressure injury prevention," which further expanded to state that social and cultural factors influence pressure injury prevention implementation in the care setting.

Conclusion: Nurses play a critical role in pressure injury prevention in China. Although they are important in the current system and consider pressure injury prevention a high priority, there are needs that could be implemented to improve compliance. There is a need for adequate resources and a supportive organizational structure in China for nurses regarding pressure injury prevention.

In nursing, research is a validated way of knowing. Prior to a more extensive use of research to validate many interventions, the nursing profession retrieved knowledge through traditions, authority, borrowing, trial and error, personal experience, role modeling, and intuition. Use of reasoning and research are foundational to delivery of care for nurses in the current evidence-based environment. Research uses a process to promote retrieval and dissemination of study results to achieve the best patient outcomes. Many questions or topics of interest arrive from the nurse's clinical practice that are the focus of the **research process**. Some may also result from reading the research of others or course work for advanced practice study (see Figure 15.1).

Research is now a driving force in nursing. Nurses at all education levels have a place in the research process. Nurses at the bedside are pivotal in identifying problems and collecting data for analyses. This serves to expand the base of nursing research. Expanding the research base for nursing also expands the amount of evidence available for use to manage patient care situations.

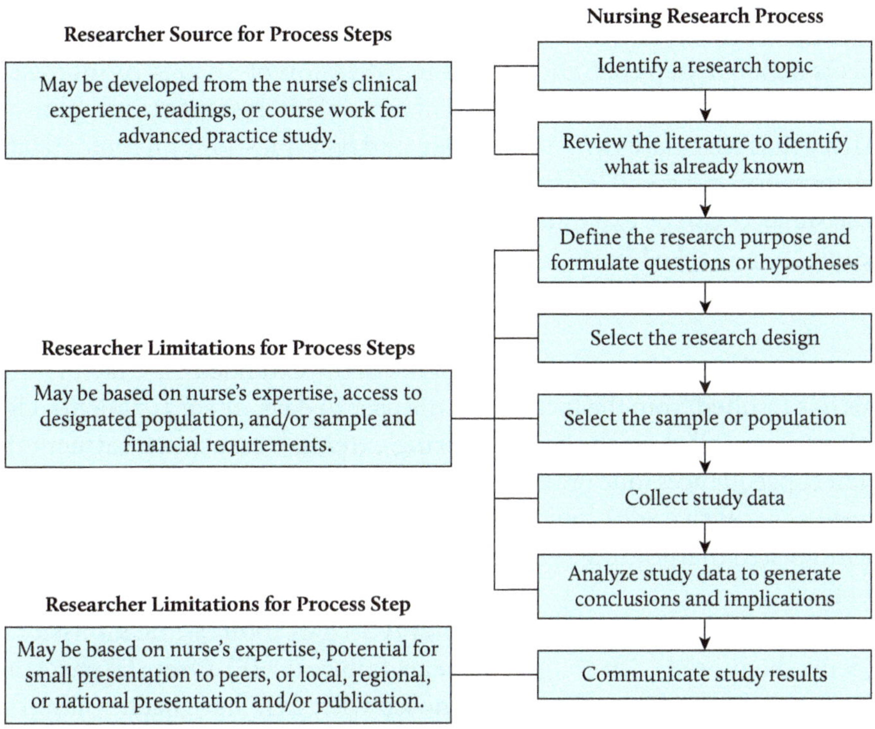

FIGURE 15.1 Stages of the Research Process With Researcher Source or Limitations

The Research Process

Research allows the movement of information from an abstract idea to the realities of knowing. It permits a researcher to test or validate responses or answer questions posed through clinical experiences or other situations. This section is intended to give you a brief introductory review to the research process in order to prompt interest and a desire to learn more. It is not comprehensive, as research is a process with many subactivities that must be completed in order to comply with regulations for initiation of the research process and the ultimate success of the project. Quantitative and qualitative research processes are not the same, but the steps in the following sections can be adjusted for either form of research.

Research is systematic inquiry. It requires adherence to a specific format for investigation to have results that meet criteria for scientific merit. Collaborative research is a good place to start when you are looking to become involved in research. This allows you to learn while doing and establishes a peer mentoring relationship that can be mutually beneficial. Use of textbooks and other material that assists with specifics of the research process, including statistical analyses, is also beneficial. Give the process enough time to allow for success. Do not expect to complete this process in a few days. A brief review of steps in the research process is identified in the following sections.

Identify the Research Topic

This is a global step that allows for identification of an area of interest in order to generate a specific question. This area of interest may result from any activity that stimulates *why*, *when*, *what*, and *how* questions on topics related to an activity that could lead to a specific outcome. Questions resulting from these subjects can be expanded to specifically address areas. Make sure that the question is asked in such a way that guides you forward in the process. This step may appear as follows.

First general area of interest: Patient falls in the extended-care facility unit. This has resulted from the fact that in the past 30 days, out of 21 patients, eight of them have fallen, with three requiring extensive care and treatment due to fall consequences (one broken hip, one broken arm, one elbow dislocation) as well as extensive additional care, causing patient and family distress. You are interested in initiating evidence-based interventions to reduce unit falls.

Let's look at another one. **Second general area of interest:** Readmission of patients diagnosed with congestive heart failure (CHF). Over the past three months, six of the nine patients diagnosed with CHF have been readmitted within 30 days of discharge due to eating foods high in sodium (salt) or not adhering to their medication regimen (i.e., not taking medications as prescribed). You are interested in developing evidence-based patient education and medication adherence strategies.

Third general area of interest: Asthma in children. Asthma is a common childhood disease that affects children's quality of life. You work in a pediatrician's office where children appear to be disinterested in the current asthma care program. You are interested in developing a program that is of interest to these children with asthma in an effort to promote quality of life.

Review the Literature to Identify What Is Already Known

Now you need to explore what others had to say about your specific area of research interest. Find out if there are similar studies to support your research topic. You can do this by looking in the research literature to identify what research has been done in the past by individuals interested in these topics. This is called the *literature review.* You may find a completed supporting study that you can replicate for your specific area. All the literature review news may not be good news. You may also find that the literature does not support your original thought or question. It has been thoroughly investigated in the research and been found to be detrimental to patient outcomes. If this is the case, it will require you to rethink and restructure your research study.

The literature review is a critical part of defining the research process. Give preference to literature that is current or within the past five years. This step usually requires a significant outlay of time and effort. This is where a collaborative effort may be helpful. If you have a peer in an advanced educational nursing program looking to do a project for a specific course, this may be an ideal way to get some much-needed assistance to retrieve and critique research as well as help with the entire research process. A relationship involving this person in the research study may be mutually beneficial.

When performing the literature review, be sure to keep notes on what has been retrieved. Keep a log of keywords used in searches to prevent duplication of this work. Use databases that will give you access to research-based articles and not just general information articles. Look for articles that are in peer-reviewed journals. This means that the articles have been evaluated by a group of peer nurse researchers for quality and relevance. They also evaluate the articles' adherence to the research process. Identify specific search categories to reduce retrieved relevant articles to a manageable number. When you come across an article that you think might be useful, immediately retrieve it for later reference and add it to a computer folder for later review. This can save you significant time later in searching for "that article I saw two days ago that would be perfect."

One mechanism to use to validate an exhaustive literature review is to critically analyze the reference list of appropriate research studies. These can give you a lot of information regarding other relevant research on your topic. Once you start to see duplication of research in the reference lists and do not identify new articles in these lists compared with your own list of articles reviewed, you know that your literature review phase has come to a close. Articles that review research literature on the topic can save you time critiquing articles for relevance. These are called *systematic reviews of the literature* and can be an excellent source of information regarding types of research on your topic along with study quality.

Define the Research Purpose

Your next move is defining the purpose. Leaving the topic general can be overwhelming and keep you from addressing what you are really interested in finding out. What do you really want to know? What question will allow you to address specific areas of true interest? Looking at the first general area of general interest mentioned earlier, you might develop a question that addresses prevention of hospitalized patient falls. The question may appear as "What is the best intervention to prevent patient falls on my C4-East Wing unit of the extended care facility?" Looking at the second general area of interest, you might develop a question that addresses readmission of CHF patients. The question may appear as "Does the educational intervention we are giving patients with congestive heart failure make a difference in readmission rates for these patients?" Looking at the third general interest area, you might develop a question directed at obtaining the perspective of children between ages 7 and 10 years of age with asthma about what they see as important to include in an educational program. The question may appear as "How do children describe their asthma experience, and based on this, what do they want to know about caring for themselves?"

Select the Research Design

Now you need to select the research design. The design is the study blueprint. Here, you will identify whether you will complete a quantitative research study or qualitative research study. This will guide the selection of individuals for the study and the data collection tools. This step can be affected by nurses' level of expertise, access to the designated population, and/or sample and financial requirements (e.g., costs associated with data collection tools, paid time off to complete the research process, and/or costs required for statistical analyses).

There are many other components to consider in this phase, but for the sake of simplicity, this is the only component presented in this textbook. It is recommended that you consult a formal research textbook for specifics regarding this phase of the research project. This will facilitate how you progress to identifying tools needed for the research study. A detailed textbook can assist you in identification of questionnaires as well as the format for data collection.

Select the Sample or Population

Selecting the sample involves identifying specific individuals who will be invited to participate in the study. This may be governed by access and permissions, which are part of the required review by a committee called an *Institutional Review Board* (IRB). An IRB is an independent ethics committee established by organizations to protect the rights of individuals being invited for the study (called *subjects*). These rights and explanations are displayed in Table 15.3.

A *population* is defined as all elements who meet designated criteria for inclusion in your study. This number can be extremely large and costly to incorporate. Your study may use a sample, which is a subset of the entire study population. All permissions and consents are required to be obtained prior to any data collection.

TABLE 15.3 Individual Rights in Research

Research Right	Explanation
Right to self-determination	This right is based on the ethical principle of respect for others. This means that subjects should have the right to determine whether they desire to participate in a study. Special considerations are made for individuals who are (a) legally or mentally incompetent; (b) younger than age 18 years (i.e., neonates, children, and teenagers); (c) have diminished capacity (e.g., mentally ill or have a disease process that impairs their cognitive abilities, such as Alzheimer's disease or they are in a coma); or (d) are confined to an institution (e.g., mental hospital, prison).
Right to privacy	This right means that an individual can determine the circumstances for disclosure or sharing of personal information with other people.
Right to autonomy and confidentiality	*Autonomy* means that subject identity cannot be linked to any information in the study. *Confidentiality* means that the researcher responsibly manages data and protects private information shared by subjects.
Right to fair treatment	This right is based on the ethical principle of justice, which states that each individual should have fair treatment and receive what they are due or owed.
Right to protection from discomfort and harm	This right is based on the ethical principle of beneficence, which states that an individual should do good and, above all, do no harm to subjects in the research study.

Collect Study Data

Collection of study data involves interaction of the researcher with subjects in order to collect information through observations, interviews, or completion of specific hard-copy or electronic questionnaires. Study assistants may be used to collect data when a large number of participants must be contacted or when information retrieval exceeds the researcher's capacity. They may also assist in data collection when participants are geographically dispersed or located outside the researcher's immediate area. It is important that all individuals collecting data be familiar with the study. They should be given specific information on how to collect information, and this knowledge base should be verified for accuracy of the data collection process and actual data retrieved. Inaccurate data collection can affect study results and, ultimately, lead to invalid results. Data collectors must be familiar with the rights of study subjects and adhere to protocols to protect these rights.

Analyze Study Data

Analysis of study data involves differentiation of the data, data entry, and analyses. Measurement strategies in the data collection step are used to find an answer to the questions and/or hypotheses posed earlier in the process. This can appear to be an overwhelming task. It is important to perform the correct statistical tests; otherwise, the study will not be valid. Results will not represent accurate outcomes from data collected, and the research study will not present "true" results regarding answers or responses to initial questions or hypotheses. If you have a collaborative team of individuals, a statistician may be among them. This individual can help with quantitative research analyses. If you are doing qualitative research, you will need someone skilled in this type of data analysis. In qualitative research, there can be thousands of words to analyze and reduce to themes from subjects interviewed for data retrieval. It is important to solicit assistance and use experts to assist in determining numerical outcomes in quantitative research or themes from analysis of words collected in qualitative research.

Analyses of research findings allow for identification of study conclusions. Study findings are discussed, and information is presented to show how these findings build on and add to the body of knowledge identified in the review of the literature. This allows for identification of whether the study supports or does not support previous research findings. This area will also allow the discussion of implications and relevance to clinical practice. Specific contributions to the body of knowledge can be presented along with areas for future research on the topic.

Communicate Study Results

Communicating your results is the final step in the research process. This allows others access to your research for use in EBP for care delivery to patients, families, and communities. A research report will be written, and appropriate venues will be identified for dissemination of study findings. This may be at a local, regional, national, or international level. It may involve publishing information in journals that may be in hard-copy or electronic format. It is important to communicate findings to build the body of nursing knowledge.

Research Organizations in Nursing

National Nursing Research Organizations

National Institute of Nursing Research

Through Public Law 99-158, the Health Research Extension Act of 1985, the National Center for Nursing Research (NCNR) at the National Institute of

Health (NIH) was authorized following a presidential veto override by U.S. Congress. In 1986 the Department of Health and Human Services officially announced establishment of the NCNR at NIH with Doris Merritt, a research physician, appointed as the acting head. She served until Ada Sue Hinshaw was appointed as the first nursing director. The NCNR supported not only research initiatives but also research training and career development in health promotion and disease prevention, acute and chronic illness, and nursing systems. The center also supported strategies to improve patient outcomes. Through research training grants, beginning and advanced nurse researchers engaged in predoctoral, postdoctoral, and senior fellowships to increase individuals prepared to engage in research activities.

In 1992, through the collaborative efforts of multiple nursing organizations and with support from Congress and the Executive Branch, the NIH Revitalization Act of 1993 elevated the NCNR to institute status, thereby establishing the **National Institute of Nursing Research (NINR)**. The NINR has as its mission "to lead nursing research to solve pressing health challenges and inform practice and policy—optimizing health and advancing health equity into the future" (NIH, 2023). In promoting the mission, NINR supports clinical and basic research training on health and illness across the lifespan. Its research lenses, based on the 2022–2026 NINR strategic plan, include health equity, social determinants of health, population and community health, prevention and health promotion, and systems and models of care. Through NINR support, research in nursing has increased, and recognition has been achieved and promoted to the public through press releases. Technology has also given nursing research a boost with an avenue for nurse researchers to communicate and disseminate findings on a worldwide scale.

Council for the Advancement of Nursing Science

The American Nurses Association restructured and disbanded the Council of Nurse Research in the late 1990s. Members quickly recognized the need to create a national nursing research-based organization. As a result, the council established the **Council for the Advancement of Nursing Science (CANS)** as an open membership entity of the American Academy of Nursing in 2000. This national organization strives to be recognized as a collective national voice for nursing science, and its mission is to promote better health through this science. In order to accomplish this mission, the organization serves as a strong voice for nursing science at both the national and international levels. Goals are accomplished by developing, conducting, and using nursing science; disseminating research findings; and facilitating lifelong learning opportunities for nurse scientists. The organization serves to integrate nursing science into wellness, health, and policy decisions. Organization-specific information can be retrieved at https://aannet.org/page/cans.

Regional Nursing Research Institutes/Societies

Several regional organizations exist in the United States to promote nursing research that affects the profession of nursing and overall patient health and outcomes (see Figure 15.2).

These organizations were established between 1975 and 1986. They promote research on special topics based on organizationally identified research initiatives. Many offer journals to disseminate research and encourage collaborative interactions. They also offer financial support on topics of special interest to the organization. Member communication is further augmented electronically. All have online information sites that are identified, along with specific information in the following sections. They are presented in the order in which they were established.

Midwest Nursing Research Society

The **Midwest Nursing Research Society (MNRS)** was established in 1975 by a group of nurses working on a research project entitled the *Nursing Faculty Research Development in the Midwest*. This research project was for the U.S. Department of Health and Human Services, the government's principal agency for protection of the health of U.S. citizens and provider of essential human services. During this collaborative research-based activity, these nurses discussed the need for a specific organization dedicated

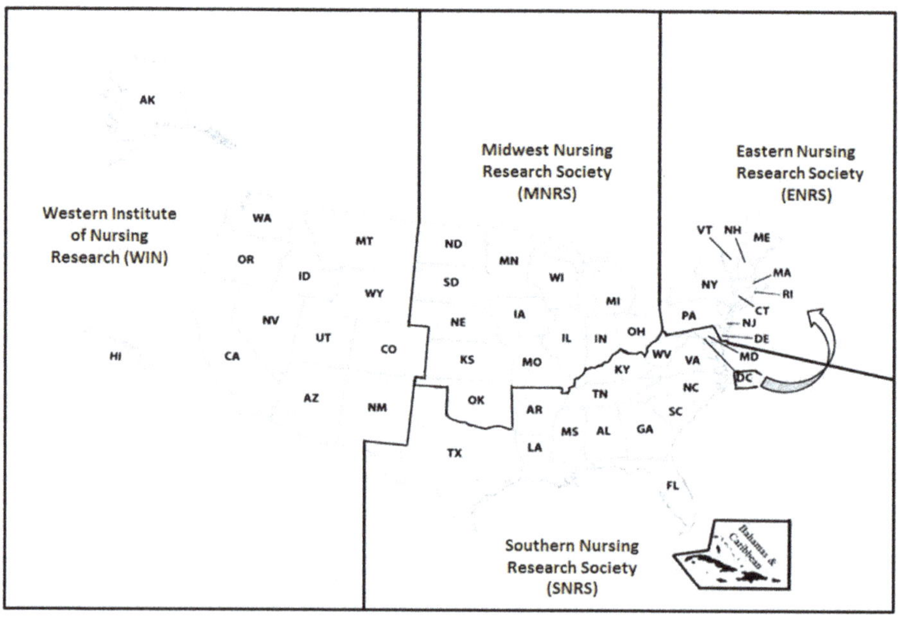

FIGURE 15.2 Regional Nursing Research Organizations

to nursing research. With continued effort, these initial communications formed this research-based organization. MNRS membership is drawn from nurses and nursing students living in Illinois, Indiana, Iowa, Kansas, Michigan, Minnesota, Missouri, Nebraska, North Dakota, Ohio, South Dakota, Oklahoma, and Wisconsin. The MNRS is committed to advancing science, transforming practice, and enhancing careers through a network of scholars. The MNRS offers numerous grant opportunities that include several types of dissertation grants and seed grants. Research areas include a multitude of topics (e.g., acute care, family health, nursing education, nursing informatics, pediatric nursing, women's health). The *Western Journal of Nursing Research* is the official journal of the MNRS. This journal disseminates research studies, book reviews, discussions and debates, meeting dates, and calendars for events. Specific information regarding initiatives can be obtained from the organization's website: https://www.mnrs.org.

Western Institute of Nursing Research

The **Western Institute of Nursing Research (WIN)** is a western regional nursing research organization that was formed in 1985. This organization succeeded formation of the Western Council on Higher Education for Nursing following deliberation by special committees to create a research-based, autonomous, self-supporting organization. The WIN consists of 13 states: Alaska, Arizona, California, Colorado, Hawaii, Idaho, Montana, Nevada, New Mexico, Oregon, Utah, Washington, and Wyoming.

The WIN's mission is to connect a diverse community of nurses in the West to improve health through nursing research, practice, and education excellence. It supports research that advances the nursing profession and improvements in practice, outcomes, and cost in health care. It supports a diverse community of nurses in their research initiatives. This organization supports research through an annual fund drive to support WIN awards and joint research grants. These initiatives are further supported in organizational goals. Additional organization information can be obtained at https://www.winursing.org/.

Southern Nursing Research Society

The **Southern Nursing Research Society (SNRS)** was founded in 1986 by a group of 60 nurses who collaborated to establish an organization for nursing researchers in the southern region of the United States. The SNRS was officially identified as an independent organization in 1987. The original organizational membership of 14 states (Alabama, Arkansas, Florida, Georgia, Kentucky, Louisiana, Maryland, Mississippi, North Carolina, South Carolina,

Tennessee, Texas, Virginia, and West Virginia) was expanded in 1991 to include the Caribbean, Latin America, and the Bahamas. The SNRS has an organizational vision that values leading the transformation of health outcomes through nursing research. An annual conference allows dissemination of research for this organization. Research interest group topics allow discussion and collaborative research initiatives by individual members through the organization. The SNRS offers 13 different discussion areas for research, including aging/gerontology, education, health systems/policy, military and veteran health, psychiatric nursing, parent/child, and minority health. A listing of all special interest research groups is located at https://snrs.org/riigs.php. Additional organization information can be obtained at https://www.snrs.org.

Eastern Nursing Research Society

The **Eastern Nursing Research Society (ENRS)** was established in 1988 as the research arm of two existing organizations: the Mid-Atlantic Regional Nursing Association and the New England Organization for Nursing. The purpose of this organization was to create a community for nurses interested in research in the eastern region of the United States. This organization includes 10 states (Connecticut, Delaware, Maine, Massachusetts, New Hampshire, New Jersey, New York, Pennsylvania, Rhode Island, and Vermont) and Washington, D.C. The ENRS mission is to advance innovative nursing science. Its vision is to promote health through nursing science and a commitment to promoting diversity in all forms in nursing research through the establishment of an inclusive environment. The organization is committed to knowledge and evidence generation, translation and implementation. The ENRS provides a networking forum for nurse scientists through conferences and online interest groups, nursing science development, translation of evidence to guide nursing practice and education as well as influence policy in these areas, and mentoring nurse scientists. They have a student discovery network to link students to the nurse research community. The organization has established research interest groups on aging; criminal justice; trauma and violence; early-career nurse scientists; EBP improvement; family- and community-based participatory; global health; health services; LGBTQIA+ health and health disparities; mental health and substance abuse and use; military and veteran, nursing education; nurse scientists: advancing research; palliative care; precision health; qualitative research; and theory development. Additional organization information can be obtained at https://www.enrs-go.org/.

Specialty Nursing Organizations

Specialty organizations are numerous in nursing. These range from academies to associations and societies in areas such as medical-surgical nursing, critical care nursing, gerontological nursing, rehabilitation nursing, emergency care, and long-term care (see a current listing at https://www.nurse.org/orgs.shtml). Many have research as part of their organization's mission and/or goal. They may set research-based initiatives or priorities that identify research topics of interest to the organization. Some have funds that range from a few hundred to several thousand dollars that may be obtained through an application process. These grants may be available on an annual basis. They may allow several years of research in order to address a topic of interest and allow for data collection, analysis, and dissemination of the results. Many of these organizations promote research of specialty initiatives, based on their healthcare focus, that increase evidence validation for clinical patient management.

Summary

The abilities to critically analyze, use, and conduct research are becoming key skills for individuals in nursing practice. Use of research promotes high-quality care provision for patients. Use of EBP in practice gives nursing a professional base of support. It is important to continue the quest to research those specific nursing issues that are important to the development of care modalities and promote the best patient outcomes. As health care changes, it is important for nurses to respond with current management that is systematic and based on empirical and observable evidence.

References

Alay-odao, E. M., Cruz, J. P., & Almazon, J. U. (2024). Consequences of the hospital nursing research culture: Perspective of staff nurses. *International Journal of Nursing Sciences*, *11*(2), 233–240. https://doi.org/10.1016/j.ijnss.2024.03.007

Chien, L. Y. (2019). Evidence-based practice and nursing research. *Journal of Nursing Research*, *27*(4), e29. https://doi.org/10.1097/jnr.0000000000000346

Cardoso, D., Couto, F., Cardoso, A. F., Bobrowicz-Campos, E., Santos, L., Rodrigues, R., Coutinho, V., Pinto, D., Ramis, M. A., Rodrigues, M. A., & Apóstolo, J. (2021). The effectiveness of an evidence-based practice (EBP) educational program on undergraduate nursing students' EBP knowledge and skills: A cluster randomized control trial. *International Journal of Environmental Research and Public Health*, *18*(1), 293. https://doi.org/10.3390/ijerph18010293

Flemming, K. (1998). Asking answerable questions [editorial]. *Evidence-Based Nursing, 1*, 36–37.

Gray, J. R., & Grove, S. K. (2021). *The practice of nursing research: Appraisal, synthesis, and generation of evidence* (9th ed.). Elsevier Saunders.

Li, Z., Marshall, A. P., Lin, F., Ding, Y., & Chaboyer, W. (2022). Registered nurses' approach to pressure injury prevention: A descriptive qualitative study. *Journal of Advanced Nursing, 78*(8), 2575–2585. https://doi.org/10.1111/jan.15218

National Institutes of Health. (2023, June 30). *National Institute of Nursing Research*. https://www.nih.gov/about-nih/what-we-do/nih-almanac/national-institute-nursing-research-ninr

Rivera, J., Donohoe, E., Deady-Rooney, M., Douglas, M., & Samaniego, N. (2020). Implementing a pressure injury prevention bundle to decrease hospital-acquired pressure injuries in an adult critical care unit: An evidence-based, pilot initiative. *Wound Management & Prevention, 66*(10), 20–28.

Straus, S. E., Richardson, W. S., Glasziou, P., & Haynes, R. B. (2011). *Evidence-based medicine: How to practice and teach it* (2nd ed.). Churchill-Livingstone.

Image Credits

Fig. 15.2: Generated using Adobe Firefly.

CHAPTER 16

I Am a Nurse

Transitioning to the Profession

Objectives

Upon completion of this chapter, the learner will be able to do the following:

1. Implement selective coping strategies for transitioning from school to work.
2. Understand the steps for a successful transition from the educational process to the nursing profession.
3. Develop an evidence-based résumé/portfolio for successful transition to a nursing job.
4. Understand the importance of identifying work preferences in nursing.
5. Explain the importance of nursing professional development.

Key Chapter Terms

- Licensure
- National Council Licensure Examination (NCLEX)
- National Council of State Boards of Nursing (NCSBN)
- Computerized adaptive testing (CAT)
- Next-generation (next-gen; NGN)
- Interview
- Professional portfolio
- Professional goals
- Nursing philosophy statement
- Graduate nurse/intern
- Work environments
- Continuing education
- Reflective practice
- American Nurses Credentialing Center (ANCC) Magnet Recognition Program

I Am a Nurse: Transitioning to the Profession

> My job as a nurse is hard but extremely rewarding. It requires that I physically and emotionally support patients and families in my care. I must have a base of knowledge that is continually challenged and requires that I remain ever vigilant about new innovations in patient care delivery. I feel like I am always learning in order to teach my patients and peers. I truly love my patients and thoroughly enjoy helping them work to achieve a good quality of life. They hold a special place in my heart. They are the reason I love what I do. They are the reason I am a nurse.

These words spoken by one nurse relay the fundamental reasons why many individuals choose nursing as a profession. The nursing profession supports a caring attitude in administering care activities and, at its core, promotes working with people to improve their health.

Transitioning From Classroom to Job

New-Graduate Status

Following graduation from an accredited nursing program, you still are not allowed to use the initials *RN* (registered nurse) or *LPN* (licensed practical nurse)—not even on the mortarboard (i.e., cap) at the graduation ceremony! These initials are authorized only after successfully passing a **licensure** examination. Following graduation, you move from studying for course grades to continuing a study regimen to be successful at the **National Council Licensure Examination (NCLEX)** for Registered Nurses (NCLEX-RN) or the National Council Licensure Examination for Practical Nurses (NCLEX-PN). This will give you the right to use the licensure abbreviation *RN* or *LPN* following your name. Your signature line in validating orders or notes would be your name followed by *RN* or *LPN*. Some organizations encourage you to include your terminal degree or educational preparation initials as well. The proper format would be as follows: name (first initial and last name), degree conferred, and licensure. This would translate to the following examples: B. Smith, BSN, RN (for a bachelor's degree) or B. Smith, ASN, RN (for an associate's degree). As you progress to include certifications, these can be added to your standard signature format, and your certification should follow your licensure initial. Be sure to check with your organization to validate the format for proper initials to use for this purpose. Movement into a management-type position may require that you alter your signature to include more information. You may also need business cards with specific information. Always comply with the regulations of the organization, but for presentations or publications, you might use this format: *name (first initial and last name), degree conferred, licensure, certification, and job title*. This could translate to the following example: *B. Smith, BSN, RN, CCRN, Clinical Nurse Manager for SICU*. Be sure to check with the specific organization to identify proper signature format (whether or not to use your degree conferred and the official citation for any position). This information is generally disclosed during organizational orientation periods. If you are using an electronic signature, this may be set and linked to your computer sign-on code, so there is no need to add any additional identifiable information to notes or comments entered via the computer terminal.

Often graduates ask when they can wear their pin purchased from their school or college of nursing. The pin can be worn while working as a new-graduate nurse. It symbolizes graduation from an academic institution, not licensure.

Preparing for Licensure

Upon graduation from an academic institution, graduate nurses have successfully completed a program of academic study and earned a degree but are still not licensed to practice as a RN or LPN. The initials *RN* or *LPN* cannot be used until the licensure examination called the *NCLEX-RN* or *NCLEX-PN* has been successfully passed. It is important to successfully navigate the examination process from preparation to completion (see Box 16.1).

Box 16.1

1. Apply for licensure to the board of nursing in the state or territory in which you desire to be licensed. Review the board's website regarding its requirements.
2. Register for the NCLEX and pay the examination fee online (https://www.pearsonvue.com/us/en/nclex/contact.html) or by calling Pearson VUE at (866) 496-2539. There are no refunds of NCLEX fees for any reason.
3. You will receive an NCLEX registration acknowledgement from Pearson VUE.
4. You will receive eligibility from the nursing regulatory body (NRB) in the state or territory in which you desire to be licensed, and you must follow up within 365 days of registration and payment.
5. You will receive authorization to test (ATT) from Pearson VUE. You must test within validity dates (an average of 90 days). Your identification's (ID) printed name must exactly match that which ATT received. Legal documents accepted for validation of a name change at the test center include marriage license, divorce decrees, or court action legal name change. Documents must be in English.

6. Visit https://www.nclex.com/ or call Pearson VUE NCLEX Candidate Services to schedule a testing appointment.
7. Arrive at the testing center on the examination day and present an acceptable form of ID and the ATT. Acceptable forms of ID for domestic centers include passport books and cards, a driver's license, a provincial/territorial or state ID card, a permanent residence card, and a military ID card. All international testing centers accept only passport books or cards. All forms of ID must be valid and meet the following requirements: government-issued, nonexpired, and physical (i.e., nondigital) and have your name (in Roman characters), a recent photograph, and a signature.
8. Candidates seeking licensure in the United States can receive unofficial "Quick Results" in two business days, if purchased, but this does not authorize candidates to practice.

The **NCSBN** is exploring the potential for candidates to take the NCLEX at home. It is anticipated that advanced artificial intelligence security measures will be in place for this remote testing. This is anticipated in 2026 and will offer increased flexibility, greater comfort, more testing choices, and easier access to the test without travel.

It is important to prepare for the NCLEX. Start by reviewing information on the NCSBN website, which has a wealth of information, including the NCLEX test plan, sample questions, and an examination preview. Preparation may include self, group, and/or formal study scenarios. Self and group study sessions afford structured preparation for taking the computerized licensure examination. A formal review course may be taken in an effort to obtain intense concentrated review time. Formal review courses are not a requirement to take the examination and should be viewed as a point of decision for the nurse candidate. Just as for any examination, arrive early (at least 30 minutes prior to test time), eat a good breakfast following a good night's sleep, and dress comfortably. Usually, dressing in layers will allow more flexibility in adjusting body temperature. Outside materials cannot be used during the testing session, but the opportunity to make notes is available as an erasable board and marker will be provided, as will access to an on-screen calculator, if needed. Biometrics will also be retrieved prior to being admitted to test, which will include a signature, photograph, and palm vein scan.

The NCLEX is offered in a **CAT** format (NCLEX, n.d.). This means that the computer will vary test item difficulty around a baseline required passing score. When an item is answered incorrectly, the computer re-estimates the candidate's ability based on all prior test item answers and the difficulty of those items. The computer will then select the next item that is most optimal

TABLE 16.1 NCLEX Pass-or-Fail Rules

Rule	Explanation
95% confidence interval rule	The most common for candidates. The computer will stop giving items when it is 95% certain that a candidate's ability is clearly above or below the passing standard.
Maximum-length exam rule	When the person's ability is very close to the passing standard, the computer will continue to issue items until the maximum number is reached. The computer will disregard the 95% rule and consider the final ability estimate on all exam items, according to the following: • If the final ability estimate is at or above the passing standard, the person passes. • If the final ability estimate is below the passing standard, the person fails.
Run-out-of-time rule	If a person runs out of time before reaching the maximum number of items and the computer has not determined with 95% certainty that the person has passed or failed, the following alternate criteria are used: • If the number of required items has not been answered, the person automatically fails. • If at least the minimum number of required items has been answered, the final ability estimate is based on all responses taken before the exam time expired. If the final ability estimate is at or above the passing standard, the person passes. If not, the person fails.

for the candidate based on its estimation of previous responses. Each item is targeted to the candidate's ability, and items are ensured to be not too hard or too easy. This allows the examination to obtain maximum information about the candidate's ability. Passing is determined based on one of three rules (NCSBN, 2024; see Table 16.1).

There is a maximum testing period of five hours, but there is no time limit for each test item. The current NCLEX is a **next-generation (next-gen; NGN)** format, which was updated and initiated in April 2023, meaning that it still includes multiple-choice, select-all-that-apply, hot-spot, fill-in-the-blank, drag-and-drop, chart or graphics, graphic answer multiple-choice, and audio or video question types from the prior version. The next-gen format incorporates case scenario, extended multiple-choice, extended drag-and-drop, highlight-text, matrix/grid, and trend question types. There are 70 to 145 questions with 15 pretest questions that are not calculated into the final score but are used for future question development. A test plan for the NCLEX is posted to the NCSBN website at https://www.nclex.com/test-plans.page.

Seeking Employment: The Interview

Seeking employment is always a challenge for many nurses, as this is the first time many have engaged in the **interview** process for a working position. Nursing school offers a unique opportunity that is not afforded to many other academic programs. While in clinical locations, students may identify a specific organization they are truly interested in as a first work experience following graduation. Demonstration of skill level and the ability to eagerly learn can identify individuals who may be sought out by organizations looking to hire new graduates with these traits. The formal interview will often not take place until the program of study has been completed. When seeking employment, use common-sense skills and courtesies. See interview tips in Table 16.2.

TABLE 16.2 Interview Tips

Tip	Successful Interview Techniques
1. Prepare for the interview.	• Have a professionally prepared résumé. • Practice for the interview. This is like any other skill and takes rehearsal and repetition. • Know the organization. Investigate its mission, philosophy, and goals as well as other information that can relate to the foundation for working there (e.g., annual report). • Know the interview time frame and format.
2. Dress for a successful outcome.	• This is the first visual impression. • Dress professionally, using the following guidelines: ▹ For men, this could include a solid-color suit (usually black or navy) with a white or coordinated shirt, conservative shoes, light jewelry and use of perfumed odors, professional hairstyle, and portfolio or briefcase (see Figure 16.1). ▹ For women, this could include a solid-color suit (usually black or navy) with a skirt that allows comfortable and discreet sitting with a coordinated blouse, conservative shoes, limited jewelry, professional hairstyle, light makeup and perfume, and portfolio or briefcase (see Figure 16.1).
3. Leave early enough to arrive on time.	• Know your method of transportation. ▹ Car travel: Address any issues at least 24 hours prior to the time proposed to leave for the interview (e.g., low gasoline, engine issues). ▹ Bus travel: Know route times and potential transfers. ▹ Uber/taxi travel: Contact the company in advance to identify proper time for pickup in order to arrive on time. Some outlying areas require 24-hour notice for pickup appointments. • Know the route and identify potential times that have heavy traffic, which can impede travel.

Tip	Successful Interview Techniques
4. Stay calm.	• Take a deep breath prior to entering the interview room. • Remain as calm as possible during the interview. • Ask for clarification, if necessary, in order to address the specific question asked. • Take a moment or two to frame your response before speaking. • Fully address questions.
5. Use a recognition form that relays confidence and authority.	• Respect alternative greetings. • If a handshake is used, it should be firm but not viselike. • If a fist bump is used, it should be a touch. • If no hand is extended, you might use a head nod to validate recognition. • Stand firmly on two feet and upright during recognition. • If a hand is extended while you are seated, stand and move into the hand-recognition component (handshake or fist bump). If you are uncomfortable with shaking hands, you can identify that you prefer not to do so. You might say, "I am sorry, but I prefer not to shake hands. It is great to meet you."
6. Professionally present yourself.	• Carry a professional portfolio that contains information. • Use business cards to identify yourself for future contact. • Take extra copies of your résumé to the interview.
7. Take the time to say thank you upon exiting.	• Verbally thank the interviewer. • Use a follow-up thank-you letter to address any issues and concerns that may have come up during the interview.

Modify the tips in Table 16.2 and Figure 16.1 for phone- or video-based interviews. These are just as important and carry the same potential outcome. Be sure to get any required or requested information to individuals conducting the interview in a timely manner, regardless of format.

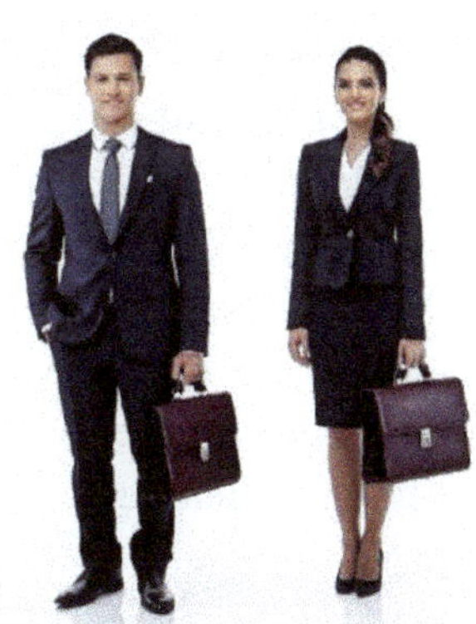

FIGURE 16.1 Dressing for a Successful Interview Outcome—Male and Female

The Portfolio

Like other professionals, nurses need evidence of their growth and achievements over time, which includes the college years. The **professional portfolio** is a method of collecting and presenting this evidence. You need to carefully select your best work over a period of time and use this to demonstrate how much you have learned and done in the profession. The portfolio allows reflection on one's professional life and encourages active engagement in purposeful decisions regarding growth and achievements (Ball, n.d.). A résumé is a one to two-page summary of skills, experiences and achievements (ResumeGiants Team, 2024).

The Portfolio Process

The portfolio is a tool that showcases your professional work and provides evidence of career growth and accomplishments. It should not be something simply thrown together but rather a purposefully crafted document. It must be meticulously constructed and demonstrate a relationship between information collection, selection, and reflection (William & Jordan, 2007).

The portfolio is a representation of a career over time (Cope & Murray, 2018). Updates can be done on an annual basis, so collect artifacts over time. Keep these in a safe place and organize them in folders with portfolio headings for careful selection later. Make sure to date all items added to the growing resource of information in order to verify the time frame in which to reference them. This will allow sequential placement of information in the portfolio. Use a mentor to help with review and critique of the portfolio. This individual should be experienced in the profession in order to give the best feedback. Don't take comments personally, and work with the mentor to make the portfolio the best professional representation possible. Carefully review the document. This will allow you to look at your personal career in a reflective mode. Answer the following questions:

- Does the document accurately reflect my career to this point? If not, why not, and what can I do to change this representative document? (A mentor may be able to assist with this.)
- Am I where I want to be at this point in my career?
- What has contributed to my successes?
- What has not allowed me to progress to the degree I desire?
- What are some future activities that will promote continued growth toward identified goals?

Things to Include in the Portfolio

There are many ways to maintain and organize a portfolio. These usually begin with a combination of hard-copy and electronic information. They often transition fully to an online format as a website or digital design program that can be downloaded. Some programs are free, while websites generally cost a fee to originate, upgrade, and maintain. The key is to identify a cost-effective format that is long-lasting. Be sure to keep a copy of all uploaded files to any cloud portfolio system. Keep your copies safe and in a format that allows long-term management.

Online portfolios may lock you into a specific format, but if not, you can use a general setup. Portfolios generally start with a title page that includes your name, address, telephone number, email address, program name, and degree (working to complete and projected date of graduation or degree completion, if prior to graduation). The initial page design for any online portfolios should be tasteful and professional. A table of contents and introductory statement may follow this section. The introductory statement should include an overview of the portfolio. Major components are identified in brief in Box 16.2. Use this outline to collect information and place it in electronic format (scan) in preparation for online inclusion.

Box 16.2

Brief Portfolio Outline

1. Name and demographic information
2. Education, license(s), certification(s)
3. Continuing education certificates (conferences, workshops, or self-directed independent learning activities)
4. Professional organization memberships (academic, local, state, or national)
5. Nursing philosophy
   a. Rationale for choosing nursing as a profession
   b. Inspirational people or experiences for entering the profession
6. Committees and professional projects
7. Community service (name of the organization, city and state of the organization, purpose of the organization, and your role in the organization)
8. Annual performance appraisals
9. Professional awards and achievements (copies of actual letters or awards received)
10. Scholarly publications
11. Professional presentations
12. Appreciation communications (emails/letters; from supervisors, peers, patients)
13. Future career goals:
    a. Short-term goals (two to four years)
    b. Long-term goals (five to 10 years)
    c. Ultimate career goal

Box 16.3

Goal Statement Examples

Short-Term Goals (Two to Four Years)

- To ultimately promote and implement the standards of nursing practice as established by the profession in the care of geriatric patients
- To secure a position in an area of nursing that will allow promotion of health for laboring women and their newborn infants
- To secure a clinical position in an acute care facility in an area that emphasizes critical care nursing
- To promote health and wellness for children through a position as a school nurse

Long-Term Goals (Five to 10 Years)

- To obtain a graduate degree with a focus in administration in preparation for a management position in nursing in an extended care facility
- To obtain a graduate degree with a focus in teaching to prepare myself for a position in an academic setting to promote the educational process for others interested in the nursing profession
- To obtain a challenging position within a healthcare organization that will allow me to expand my knowledge and increase my skills in management of acute care patients
- To obtain a position in a health-related organization that focuses on research and health promotion for children with cancer

Specifically state **professional goals** succinctly, clearly, and directly (see Box 16.3 for examples). Describe goals in detail. Find a theme for this information. If the theme is to help people, be specific in identifying which people (e.g., children, adults, older adults). Expand on this theme to include which specific category (e.g., children with cancer, adult critical care patients, older adults in the community). Use specific personal experiences to illustrate the theme's evolution.

Information should be presented from a professional perspective in the portfolio. It is not appropriate to include personal goals, such as getting married or moving to a specific part of the country. Goals should be well thought out and presented in a coherent manner that reflect precision and specifics. Based on the online format allowed, you may be able to arrange information in paragraph format, which demonstrates thought and active reflection.

Organize information in an easy-to-read format that is grammatically correct. Guide the reader with all information included in the portfolio.

Examples of academic papers should follow a specific form of writing style, such as the American Psychological Association or Modern Language Association, throughout. Use examples of the best work completed during the academic pathway (e.g., papers written) and work-quality reviews (e.g., annual evaluations).

Your **nursing philosophy statement** should be developed carefully in a stepwise fashion (see Figure 16.2). The opening statement should introduce the reader to you as an individual. The ending statement should be a powerful conclusion to this philosophy. Make the final sentence memorable for the reader. The philosophy should reflect personal beliefs and justification for them.

Assemble all information in documents that are easy to read and do not have too many pages for each area. Adhere to the template format save documents in PDF for ease of uploading and to preserve formats for the reader regardless of the type of computer system used for review and retrieval. Don't forget to date all your information for accurate sequencing. This can be done by adding the date to the name of the saved file, which will allow you to eliminate altering any original work or uploading duplicates to your portfolio. Give the documents names that also allow for easy identification from your folder review (e.g., annual evaluation 2023, CPR 2024).

Proofread all information. Correct grammar and sentence structure are important to making a favorable impression. Structurally organize content to create a memorable impression. It is good to read information over a period of time in order to verify that all information has been included for a professional presentation with personal reflection and enthusiasm. Review and update the portfolio as personal and professional goals change over the years.

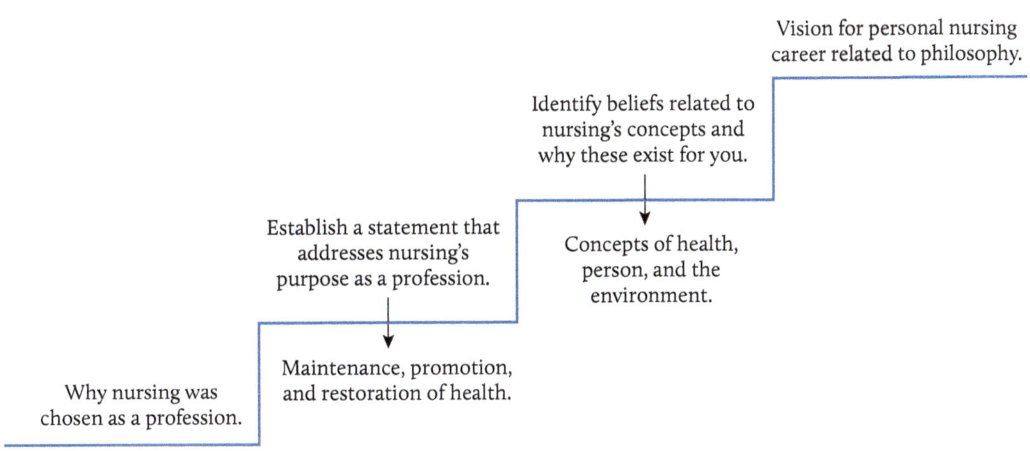

FIGURE 16.2 Steps to Developing a Nursing Philosophy

The First Job

New graduates may look to facilities used for educational clinical sites as a potential first job (AMN Healthcare, 2025). This has advantages for organizations and nurse graduates. Organizations have an opportunity to evaluate skills and potential for continued learning of graduate nurses, and graduates have the opportunity to evaluate compatibility with an organization's goals and philosophy.

Some organizations allow the new graduate to work as a **graduate nurse or intern** in a residency program within limitations on role responsibility and accountability. These depend on state regulations, which are not the same in all states. Salaries for these positions are often reduced, with salary and position increase occurring upon verification of licensure. Following your successfully obtaining licensure, the initials *RN* or *LPN* may be used to designate that nurse status has been achieved and approval has been granted by the state board of nursing. Patient care, legal responsibility, and accountability will also increase following licensure. This usually starts with an orientation to the organization and the validation of skills to be used in the specific area of employment (acute or extended care). This begins annual events training, which many organizations require (e.g., fire management training, cardiopulmonary resuscitation training and certification, medication administration protocols). This orientation will include timed instructional sessions that will educate new nurses about computerized organizational components, such as electronic patient records, the computerized medication administration system, and the laboratory/radiological data retrieval system. Orientation will include retrieval of computer access codes and log-on components, which should be kept confidential and not shared with anyone. These are unique to each nurse and may time-stamp and electronically sign information entered

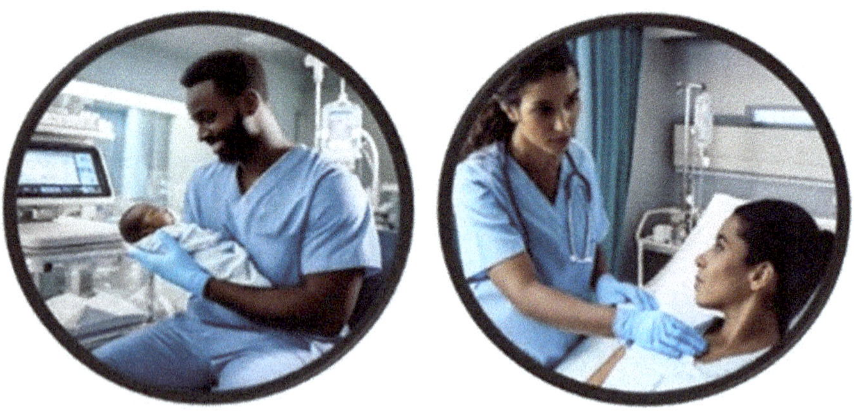

IMAGE 16.1 First Nursing Job

into the system following login. They are also geographic maps within the computerized system of where you go and when, for system audit purposes.

New-employee orientation is usually performed in a classroom format. Information regarding care area specifics will usually be taught following new-employment orientation. This is where new nurses enter the care area for orientation related to specialized equipment and skills that may be needed. At this time, new nurses may be paired with an experienced nurse to promote continued learning of area specifics. This time frame and peer collaboration situation is given different names by various organizations. It may be called *preceptorship*, *mentorship*, or *nurse residency*. The length of time for this orientation program can vary based on the care area complexity and progression of new graduates along the learning continuum. It may range from a few weeks to several months for more complex areas such as critical care or the emergency department.

This is an exciting time for new RNs and LPNs. It is the culmination of months and years of study and work. It validates success and is just the beginning of a professional course of learning as health care continues to evolve.

Work Environments

What to Consider in a Work Environment

Work environments vary greatly from organization to organization based on type, structure, goals, and philosophical base. Choosing an environment that augments your personal philosophy is important. Many organizations have online information that provides the organization's history, organizational structure, philosophy, purpose, aim, departments for patient care delivery, and employee information, among others. Take the time to go through the information available for review. Demonstration of some knowledge related to the organization validates true interest in employment during an interview. It also allows you to identify questions that may need to be clarified prior to employment. For example, if you are interested in returning to school during the first two years of employment and you plan on working for this organization for a minimum of six years, identifying educational benefits would be important.

Salary is an important component to consider. Don't assume that salary is nonnegotiable. Of course, the more experience you have in an area of specialty, the more bargaining power you have. The key is to do your homework. Take a look at posted salary ranges for your position of choice in the geographic and professional areas in which you are interested for employment. Request the range and which components are considered when discussing this topic.

Don't be shy. It is important to get this right the first time. Opportunities to discuss salary prior to beginning employment end when the contract is signed. Following acceptance of the contract, salary increases may only be based on strictly identified components for the organization (e.g., obtaining certification in a specialty, cost-of-living raises, moving up to a new salary level on a structured position ladder).

Know yourself and which characteristics are important to personally augment in an organization for you to achieve professional satisfaction. You chose nursing because it fits certain personality traits. Preferences regarding a work environment can be just as important as choosing a career. Work to identify organizations that will allow you to continue and achieve identified career goals. Use the form in Table 16.3 to help you with this.

TABLE 16.3 Know-Your-Work-Preference Questionnaire

Instructions: Respond to the following items in the table.

Questions	Rationale	Rank the Order of Importance by Number (1, 2, or 3)
1. In which city and state would you like to work?	Why did you select these areas of the country?	
2. In what type of organization do you want to work?	Why did you select this type?	
3. Is distance from employer important?	Why?	
4. Are employment hours of work important?	Why?	
5. What hours would you prefer to work if the organization offers shift work for nurses (e.g., two 12-hour shifts: 7 a.m. to 7 p.m., or 7 p.m. to 7 a.m.; three 8-hour shifts: 7 a.m. to 3 p.m., 3 p.m. to 11 p.m., or 11 p.m. to 7 a.m.)?	Why did you select these hours?	
6. In which specific area in the organization would you like to work?	Why this area?	
7. Do you have any convictions that would be a dealbreaker when it comes to seeking employment?	What is the source of your convictions?	
8. Do you have any specific personality traits that are important to augment in your work area?	What are these?	

Questions ranked #1 ______________________

Questions ranked #2 ______________________

Questions ranked #3 ______________________

The know-your-work-preference questionnaire can give you a start to identifying what you are looking for in an organization for employment and facilitate looking in the right place for the right job. For example, if you completed the questionnaire as follows (see Table 16.4), you would look for a job in Atlanta because it would be close to family and friends. You would give preference to job openings in an organization that did surgeries but did not perform procedures that were against your religious convictions.

TABLE 16.4 Example of Completed Work Preference Questionnaire

Instructions: Respond to the following items in the table.

Questions	Rationale	Rank the Order of Importance by Number (1, 2, or 3)
1. In which city and state would you like to work? **ATLANTA**	**CLOSE TO FAMILY AND FRIENDS**	**1**
2. In what type of organization do you want to work? **HOSPITAL OR FREESTANDING SURGICENTER**	**WANT TO WORK IN SURGICAL AREA**	**1**
3. Is distance from employer important? **NO**	**HAVE OWN TRANSPORTATION**	**3**
4. Are employment hours of work important? **NO**	**SINGLE**	**3**
5. What hours would you prefer to work if the organization offers shift work for nurses (e.g., two 12-hour shifts: 7 a.m. to 7 p.m., or 7 p.m. to 7 a.m.; three 8-hour shifts: 7 a.m. to 3 p.m., 3 p.m. to 11 p.m., or 11 p.m. to 7 a.m.)? **DAY SHIFT**	**PREFER DAYTIME WORK**	**3**
6. In which specific area in the organization would you like to work? **RECOVERY ROOM**	**LIKE TO WORK WITH PATIENTS AFTER SURGERY**	**3**
7. Do you have any convictions that would be a dealbreaker when it comes to seeking employment? **YES**	What is the source of your convictions? **RELIGIOUS**	**1**
8. Do you have any specific personality traits that are important to augment in your work area? **YES**	What are these? **CONSCIENTIOUSNESS, OPENNESS, EXTROVERSION**	**2**

Just remember that it is important to work in an area that fulfills professional goals and personal needs. This will increase your success and enjoyment as a nurse.

Professional Development

Continuing Education

Continuing education is critical for nurses to engage in as it ensures that they remain competent and up to date with practice standards and care components. Health care is continually evolving with new technologies, treatments, and care practices. In order for nurses to remain current with knowledge and skills, they must practice lifelong learning and engage in educational activities, which can include workshops, seminars, and formal education. These activities can result in additional academic degrees and certifications. These efforts allow nurses to remain current and deliver safe, high-quality patient care. Continuing education benefits not only the nurse but also patients and healthcare organizations.

Many states and nursing boards require nurses to complete a certain number and some specific types of continuing education units to maintain licensure. These courses can cover a variety of subjects, which include the latest advancements in medical treatments, patient safety protocols, and subjects, including the latest advancements in medical treatments, patient safety protocols, and leadership skills. These courses allow nurses to make informed decisions and remain current in their specific field, which is a plus when looking for employment, as these courses can be added to the professional portfolio.

Mentoring, networking, and leadership opportunities also promote professional development. Mentoring relationships allow experienced nurses to share their knowledge and insights with less experienced colleagues, fostering a culture of collaboration and continuous improvement. Networking through professional organizations provides nurses with access to a community of peers who share best practices and advocate for the profession. Leadership development helps nurses take on supervisory roles and influence healthcare policy and decision-making.

Nurses who invest in their own growth are better equipped to provide high-quality, patient-centered care, which leads to improved patient outcomes, increased job satisfaction, and lower turnover rates. Well-prepared nurses are more adept at handling complex cases and implementing innovative strategies for patient care. By making professional development a priority, nurses can ensure they remain valuable contributors to the healthcare system and the profession.

Reflective Practice

Reflective practice promotes self-assessment and improvement. Reflection allows nurses to critically examine their own practices, behaviors, and decision-making processes to identify areas for additional growth. This introspective approach helps nurses evaluate how their actions align with best practices and professional standards, fostering a deeper understanding of their strengths and weaknesses. By incorporating reflection into the daily routine, nurses can continuously refine their skills and enhance the quality of patient care they provide (Koshy et al., 2017).

There are various models (see Table 16.5) and many forms of reflective practice.

Reflective practice can include journaling to identify progress and patterns of behavior to art if it is used as a method of reviewing one's actions. Reflective practices build confidence, encourage innovation and engagement, and make you more responsible for yourself.

Reflection promotes professional development and allows nurses to engage in continuous self-improvement. It allows for the identification of gaps in knowledge and promotes proactive learning. It encourages one to view challenges and mistakes as opportunities for learning rather than failures. By incorporating reflection into practice, nurses not only enhance their own

TABLE 16.5 Models of Reflective Practice

Name	Author	Components	Comments
ERA cycle	Jasper (2013)	• Experience • Reflection • Action	The simplest model to use
Driscoll's What Model	Driscoll (1994)	• What? • So what? • Now what?	Focuses on three key questions
Kolb's experiential learning cycle	Kolb (1984)	• Concrete experience • Reflective observation • Abstract conceptualization • Active experimentation	Centers on developing understanding through actual experiences
Gibbs reflective cycle	Gibbs (1998)	• Description • Feelings • Evaluation • Analysis • Conclusion • Action plan	A more complex model

competence but also contribute to better patient care, as they are more likely to engage in critical thinking and apply evidence-based practices to improve outcomes.

Magnet Hospital Recognition Program Work Environments

One designation for excellence in organizations is the **ANCC Magnet Recognition Program** (Wolters Kluwer, 2022). This program grew out of a study to identify hospital work characteristics. The American Academy of Nursing Task Force on Nursing Practice in Hospitals conducted this study in 1983 to identify work environments that were nursing and patient care–focused. It looked to identify organizations that attracted as well as retained well-qualified nurses who promoted quality patient care. In this study, 163 hospitals participated, and of that number, 41 possessed qualities identified to have a greater capacity to attract and retain nurses. These hospitals were described as "Magnet" hospitals.

Characteristics that distinguished these 41 hospitals from their counterparts are known as the *Forces of Magnetism* (ANCC, 2022; see Table 16.6). In 1990, the American Nurses Association Board of Directors approved a proposal for the Magnet Hospital Recognition Program for Excellence in Nursing Services. This program was directly built on the 1983 study results that form the framework for the appraisal process.

TABLE 16.6 Forces of Magnetism

Force	Explanation
1. Quality of nursing leadership	Knowledgeable, strong, risk-taking nurse leaders follow a well-articulated, strategic, and visionary philosophy in the day-to-day operations of nursing services. Nursing leaders, at all organizational levels, convey a strong sense of advocacy and support for the staff and patients. The results of quality leadership are evident in nursing practice at patients' side.
2. Organizational structure	Organizational structures are generally flat rather than tall, and decentralized decision-making prevails. The organizational structure is dynamic and responsive to change. Strong nursing representation is evident in the organizational committee structure. Executive-level nursing leaders serve at the executive level of the organization. The chief nursing officer typically reports directly to the chief executive officer. The organization has a functioning and productive system of shared decision-making.

Force	Explanation
3. Management style	Healthcare organization and nursing leaders create an environment supporting participation. Feedback is encouraged, valued, and incorporated from the staff at all levels. Nurses serving in leadership positions are visible, accessible, and committed to effective communication.
4. Personnel policies and programs	Salaries and benefits are competitive. Creative and flexible staffing models that support a safe and healthy work environment are used. Personnel policies are created with direct care nurse involvement. Significant opportunities for professional growth exist in administrative and clinical tracks. Personnel policies and programs support professional nursing practice, work-life balance, and the delivery of quality care.
5. Professional models of care	There are models of care that give nurses responsibility and authority for the provision of direct patient care. Nurses are accountable for their own practice as well as the coordination of care. The models of care (i.e., primary nursing, case management, family-centered, district, and wholistic) provide for the continuity of care across the continuum. The models take into consideration patients' unique needs and provide skilled nurses and adequate resources to accomplish desired outcomes.
6. Quality of care	Quality is the systematic driving force for nursing and the organization. Nurses serving in leadership positions are responsible for providing an environment that positively influences patient outcomes. There is a pervasive perception among nurses that they provide high-quality care to patients.
7. Quality improvement	The organization possesses structures and processes for the measurement of quality and programs for improving the quality of care and services within the organization.
8. Consultation and resources	The healthcare organization provides adequate resources, support, and opportunities for the utilization of experts, particularly advanced practice nurses. The organization promotes involvement of nurses in professional organizations and among peers in the community.
9. Autonomy	Autonomous nursing care is the ability of nurses to assess and provide nursing actions as appropriate for patient care based on competence, professional expertise, and knowledge. Nurses are expected to practice autonomously, consistent with professional standards. Independent judgment is expected within the context of interdisciplinary and multidisciplinary approaches to patient/resident/client care.
10. Community and the healthcare organization	Relationships are established within and among all types of healthcare organizations and other community organizations to develop strong partnerships that support improved client outcomes and the health of the communities they serve.

(Continued)

TABLE 16.6 (Continued)

Force	Explanation
11. Nurses as teachers	Professional nurses are involved in educational activities within the organization and community. Students from a variety of academic programs are welcomed and supported in the organization; contractual arrangements are mutually beneficial.
12. Image of nursing	The services provided by nurses are characterized as essential by other members of the healthcare team. Nurses are viewed as integral to the healthcare organization's ability to provide patient care. Nursing effectively influences systemwide processes.
13. Interdisciplinary relationships	Collaborative working relationships within and among the disciplines are valued. Mutual respect is based on the premise that all members of the healthcare team make essential and meaningful contributions in the achievement of clinical outcomes. Conflict management strategies are in place and used effectively, when indicated.
14. Professional development	The healthcare organization values and supports the personal and professional growth and development of staff. In addition to quality orientation and in-service education addressed in Force 11, Nurses as teachers, emphasis is placed on career development services. Programs that promote formal education, professional certification, and career development are evident. Competency-based clinical and leadership/management development is promoted, and adequate human and fiscal resources for all professional development programs are provided.

Source: Dumpel, 2008.

Since 2008, the magnet program has evolved into five components that contain the 14 Forces of Magnetism. These components represent the framework that serves to distinguish Magnet organizations. They include the following:

1. **Transformational leadership.** Leaders are required to transform their organizations, beliefs, and behaviors. This leader leads people to where they need to be in order to meet organizational future demands. The transformational leader must have vision, influence, clinical knowledge, and strong nursing practice expertise. This component represents Forces of Magnetism 1, Quality of nursing leadership, and 3, Management style.
2. **Structural empowerment.** Solid structures developed by influential leadership provide an innovative environment in which the organizational mission, vision, and values achieve outcomes. The organization's

strategic plan, structure, systems, policies, and programs develop, direct, and empower staff to achieve desired outcomes. This component represents Forces of Magnetism 2, Organizational structure; 4, Personnel policies and programs; 10, Community and the healthcare organization; 12, Image of nursing; and 14, Professional development.

3. **Exemplary professional practice.** The essence of a Magnet organization is based on exemplary professional nursing practice. This entails role understanding; role application with patients, families, communities, and the interdisciplinary team; and new knowledge and evidence application. This component represents Forces of Magnetism 5, Professional models of care; eight, Consultation and resources; nine, Autonomy; 11, Nurses as teachers; and 13, Interdisciplinary relationships.
4. **New knowledge, innovation, and improvements.** Magnet-recognized organizations demonstrate strong leadership, empowered professionals, and exemplary practice. Magnet organizations have an ethical and professional responsibility to contribute to new knowledge, innovations, and improvements that contribute to patient care, the organization, and the profession. This component represents Force of Magnetism 7, Quality improvement.
5. **Empirical quality results.** This component represents Force of Magnetism 1, Quality of nursing leadership.

Hospitals must meet all components in order to be considered for Magnet status. Following designation, the organization must maintain quality patient care, nursing excellence, and innovations in professional nursing practice in order to meet redesignation criteria. Characteristics of these facilities include a high number of nurses with bachelor/university degrees or higher (72.39%). Many hospitals report longevity of nurses, with an average length of employment identified as 12 years. Turnover rates were 12.47%, with a clinical nurse vacancy of 2.72%. Organizations that have achieved Magnet recognition are reported to have satisfied nurses who foster collaborative environments between nurses and among other healthcare members.

Summary

Nursing is a profession of tremendous possibilities and opportunities. Knowledge of initiatives and current care activities promotes safety for patients and providers. The profession uses a dynamic process of communication that allows nurses to make a significant difference in the lives of the patients for whom they care. This unique profession is rewarding and allows growth and expansion of an individual personally and professionally. It is rewarding to hear yourself say, "I am your nurse today."

References

American Nurses Credentialing Center. (2022, May). *Characteristics of Magnet organizations.* https://www.nursingworld.org/organizational-programs/magnet/about-magnet/why-become-magnet/characteristics-of-magnet/

AMN Healthcare. (2025). *Explore top nursing jobs: Travel, per diem, and crisis.* https://www.amnhealthcare.com/careers/nursing/

Ball, W. S. (n.d.). *Build a nursing portfolio: The record of your career.* Nurse Plus Academy. https://nurse.plus/become-a-nurse/nursing-portfolio/

Cope, V., & Murray, M. (2018). Use of professional portfolios in nursing. *Nursing Standard (Royal College of Nursing (Great Britain), 32*(30), 55–63. https://doi.org/10.7748/ns.2018.e10985

Dumpel, H. (2008). *The true forces behind Magnetism: CAN/NNOC's position statement on hospital magnet status.* Joint Nursing Practice Commission. https://nostrikefornurses.wordpress.com/wp-content/uploads/2010/10/2008-05-01_cal-nurses_trueforcesofmagnetism_article11.pdf.

Koshy, K., Limb, C., Gundogan, B., Whitehurst, K., & Jafree, D. J. (2017). Reflective practice in health care and how to reflect effectively. *International Journal of Surgery Oncology, 2*(6), e20. https://doi.org/10.1097/IJ9.0000000000000020

National Council of State Boards of Nursing. (2024). *Computerized adaptive testing (CAT): A look into the NCLEX scoring method.* https://www.nclex.com/computerized-adaptive-testing.page

NCLEX. (n.d.). *Computerized adaptive testing (CAT).* https://www.nclex.com/computerized-adaptive-testing.page

ResumeGiants Team. (2024, August 5). *The professional work portfolio and how to create a great one.* https://www.resumegiants.com/blog/professional-portfolio/

Williams, M., & Jordan, K. (2007). The nursing professional portfolio: A pathway to career development. *Journal for Nurses in Staff Development, 23*(3), 125–131. https://doi.org/10.1097/01.NND.0000277181.24959.3b

Wolters Kluwer. (2022, September 13). *History of the ANCC Magnet* Recognition *Program.* https://www.wolterskluwer.com/en/expert-insights/history-of-the-magnet-recognition-program

Image Credits

Fig. 16.1: Generated using Adobe Firefly.
IMG 16.1: Generated using Adobe Firefly.

CHAPTER 17

Selected Nursing Careers

Objectives

Upon completion of this chapter, the learner will be able to do the following:

1. Explain a range of career options for nursing professionals based on educational level of entry.
2. Explore educational pathways and licensure and certification requirements for various levels of nursing.
3. Assess specific duties, responsibilities, and scopes of practice for different nursing career options.
4. Formulate a personal career development plan based on interests.

Key Chapter Terms

- Agency nurse
- Critical care nurse
- Emergency department (ED) nurse
- Flight nurse
- Geriatric nurse
- Home health nurse
- Military nurse
- Neonatal nurse
- Occupational health nurse (OHN)
- Office nurse
- Oncology nurse
- Pediatric nurse
- Perioperative nurse
- Psychiatric nurse
- Public health nurse
- School nurse
- Transplant nurse
- Trauma nurse
- Travel nurse
- Urology nurse
- Women's health nurse
- Certified registered nurse anesthetist (CRNA)
- Clinical nurse specialist

- Nursing instructor
- Forensic nurse
- Holistic nurse
- Informatics nurse
- Legal nurse
- Nurse-midwife
- Nurse practitioner
- Research nurse
- Telehealth nurse

A Nursing Career

Selecting to enter the nursing profession is just the beginning. It will take time to transition through all requirements to be licensed as a nurse (see Figure 17.1). The initials that represent licensure (*RN* [registered nurse] and *LPN* [licensed practical nurse]) can be legally used only after one has passed the licensure examination and holds a valid and current license to practice.

After graduation, it is important to determine an area of focus as a career choice. There are many areas from which to choose, and personal interests will determine the final choice. You can also transition between several nursing areas during a professional career, working in one area for several

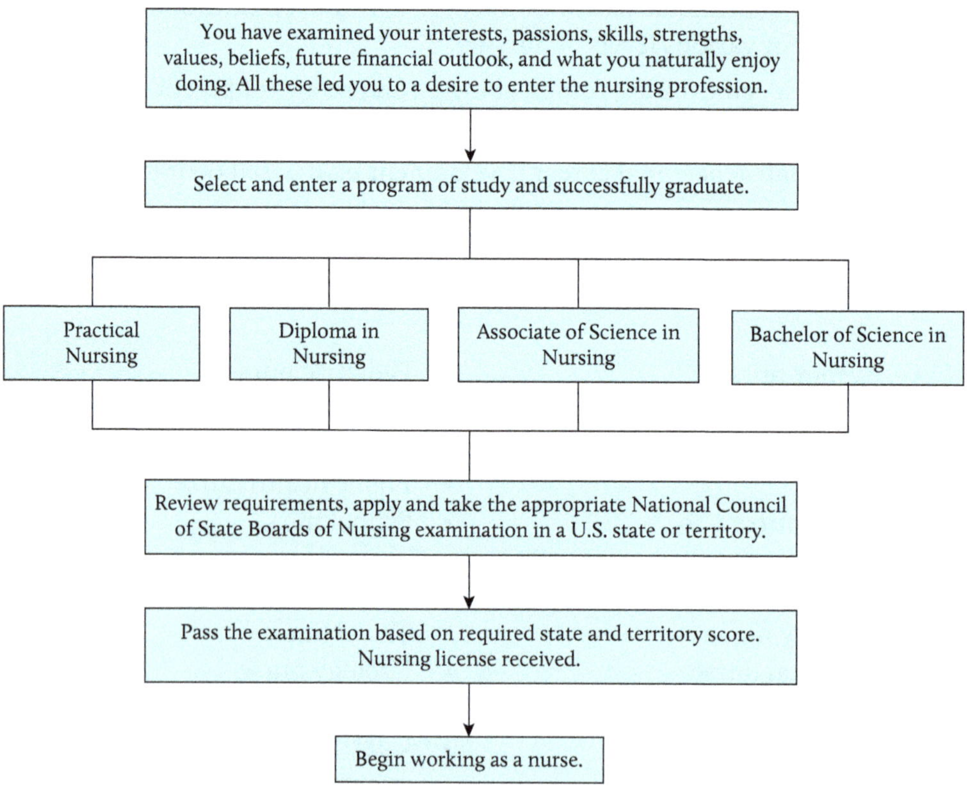

FIGURE 17.1 Transitioning to Nursing Licensure

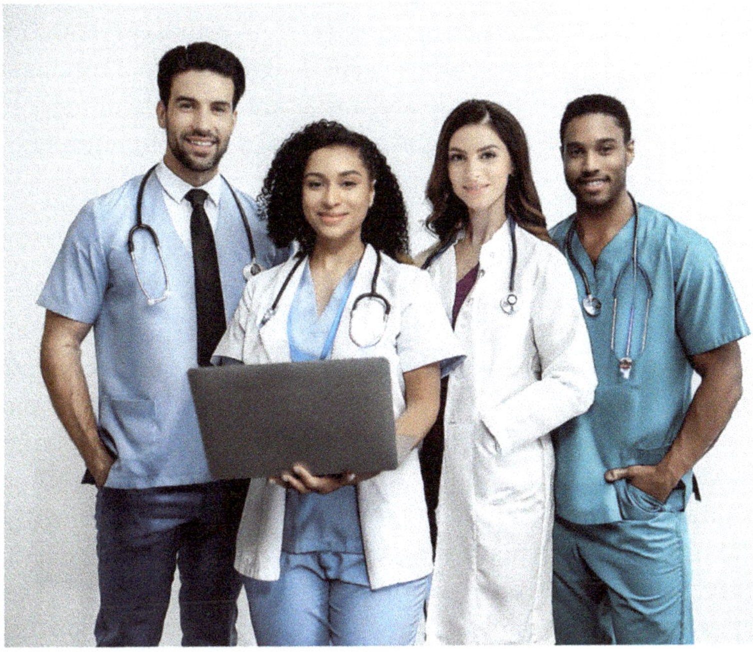

IMAGE 17.1 Various Nursing Career Options

years and then deciding, after advanced education, to focus on another. So, how do you make the first choice? Many find that clinicals during the program of study are a good place to start. Working in various focus areas while on the educational path introduces you to selecting an area as a professional choice for one's career. This chapter will introduce you to several options for career choices.

Select Nursing Career Options

Nursing offers a variety of professional pathways. Upon completion of a nursing educational program, it is important to select an employment area of interest, one that you feel can promote the best process for socialization into the profession. Many new graduates start out in hospitals in an area of interest. As you progress through the years of educational preparation, it is important to identify areas with which you find a match—the ones that just feel right. This can give you a clue regarding areas that may be a good personal and professional complement.

Organizations differ, and all career options are not available in all institutions. Some companies validate the expertise of individuals who apply for work through an agency. Some require satisfactory demonstration of knowledge, such as acquiring a specific score on a pharmacology test or an assessment that evaluates basic nursing care. As your experience and education increase, your career options expand significantly. This chapter will give you an introduction to some areas that are available to new-graduate nurses. It is not a complete listing of all potential areas in nursing.

Potential Career Options for New Graduates

Agency Nursing

Nurses who work in agencies register or sign up for a specific company that is usually outside of a healthcare organization. The company will designate areas of potential work based on experience. As an **agency nurse**, you may work in one of several healthcare organizations (e.g., clinic, acute care hospital, extended care facility, rehabilitation hospital) with which the company has a contractual agreement to supply nurses at times of shortage (e.g., employees on vacation, maternity leave, illness). These jobs are temporary and can range from a few days to several months. As an agency employee, you are paid directly by the company. It is important to familiarize yourself with policies and procedures for both the company and organization. If you travel to other parts of the country or world, this is called *travel nursing*.

Critical Care Nursing

Critical care nurses provide care for patients who are acutely and critically ill. Knowledge of advanced care management usually requires extended orientation times for organizations who hire new graduates into this area. Orientation to work as a critical care nurse may be from six months to one year in order to build knowledge and confidence to manage patients experiencing life-threatening situations (e.g., cardiac or respiratory arrest). More specific areas in critical care include those specifically devoted to care of cardiac patients (coronary care unit), surgical patients (surgical intensive care unit [ICU]), and neurological patients (neurological ICU), among others. Additional information can be obtained from the American Association of Critical Care Nurses (AACN) at https://www.aacn.org/.

Emergency Department Nursing

Nurses who work in the ED see patients who present due to various complications, from minor complications to life-threatening ones. As an **ED nurse,** one must be able to quickly assess patients, provide independent and interdependent interventions, and evaluate patient outcomes. Nurses work with patients and families as they experience illness, injury, and crisis. This area can be a high-intensity area in which to work. Some EDs manage trauma patients who arrive in critical condition by helicopter and require intense life-saving measures. Additional information can be obtained from the Emergency Nurses Association at https://www.ena.org.

Flight Nursing

Flight nurses are RNs with intensive/critical care nursing experience as well as emergency nursing. This type of care deals with patients who have a variety of emergencies under some very difficult situations. Transport may require initial treatment in remote areas under treacherous conditions in various parts of the country. Collaborative patient management may include teams of nurses and physicians while in flight as well as ground healthcare members. Flight nurses respond to transport critically injured individuals by helicopter or plane to trauma centers. These critical patients are aggressively managed during transport. Flight nurses are key members of medical disaster teams. Additional information can be obtained from the Air & Surface Transport Nurses Association at https://www.astna.org/.

Geriatric Nursing

Geriatric nurses care for older patients in a number of settings, which include patients' home, extended care facilities, and hospitals. Geriatric nurses work to improve overall health and quality of life for older individuals while working to maintain independent care. They work directly with patients who are experiencing health concerns that are age-related. Many older patients have multiple complex disease processes that pose a challenge to this type of nursing care. Patient education and management of care are essential to this population. Geriatric nurses are committed to providing high-quality, culturally sensitive care. Additional information can be obtained from the American Geriatrics Society at https://www.americangeriatrics.org/.

Home Health Nursing

Home health nurses provide intermittent care services to patients at home. These nurses travel to urban and rural sites to give care to individuals who do not require institutional care on a constant basis. Home health nurses work with individuals who are being managed at home due to illness, accident, or childbirth. These may be individuals who are restricted to their homes and cannot travel for care. Home health nurses work collaboratively with other care providers and may directly supervise assistants. Additional information can be obtained from the National Alliance for Care at Home (the Alliance) at https://allianceforcareathome.org/.

Military Nursing

Military nurses work in a variety of settings, ranging from providing family practice at a homeland military base to providing emergency care for the wounded in the field during time of war. All services currently have a branch that includes nurses. These branches are called *corps*. A *corps* is a military command whose members share a common mission and are grouped together. These nurses serve in the military and hold military rank. Military nurses serve in the U.S. Army, Navy, Air Force, and Coast Guard. Additional information can be obtained about the U.S. Army Nurse Corps from https://www.registerednursing.org/military/army-nurse-corps/, the Navy Nurse Corps Association from https://www.nnca.org/, the Air Force Nurse Corps from https://www.airforcemedicine.af.mil/About-Us/Medical-Branches/Nurse-Corps/, and the Coast Guard from https://www.gocoastguard.com/careers/officer/healthcare.

Neonatal Nursing

Neonatal nurses provide care for newborn infants until they are discharged from the hospital while supporting the family. The neonatal period is usually considered the first month of life, but neonatal nurses may work with newborns who are sick for several months. Neonatal nurses must have astute assessment skills and knowledge of the care required for well and ill infants. Some organizations assess nursing skill abilities and pharmacological skills, including medication calculation, knowledge of intravenous lines, and cardiopulmonary resuscitation (CPR) in the newborn population following an extensive orientation period. Neonatal nurses critically assess the patient to ensure good health and provide preventive care to prevent illness and care for ill infants. Neonatal nurses are responsible for anticipating, preventing, diagnosing, and minimizing illness in newborns. There are various levels of the nurseries in which neonatal nurses may work. These include Level I: well newborn nursery, Level II: special care nursery, Level III: neonatal intensive care unit (NICU), and Level IV: regional NICU. Additional information can be obtained from the National Association of Neonatal Nurses at https://www.nann.org/.

Occupational Health Nursing

Occupational health nurses (OHNs) are also called *employee health nurses* and *health promotion nurses*, among other names that may be specific to an organization. This type of nurse is responsible for maintaining the health and wellness of employees in an organization. They focus on the health, safety, and productivity of employees. They not only treat illnesses that affect employee productivity but are often responsible for maintaining wellness programs and activities for a business. Depending on the employer, OHNs may provide emergency care, prepare accident reports, and arrange for further care if necessary. They can offer health counseling, assist with health examinations and immunizations, and assess work environments to identify potential health or safety problems. OHNs are responsible for improving, protecting, maintaining, and restoring the health of employees. By providing this care, OHNs are able to influence the health of the business. Additional information can be obtained from the American Association of Occupational Health Nurses at https://www.aaohn.org/.

Office Nursing

Office nurses may also be called *medical assistants*. Office nurses are responsible for assisting in the delivery of health care and patient care management based on the specific office specialty, which is governed by the physician or nurse practitioner. This includes retrieval of historical information that can assist in physician management. Office nurses obtain vital signs and other laboratory or demographic patient information (e.g., height, weight). They can assist in the preparation of patients for examination. They also perform activities to facilitate care, which can include administering injections; assisting with minor surgical procedures, wound care, biopsy, or skin removal; drawing blood for laboratory tests; and performing electrocardiograms, based on practice specialty. Patient education, connecting with patients for follow-up to evaluate patient status after procedures, and scheduling future appointments may also be part of their responsibilities. Administrative tasks can include managing office supplies, budgeting, addressing patient concerns, ensuring accurate recordkeeping, and developing and implementing nursing office policies.

Oncology Nursing

Oncology nurses provide health care for cancer patients of all ages and during all stages of treatment, from diagnosis to remission or death (Rieger & Yarbro, 2003). The spectrum of care these nurses provide includes direct care delivery to the education of patients and families. Oncology nurses not only focus on patient physical needs but also on patients' emotional status. They assess patients' understanding of their disease process and proposed treatment options to allay anxiety and facilitate their involvement in care plan development. Oncology nurses also work to coordinate care between the many healthcare team members who may be necessary to promote quality of life for the oncology patient. They work to develop treatment plans with realistic goals and objectives for patient outcomes and are usually involved in patient education to assist with management of the side effects of interventions for patients' specific type of cancer treatment. Additional information can be obtained from the Oncology Nursing Society at https://www.ons.org/.

Pediatric Nursing

Pediatric nurses care for infants, children, and adolescents in all aspects of health care (Harrison, 2010). This care is specialized because this is a unique population with different needs. Pediatric nurses must deal with growth and development as well as illness and injury. They must be familiar with laws governing confidentiality and disclosure of information for adolescents, which can vary by state. They must be skilled at communicating and working with children to reduce confusion and fear. Pediatric nurses work with families as well as infants, children, and adolescents. They also serve as educators to families in an effort to promote wellness in children. Pediatric nurses practice in a variety of settings, including hospitals, clinics, schools, and the home. Additional information can be obtained from the Society of Pediatric Nurses at https://www.pedsnurses.org/.

Perioperative Nursing

Perioperative nurses work in preoperative, intraoperative, and postoperative areas in tertiary care hospitals, community and rural hospitals, day surgery units, and specialized clinics with a multidisciplinary team of healthcare providers. They often provide total care in preoperative and postoperative areas. Perioperative nurses may have specialized positions in the operative suite and serve as scrub nurses or individuals who are dressed to handle sterile instruments and supplies and pass them to the surgeon during the actual procedure or as circulating nurses who work outside the sterile field, serve to manage overall patient care, and help maintain a safe, comfortable patient environment. Preoperative functions of perioperative nurses are aimed at preparing the patient for a surgical procedure, and postoperative functions deal with patient care following the procedure. This is the recovery phase of care through discharge to a specific care area or home. Additional information can be obtained from the Association of periOperative Registered Nurses at https://www.aorn.org/.

Psychiatric Nursing

Psychiatric nurses serve as integral members of a mental health interdisciplinary team for patient management. They provide care for patients and families with acute or chronic psychiatric and mental illnesses. This complex type of care requires nurses to administer medications, monitor treatment interventions, and be an active participant in patients' treatment plan. Psychiatric nurses can work within institutions to reduce aggression and promote safety to include "preventative assessment through observations, consumer engagement, and medication management, as well as promoting the use of emotional regulation skills with service users" (Hurley et al., 2022, p. 800). They promote suicide prevention and serve in the provision of psychotherapy for individuals with complex and challenging psychiatric needs. This nursing role can include complex assessment to support physical health promotion and maintenance. These nurses practice in a variety of settings, such as hospitals and mental health institutions. Additional information can be obtained from the American Psychiatric Nurses Association at https://www.apna.org/.

Public Health Nursing

Public health nurses provide comprehensive nursing services in preventive health, home health, and clinic programs to individuals, families, and communities. They work with entire populations improving health and preventing disease. They travel to patient homes in urban and rural settings to collect referral information and conduct home visits to determine client needs. Public health nurses develop individualized plans of care based on needs assessments and manage and coordinate community services to provide a multidisciplinary approach to resolution of needs. They work with individuals, families, and communities to find viable, accessible solutions to community health concerns. They identify health risks that may be unique to specific populations; educate and provide services to at-risk and vulnerable populations; and advocate for access to health services for vulnerable populations with local, state, and federal authorities. They work with local resources, expressing community health concerns to local health planners and policymakers, and assist members of the community to voice their own problems and concerns. Additional information can be obtained from the Association of Public Health Nurses at https://www.phnurse.org/.

School Nursing

School nurses work with students and school faculty, providing health care and other support in an in-school environment. The work setting extends from elementary school to university-level education. School nurses manage all student and faculty situations, which includes monitoring the environment for diseases, administering medications, assessing and intervening for illnesses and injuries, collaborating with other healthcare professionals to promote the health and educational success of students, and providing leadership and education in promoting nursing as a profession in the school environment. They also serve as health educators to promote childhood self-management of chronic diseases. School nurses work with employees and set up wellness programs for health maintenance. Additional information can be obtained from the National Association of School Nurses at https://www.nasn.org/.

Transplant Nursing

Transplant nurses work in a variety of settings and function in one of the two main areas of transplant: procurement and clinical. Procurement involves actual organ retrieval. These nurses work with an organ procurement agency and are members of an interdisciplinary team. They usually have a background in critical care. Transplant nurses coordinate care to optimize harvesting (retrieval) of various organs, functioning as a liaison to promote the best results for retrieval and delivery to patients waiting to receive an organ. Various body parts that may be retrieved for transplant include but are not limited to the liver, kidney, pancreas, corneas, heart, and lungs. Clinical positions may be nurses with skill and managerial experience. This area of transplant requires individuals to have good problem-solving skills, be detail-oriented, be able to multitask effectively, be self-motivated, and have excellent verbal and written communications skills due to the intense emotional nature of the job. Additional information can be obtained from the International Transplant Nurses Society at https://www.itns.org/.

Trauma Nursing

Trauma nurses care for patients in EDs or critical care settings who are experiencing the results of a life-threatening traumatic situation. These nurses generally care for patients who have suffered severe trauma, such as motor vehicle accidents, gunshot wounds, stabbings, assaults, or other traumatic injuries. They triage patients and administer life-saving interventions, including CPR. Trauma nurses provide compassionate care to family members as they deal with the challenging and traumatic event experienced by their loved one (Walter & Curtis, 2015). This area of nursing is high-intensity and requires immediate assessment, intervention, and evaluation on a continuous basis. Patient stabilization is a multidisciplinary team effort. These nurses need good communication skills to deal with family members during this highly emotionally charged time. Additional information can be obtained from the Society of Trauma Nurses at https://www.traumanurses.org/.

Travel Nursing

Travel nurses work for an agency and take travel assignments inside or outside of the United States. In this country, they can work in local hospitals on a shift assignment or in hospitals across the country for several months. Time periods can vary greatly. They work in hospitals that are usually experiencing an extreme nursing shortage, and working conditions can vary greatly from one assignment to the next. Travel nurses are usually highly paid and enjoy generous benefits, which can include sign-on bonuses and paid housing while on assignment since their services are in high demand. They may work flexible schedules in any specialty area for which they are qualified, which can encompass EDs, critical care units, postoperative care units, surgical areas, pediatrics, and any other nursing specialty. Additional information can be obtained from the American Travel Health Nurses Association at https://www.athna.org/.

Urology Nursing

Urology nurses provide guidance and treatment for all individuals across the lifespan in the specialty of urology (deals with the urinary system). They work in a variety of settings, from offices to clinics, retrieving patient historical information, performing examinations, interpreting diagnostic studies, and managing bladder diseases that cause dysfunction and incontinence. These include cancer, infertility, incontinence, plastic surgery, and urological repair, among others. Many nurses care for patients with end-stage renal disease, which requires that they be knowledgeable regarding hemodialysis, peritoneal dialysis, continuous renal replacement therapy, and transplant. Urology nurses are also focused on patient education, so they need good communication skills, since this system can be personal and intimate to individuals. Additional information can be obtained from the American Nephrology Nurses' Association at https://www.annanurse.org and the Society of Urologic Nurses and Associates at https://www.suna.org.

Women's Health

Women's health nurses work to facilitate health promotion and disease prevention of women in various healthcare settings. These nurses work with women in all stages of life and must adjust to incorporate family and community, since these issues affect women emotionally and psychologically. Women's health nurses work with women in obstetrics and gynecology and with health promotion activities (e.g., mammograms, Pap tests), reproductive health, and other general health issues that affect women. Nurses work to initiate gender-focused assessments and interventions. Patient education and follow-up are key components in this type of nursing. Additional information can be obtained from the AWHONN at https://www.awhonn.org/.

Nursing Career Options That Require Advanced Practice Status or Additional Education

Advanced practice nurses (APNs) have a minimum of a master's degree in nursing. These career options are marked with an asterisk* for ease of identification. Other careers require additional continuing education programs and training.

Anesthesia—Certified Registered Nurse Anesthetist*

CRNAs are APNs who specialize in anesthesia care for individuals of all ages. They collaborate with anesthesiologists, surgeons, and other healthcare professionals to deliver anesthesia for medical and surgical procedures in hospital, clinic, and office settings. They can work in specific areas, such as hospital or outpatient surgical centers, labor and delivery units, critical care units, EDs, the military, and various physician specialty offices (e.g., plastic surgeons, dentists, ophthalmologists, pain management). They administer and maintain anesthesia, monitor patients during surgical procedures, and oversee recovery from anesthesia. CRNAs manage anesthesia needs during all phases of patient care delivery. They interact with multiple care providers, patients, and families. Additional information can be obtained from the American Association of Nurse Anesthetists at https://www.aana.com/.

Clinical Nurse Specialist*

Clinical nurse specialists use case management as a collaborative interdisciplinary process for patient care. They diagnose, prescribe, and treat patients and specialty or subspecialty populations within their area of preparation across the continuum of care. Clinical nurse specialists can work in several roles that can include clinical practice, consulting, management, teaching, or research. They are skilled at using assessment, planning, facilitation, and advocacy for exercising options and services to meet individual health needs in inpatient and outpatient settings. These individually designed healthcare programs efficiently use available resources to promote quality cost-effective outcomes. Additional information can be obtained from the National Association of Clinical Nurse Specialists at https://www.nacns.org/.

Instructor/Professor*—Schools/Colleges of Nursing

Nursing instructors have advanced education in a specialty area. These individuals either are baccalaureate-prepared, have a master's degree, or are doctorally prepared and teach in areas of nursing based on their earned degree. These areas can include any course in a nursing program that is didactic (i.e., in a classroom) or clinically based. Academic programs usually require that in order to teach, nurses must have a degree one level higher than the level at which they teach (e.g., individuals teaching in a practical nursing program must have the minimum of a bachelor's degree, those teaching in a baccalaureate program must have the minimum of a master's degree, and those teaching in a master's program must have the minimum of a doctorate). Faculty must remain current in order to teach appropriate, relevant information that will assist new graduates to National Council Licensure Examination for Registered Nurses or National Council Licensure Examination for Practical Nurses success and effective transitioning to a new job. There are several organizations that promote nursing education. These include the AACN at https://www.aacn.nche.edu/, National League for Nursing at https://www.nln.org/, American Nurses Association at https://www.nursingworld.org/, and National Consortium of Academic Nurse Educators, Inc., at https://nc-ane.org/.

Forensic Nursing

Forensic nurses work in hospitals, coroner's offices, medical examiner offices, psychiatric hospitals, and community antiviolence programs. They work in a variety of fields and specialize in providing care for victims and perpetrators of crime. Forensic nurses specialize as sexual assault nurse examiners and work in areas such as sexual assault, child abuse and neglect, elder abuse, domestic violence, and death investigations. They work in corrections and can be seen working in the aftermath of mass disasters or in community crises. They collect evidence after crimes occur and provide medical care to patients within the prison system. They also provide education regarding such topics as human trafficking and mental health awareness. They are an integral part of the legal system and provide consultation to both medical and legal organizations. Forensic nurses help law enforcement build cases against suspected criminals and serve as expert witnesses in court trials. Additional information can be obtained from the International Association of Forensic Nurses at https://www.forensicnurses.org/.

Holistic Nursing

Holistic nurses engage in providing care that addresses all areas of care and incorporates traditional and alternative medicine (e.g., massage, music therapy, acupressure, therapeutic touch, guided imagery, relaxation). Holistic nurses focus on the principle that the whole person must be considered in order to effectively treat an individual (Covington, 2003). This includes physiological, psychological, and sociological factors. Holistic nurses provide care that incorporates patients' health beliefs and values. They integrate self-care, spirituality, and reflection into their daily nursing care activities to promote wellness that incorporates the whole person (body, mind, and spirit). Additional information can be obtained from the American Holistic Nurses Association at https://www.ahna.org/.

Informatics Nursing*

Informatics nursing combines nursing with information technology. This specialty integrates nursing science with information. This promotes their technology leveraging and data transformation into information to improve health and healthcare equity, safety, quality, and outcomes. They manage data repositories that may contain confidential patient information. They promote information retrieval from the organization to the end-user to assist in the delivery of patient care. **Informatics nurses** work closely with users of clinical information systems within an organization. They serve a key role in planning initiatives that relate to nurse-based systems or other software or hardware components that interface with these systems. They evaluate clinical information systems from the user's perspective in order to manage workflow in collaboration with organizational project managers and directors. They work to verify that information systems are clinically applicable and consistent with professional nursing standards. Their role is expanding as AI evolves (Nashwan et al., 2025). Additional information can be obtained from the American Nursing Informatics Association at https://www.ania.org/ and the Alliance for Nursing Informatics at https://www.allianceni.org/.

Legal Nursing

Legal nursing combines law and nursing. Attorneys rarely have knowledge of medical terminology, and, when dealing with medical malpractice and personal injury cases, they require assistance in reviewing patient chart information. **Legal nurses** assist with translating medical records, validating the significance and appropriateness of nursing interventions, and managing other healthcare issues. Many legal nurses have several years of experience and advanced degrees (master's degree or doctorate), which adds credibility to their testimony as expert witnesses regarding the standards and guidelines for care. They assist with identifying strategies for resolutions in healthcare cases, educate attorneys in differentiating key facts from general information, interview witnesses, draft legal documents, and provide support during legal proceedings. Additional information can be obtained from the American Association of Legal Nurse Consultants at https://www.aalnc.org/.

Nurse-Midwives*

Nurse-midwives have an advanced degree that has prepared them to deal specifically with childbirth and prenatal and postpartum care. They manage the physical, emotional, and mental state of mothers throughout the birthing process and work to reduce the use of adjunction devices or medications. Nurse-midwives work with women throughout labor and delivery (Combellick et al., 2023). They deal with the natural birthing process only and are not qualified to perform a cesarean section, should one be required. Following delivery, they perform postpartum examinations to validate the health status of mothers and babies. They may work in a clinic, alone, or as a member of a group of nurse-midwives in collaboration with a physician. They perform postpartum visits and educate mothers to promote ongoing health. Additional information can be obtained from the American College of Nurse-Midwives at https://www.midwife.org/.

Nurse Practitioner*

Nurse practitioners are APNs who have completed education at the master's or doctoral level. They can deliver primary care delivery for individuals throughout the lifespan (Savard et al., 2023). They can diagnose, treat (including prescribing medications), consult, and provide follow-up and referral for a variety of disease processes. Some can perform limited procedures, such as suturing open wounds. They educate patients and families about preventive care and treatments. They may work in clinics, offices, or hospitals, in some states. They may also work independently or interdependently. They can participate in the care of inpatient and outpatients. They are responsible for patient record accuracy and managing records according to standards and policies. There are many different types of nurse practitioners, including family, pediatric, adult, geriatric, women's health care, neonatal, acute care, and occupational health. Additional information can be obtained from the American Association of Nurse Practitioners at https://www.aanp.org/ .

Research Nursing

Research nurses work in hospitals or other companies with strong research initiatives (e.g., pharmaceutical companies, medical technology companies). They perform both clinical and basic research to develop a research or evidence-based approach to patient management. Research nurses need a good background in assessment and patient management in order to make changes to the plan of care based on patient responses and stabilize patient parameters that may result from side effects of the research intervention. They develop plans of care and treatment protocols that incorporate components of the research process and monitor patient responses to interventions. They work with individuals across the lifespan and with all types of illnesses in an effort to improve quality of life. Their research can focus on pain management, reduction of risks for disease and disability, and promotion of a healthy lifestyle in individuals with chronic diseases. Additional information can be obtained from the Western Institute of Nursing at https://www.winursing.org/, Midwest Nursing Research Society at https://www.mnrs.org/, Southern Nursing Research Society at https://snrs.org, Eastern Nursing Research Society at https://www.enrs-go.org/, International Association of Clinical Research Nurses at https://iacrn.org/, and National Institute of Nursing Research at https://www.ninr.nih.gov/.

Telehealth Nursing

Telehealth nurses are RNs who use telecommunication technologies to assess, triage, diagnose, and treat patients (Bulto, 2024). They use remote technologies to collect detailed information such as blood pressure, heart rate, and electrocardiograms. Telehealth nurses manage patients with chronic conditions and heart disease and offer education to promote maintaining health. Technologies include telephones or videoconferencing platforms (e.g., smartphones, tablets, computers) as well as kiosks and digital platforms that are compliant with maintaining patient information security. Through the provision of telehealth, these nurses can provide convenient care to individuals in remote locations without the need for patient travel. Telehealth nurses require the same education, training, and expertise as nurses providing in-person care. These nurses must have excellent verbal and listening communication skills for remote patient interactions. They must also have a comfort level with the use of technology for providing care. Additional information can be obtained from the Telehealth Nursing Practice Special Interest Group at https://www.aaacn.org/get-involved/special-interest-groups/telehealth-nursing-practice, International Society for Telemedicine & eHealth at https://isfteh.org/, and American Telemedicine Association at https://www.americantelemed.org/.

Summary

Nursing is a career of immense challenges and joys. It requires continued learning and effort to give the highest level of nursing care to individuals, families, and communities. Regardless of the type of nursing you decide to pursue, it will give you years of personal and professional satisfaction.

TABLE 17.1 Lifelong Learning Options

Lifelong Learning Method for Professional Growth	Advantage	YES, this option is for me.	NO, this option is not for me.
Going back to school for additional formal education	Offers the potential to earn a higher degree		
Acquiring a certification	Displays excellence in a specific area of nursing		
Joining a professional organization	Promotes collaborative and peer relationships with likeminded professionals		
Attending conferences and workshops	Allows in-person collaboration and networking		
Using self-paced online continuing education activities	Allows for flexible time management of learning activity		
Reading online articles in peer-reviewed journals to stay up to date	Allows for flexible time management of learning activity		
Using validated web-based videos/podcasts on specific procedures or healthcare activities	Allows for validation of information and flexible time management of learning activity		
Participating in a work-related project for patient care enhancement	Promotes a collaborative work environment		
Assisting a colleague in learning or perfecting a nursing skill	Promotes understanding, reinforces knowledge, and contributes to a collaborative learning environment in the work setting; improves self-confidence		
Adding a new skill to your professional list during employment (e.g., learning a new piece of equipment, focusing on interpretation of new technology results for patient care)	Expands your skillset, adds to your organizational value, promotes technological literacy, and potentially adds to skill transferability		
Participating in an internship program	Provides mentorship, offers firsthand experience, expands professional opportunities, and promotes personal growth		
Continually learning by finding learning opportunities in everyday work activities	Allows for multimodal adaptive learning; promotes learner autonomy		

Lifelong learning is self-initiated for personal and professional development. It is an intentional opportunity for self-growth. Be intentional, be deliberate, and set aside 15 to 30 minutes per week to engage in activities to promote learning. It is important to adhere to making time for learning. Set reminders on a calendar to promote maintaining your commitment to learn and grow. Knowing lifelong learning options is important to move toward achieving personal goals and objectives. Use Table 17.1 to identify which lifelong learning options you identify as appealing. Future planning is also a way to stay on track to success. Complete Figure 17.2 to identify future requirements and intentions related to your licensure path. These can help you in formulating a plan for future success.

Happy learning!

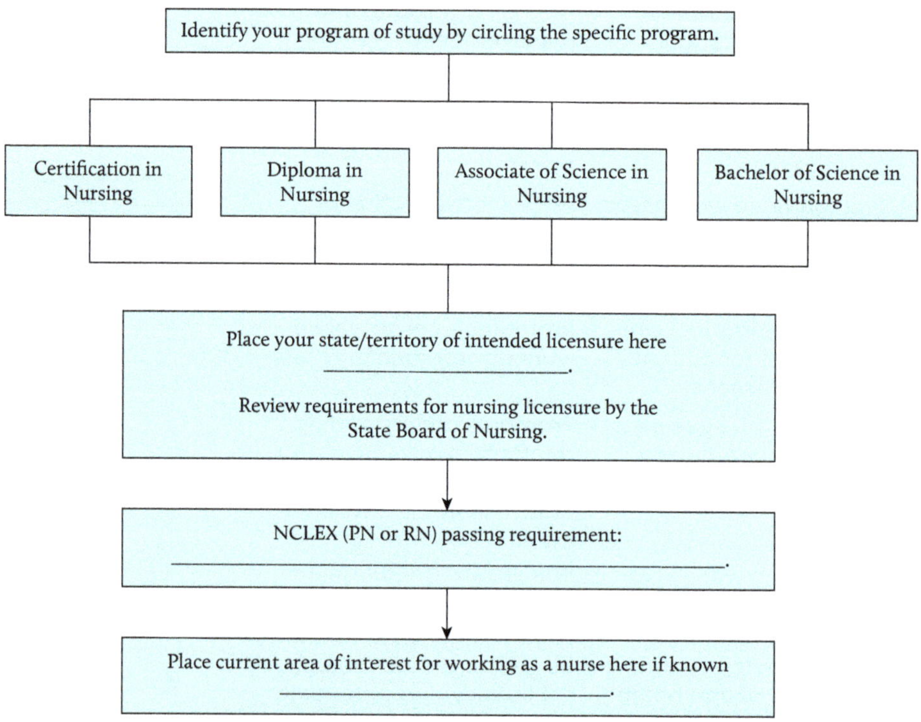

FIGURE 17.2 My Personal Licensure Path

References

Bulto L. N. (2024). The role of nurse-led telehealth interventions in bridging healthcare gaps and expanding access. *Nursing Open*, *11*(1), e2092. https://doi.org/10.1002/nop2.2092

Combellick, J. L., Telfer, M. L., Ibrahim, B. B., Novick, G., Morelli, E. M., James-Conterelli, S., & Kennedy, H. P. (2023). Midwifery care during labor and birth in the United States. *American Journal of Obstetrics and Gynecology, 228*(5S), S983–S993. https://doi.org/10.1016/j.ajog.2022.09.044

Covington H. (2003). Caring presence. Delineation of a concept for holistic nursing. *Journal of Holistic Nursing, 21*(3), 301–317. https://doi.org/10.1177/0898010103254915

Harrison T. M. (2010). Family-centered pediatric nursing care: state of the science. *Journal of Pediatric Nursing, 25*(5), 335–343. https://doi.org/10.1016/j.pedn.2009.01.006

Hurley, J., Lakeman, R., Linsley, P., Ramsay, M., & Mckenna-Lawson, S. (2022). Utilizing the mental health nursing workforce: A scoping review of mental health nursing clinical roles and identities. *International Journal of Mental Health Nursing, 31*(4), 796–822. https://doi.org/10.1111/inm.12983

Nashwan, A. J., Cabrega, J. A., Othman, M. I., Khedr, M. A., Osman, Y. M., El-Ashry, A. M., Naif, R., & Mousa, A. A. (2025). The evolving role of nursing informatics in the era of artificial intelligence. *International Nursing Review, 72*(1), e13084. https://doi.org/10.1111/inr.13084

Rieger, P. T., & Yarbro, C. H. (2003). Role of the oncology nurse. In D. W. Kufe, R. E. Pollock, R. R. Weichselbaum, R. Bast, T. S. Gansler, J. F. Holland, & E. Frei (Eds.), *Cancer Medicine* (6th ed.). BC Decker. https://www.ncbi.nlm.nih.gov/books/NBK13570/

Savard, I., Al Hakim, G., & Kilpatrick, K. (2023). The added value of the nurse practitioner: An evolutionary concept analysis. *Nursing Open, 10*(4), 2540–2551. https://doi.org/10.1002/nop2.1512

Walter, E., & Curtis, K. (2015). The role and impact of the specialist trauma nurse: An integrative review. *Journal of Trauma Nursing, 22*(3), 153–169. https://doi.org/10.1097/JTN.0000000000000126

Image Credits

IMG 17.1: Generated using Adobe Firefly.

CHAPTER 18

Nursing's Future

The Road Ahead

Objectives

Upon completion of this chapter, the learner will be able to do the following:

1. Discuss expanding roles and responsibilities of nurses.
2. Assess key nursing challenges, which include workforce shortages and burnout.
3. Evaluate strategies to create a positive workforce environment and address incivility and bullying.
4. Identify methods to navigate changes in health care related to policy implementation, varying technologies, and practice methodologies.

Key Chapter Terms

- Systemic change
- Community engagement
- Public health
- Culturally competent care
- Workforce diversity
- Data-driven solutions
- Technology integration
- Nursing leadership
- Collaborative interdisciplinary care
- Incivility
- Bullying
- Burnout
- Positive workforce environment

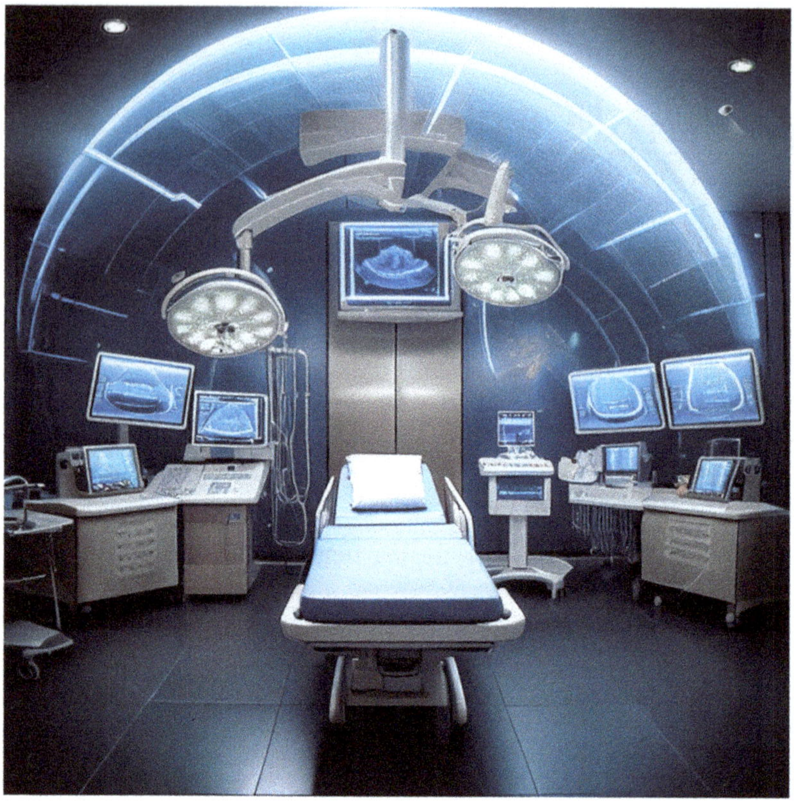

IMAGE 18.1 Futuristic View

Nursing's Future: The Road Ahead

It is difficult to envision what nursing will evolve to encompass from its past, but it will surely be an exciting and forward-moving profession. Lifelong learning through advanced educational endeavors by individuals in the profession will need to be continuous in order to address issues from a higher educational plane. Nurses will need to achieve advanced degrees to claim their rights to be at the decision-making table. As more nurses successfully achieve doctoral degrees, this trend will benefit the profession in several areas, from education to political activism.

Nursing professionalization has certainly found its niche in evidence-based patient management, and it continues to move in this direction. Nursing researchers have evolved and continue to develop foundational theoretical perspectives that give recognition to the science of nursing. They continue to study concepts related to the phenomenon of concern to nursing from a quantitative and qualitative perspective. These include research of numbers that relate to care (quantitative research) as well as attitudes that are holistic in nature (qualitative research). Results of these types of research ensure that the nursing profession will have a scientific base for care compassion and competence in patient management.

Nurses play a central role in shaping the future of healthcare systems. Their active engagement will contribute to creating a more just, inclusive, and equitable environment for all individuals and communities. The future of nursing will be characterized by expanding roles and responsibilities that promote systemic change and improvement. Key areas of focus include public health, cultural competence, nursing education, research and data-driven practice, technological advancement, leadership, and interdisciplinary collaboration, each interrelated and essential to the profession's continued evolution (see Figure 18.1). The following sections explore these emerging areas in greater depth and examine their collective impact on the nursing profession.

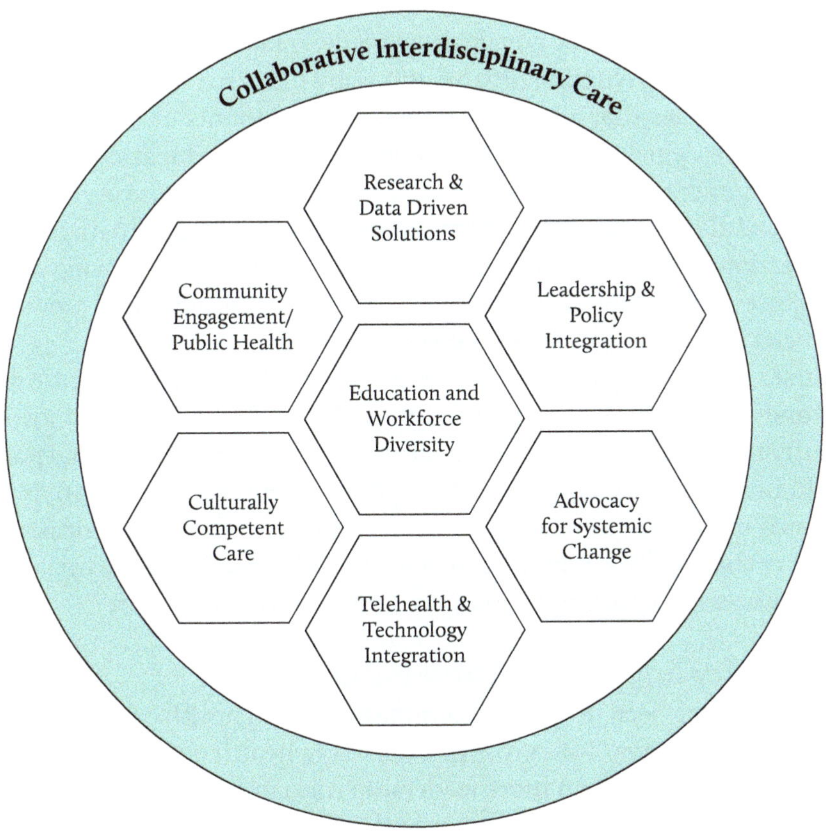

FIGURE 18.1 Future Components of the Nursing Profession

Advocacy for Systemic Change

Nursing is a values-based profession committed to high-quality patient care. The profession values the holistic nature of people and fosters health promotion across the lifespan. Nurses identify the importance of all people having a fair and equal opportunity to receive health care. Nurses are at the forefront of healthcare delivery with their first-line contact with patients and families. They can witness firsthand the impact of systemic inequities in the healthcare environment. As a result, they can effectively identify components of health equity that need to be addressed. This allows nurses to proactively and effectively advocate for policies that promote health equity and address underlying factors that contribute to disparities. Activities to accomplish this include lobbying for better healthcare access, more inclusive insurance policies, and increased funding for preventive care and community health initiatives.

In the future, nurses will be increasingly involved in leadership roles within health policy organizations. These roles will allow nurses to contribute their insights to create healthcare policies that are more equitable and inclusive. This will allow them to be engaged with policymakers to get nursing issues on a policy agenda. Nursing organizations are likely to continue advocating for health policies that address the social determinants of health (SDOH), ensuring that legislative priorities include housing, education, nutrition, and environmental factors that affect health outcomes. These organizations can extend the reach of individual nurses. Nurses can use their collective organizational voice to influence policymakers to focus on removing barriers that affect underserved communities. Nurses' presence in these arenas will be crucial to driving **systemic changes**.

Nurses will be key players in ensuring that health equity policies are developed and implemented starting at the ground level. This will require advocacy not just at the macro level but also micro-involvement in institutional policies within hospitals, clinics, and health systems (Scott & Scott, 2021). Nurses will need to work with other healthcare professionals and administrators to ensure that health equity is embedded in daily practice, including patient intake processes, treatment protocols, and resource allocation.

Community Engagement and Public Health

Nurses have long been involved in community-based health care, particularly in underserved areas. Their role in promoting health equity will continue to expand as they take on more leadership roles in community health programs. This involves working directly with vulnerable populations, providing education and preventive services, and promoting connections to healthcare resources. Community health nursing will be essential in reaching populations who are traditionally marginalized by the healthcare system, including people living in rural areas, low-income families, and communities of color.

Health literacy is a critical aspect of **community engagement**. Nurses are instrumental in educating individuals and families about managing chronic conditions, understanding medical instructions, and making informed health decisions. With the rise of chronic diseases and complex healthcare systems, the role of nurses in simplifying health information and making it accessible is more important than ever. This education empowers individuals and communities to take control of their health, reducing preventable illnesses that result in hospitalizations and improving long-term health outcomes.

Nurses also play a vital role in building trust within communities. Marginalized populations may be wary of the healthcare system due to current inequities or past injustices. Nurses often serve as the most accessible healthcare professionals. This places them in a unique position to establish relationships with these community individuals and groups, advocating for their needs and ensuring that they receive appropriate care. By working within communities and listening to identified needs, nurses help customize healthcare services to better serve diverse populations.

Culturally Competent Care

Cultural competence in nursing is crucial to delivering quality health care across culturally diverse groups. It promotes addressing health disparities and promoting equitable care. As healthcare systems become more diverse, nurses must be equipped to understand and respect patients' culture, which includes ethnicity, race, gender, education, religion, social background, sexual orientation, and physical abilities. This involves recognizing how culture affects health beliefs, communication styles, and treatment preferences and adapting care to meet these diverse needs. Educating nurses in cultural humility and competence will be essential for improving patient outcomes and delivering high-quality care in diverse populations.

Culturally competent care is based on the principles of social justice and human rights. These are important in developing a framework for implementation. Nurses will increasingly be involved in developing and implementing cultural competence programs within healthcare institutions that promote social justice and human rights. These programs will address self-awareness to identify implicit biases; improve knowledge to better understand beliefs, values, and practices associated with health based on various cultural groups; improve skills in implementing behaviors and communications that respect culture; and promote patient empowerment in various cultures. These programs may include seminars, workshops, ongoing education, and mentoring to help nurses and other healthcare professionals become more sensitive to the needs of various patient populations. Culturally competent care goes beyond language translation; it encompasses understanding a patient's worldview and values and, more importantly, how their community affects their health choices (Douglas et al., 2014). By fostering an inclusive care environment, nurses can help reduce health disparities related to miscommunication and mistrust.

In the future, nurses will also play a vital role in shaping institutional policies around diversity, equity, and inclusion. This includes advocating for the recruitment and retention of diverse staff, creating more inclusive healthcare environments, and addressing biases in clinical decision-making. Culturally competent care is not just about direct patient interaction but also about ensuring that the healthcare system as a whole is welcoming and responsive to the needs of diverse communities.

Education and Workforce Diversity

It is important for the nursing workforce itself to become more reflective of the populations whom it serves to ensure equitable care. Diversity in the nursing profession is essential for fostering trust and improving care in marginalized communities. This is important as some patients prefer to receive care from individuals who resemble them for recognition and understanding. A more diverse nursing workforce brings varied perspectives, which is critical for addressing the complex health challenges of diverse populations. Nurses from underrepresented groups can serve as role models and advocates for their communities, helping bridge gaps in care.

To achieve this, nursing education programs will need to actively recruit and support students from diverse backgrounds. One way is to use a holistic admissions strategy, which allows an educational institution to broaden an admission process to include unique experiences, qualities, and attributes in addition to traditional admission measures. Using this recruitment and retention strategy can improve diversity in the educational arena, which will ultimately increase diversity in the profession (Spencer, 2020). Other ways to improve **workforce diversity** in nursing include offering scholarships and mentorship programs and creating environments in which all students feel welcome and supported in their educational quest. By increasing the number of nurses from underrepresented groups, the profession can better meet the cultural and linguistic needs of patients, improving patient-provider communication and health outcomes. The future of health equity in nursing will depend heavily on these educational efforts to build a more inclusive workforce.

In addition to increasing diversity, it is important for nursing education to place a greater emphasis on health equity and social justice. Future nurses need to be educated not only in clinical skills but also about the broader social, economic, and environmental factors that influence health. Curricula will likely include more content on structural racism, implicit bias, and the SDOH, equipping nurses to recognize and address inequities in care. Educating nurses to be advocates for health equity will prepare them to lead initiatives that promote justice in healthcare delivery.

Research and Data-Driven Solutions

Nurses, particularly those with higher degrees in advanced practice and academic settings, are uniquely positioned to conduct research that directly addresses health disparities. Nursing research focuses on patient care, community health, and **public health**, all of which are critical areas for understanding and eliminating inequities. Even studies that do not identify statistical significance can be of value to the profession and beyond. A research study that is not statistically significant can be clinically significant. For example, a 1.5% reduction in pressure ulcers may not a represent a statistically significant difference, but it may represent 50 or more patients who did not get pressure ulcers within an organization, which is certainly clinically significant as it reduces patient suffering and overall healthcare costs.

In the future, nurses will be key players in gathering data on health outcomes, the SDOH, and the efficacy of interventions designed to reduce disparities. Their research will help identify gaps in care and develop strategies to address them.

Data-driven solutions are essential for promoting health equity. By collecting and analyzing health data, nurses can pinpoint where disparities exist, such as higher rates of chronic diseases in certain racial or socioeconomic groups. This information can be used to inform policy, guide clinical practice, and target interventions where they are most needed. The future of nursing will see a significantly increased use of technology and data analytics. Data analytics will allow for tracking of data from surveys, electronic health records, insurance claims, vital records, disease surveillance, and other registries to be retrieved by software programs to track patient outcomes and develop tailored, evidence-based interventions that reduce disparities.

Nurses will play a key role in translating research findings into practice. The goal of data analysis is to drive informed decisions in health care. Research is effective only if it leads to noticeable improvements in care, and nurses are well positioned to implement evidence-based interventions that address health disparities. These interventions could include new models of patient care delivery, variability in community health programs, or changes in hospital policies to make care more equitable in society at large. Nurses' ability to bridge the gap between research and clinical practice makes them invaluable in the fight for health equity and in addressing issues that promote wellness and quality of life for all.

Telehealth and Technology Integration

The future of nursing will be significantly shaped through continued **technology integration**, which will transform how nurses deliver care, interact with patients, and manage healthcare systems. One of the most visible shifts will be the expansion of telehealth services, which became more prominent during the coronavirus disease 2019 pandemic. Telehealth has the potential to expand access to care for people in rural areas, those with mobility challenges, or those who face financial or transportation barriers to accessing in-person health care. Nurses will play a vital role in managing and delivering care through telehealth platforms, ensuring that patients receive timely, high-quality care while also helping them navigate new technologies. The integration of telehealth and digital technologies in health care provides an opportunity to address barriers to care, particularly for underserved populations. Nurses will play a crucial role in the expansion of telehealth, especially in ensuring that these services are accessible and equitable for all populations.

Beyond telehealth, nurses will increasingly use digital tools and technologies to monitor patient health, manage chronic conditions, and predict health outcomes. Wearable devices and mobile health apps allow patients to track their vital signs, medication adherence, and overall health in real time, giving nurses valuable data to guide interventions. Remote patient monitoring systems, which enable nurses to keep tabs on patients' health from a distance, will become more widespread, helping reduce hospital readmissions and manage chronic conditions more effectively. Nurses will need to be well versed in these technologies, not only in interpreting the data they collect but also in educating patients on how to use them effectively.

Nurses will also be instrumental in overcoming the digital divide that disproportionately affects the low-income and older adult populations. As more healthcare services move online, nurses can advocate for and help implement programs that provide patients with the technology and training they need to access telehealth services. This might include assisting with digital literacy, offering technical support, or helping patients navigate telehealth platforms. Nurses' ability to work directly with patients and their families makes them ideal leaders in ensuring that telehealth does not exacerbate existing inequities.

In addition to direct patient care, nurses will be involved in developing telehealth protocols that prioritize health equity. This includes ensuring that virtual care systems are designed with the needs of all populations in mind, particularly those who may have limited access to technology. As health care continues to evolve with new technological innovations, nurses will play a key role in ensuring that these advancements are used to promote, rather than hinder, equitable access to high-quality care.

Artificial intelligence (AI) and machine learning will also transform nursing practice by enhancing clinical decision-making and improving patient outcomes. AI-driven tools can help nurses analyze large datasets, identify patterns, and make more informed decisions about patient care. For example, AI algorithms can predict patient deterioration or identify early signs of complications, allowing nurses to intervene proactively. In the future, AI could assist with everything from triaging patients to streamlining administrative tasks, freeing up more time for nurses to focus on direct patient care. However, nurses will need to maintain a balance between embracing AI and maintaining the human touch that is so essential to nursing.

Finally, the integration of technology will require a shift in nursing education and training. Nurses of the future will need to be proficient in using a range of digital tools, from electronic health records to advanced diagnostic technologies. Nursing curricula will need to adapt to this new reality, emphasizing digital literacy and data analytics alongside traditional clinical skills. Continuing education will also be critical, as technology evolves rapidly. Nurses will need ongoing training to keep pace with advancements in healthcare technology, ensuring that they can provide the best care possible in a digital age. By embracing these tools, nurses can enhance the efficiency and effectiveness of healthcare delivery, making it more personalized, data-driven, and equitable.

Leadership and Policy Influence

The future of **nursing leadership** will be defined by an increased focus on advocacy, health equity, and the SDOH. As health care continues to shift toward more patient-centered, holistic models of care, nurses will play a greater role in shaping policies that address the root causes of health disparities. Nurses are increasingly assuming leadership roles, both within healthcare institutions and in broader policy arenas. In these positions, they can influence decisions that affect the allocation of resources, the design of care models, and the priorities of healthcare systems. They have the ability to bring attention to issues such as healthcare accessibility, affordability, and cultural competence, which will be key in creating more inclusive healthcare systems. Nurse leaders will be crucial in ensuring that equity and promotion of quality outcomes are central considerations in all aspects of healthcare planning and delivery. Their advocacy can help ensure that policies focus on creating more equitable systems, from how care is provided to how it is paid for.

As nurse leaders take on more prominent roles in hospital administration, public health agencies, and healthcare organizations, they will be in a position to drive systemic changes that promote equity. They will influence policy through advocacy at the local, state, and national levels. This will involve championing new models of care that prioritize preventive services, community health, and integrated care. Nurse leaders are also likely to advocate for policies that support the needs of vulnerable populations, such as expanding Medicaid, increasing funding for community health centers, or improving access to mental health services.

Additionally, nurses will be vital in shaping the future of healthcare policy through collaboration with legislators, policymakers, and other stakeholders. They will evolve as a key force in health care through collaboration. By participating in policy discussions at the local, state, and national levels, nurses can ensure that health equity remains a top priority. Nurse-led research, advocacy, and leadership will continue to influence the development of policies that promote fair and just access to health care for all populations.

Collaborative Interdisciplinary Care

Changes in health care and ways to achieve health equity cannot be achieved by any one profession alone. Nurses will increasingly collaborate with a range of healthcare professionals, including social workers, community health workers, physicians, and mental health specialists, to address the complex needs of patients. This interdisciplinary approach is essential for providing holistic care that considers both medical and nonmedical factors, such as housing, nutrition, and mental health, that influence health outcomes.

In **collaborative interdisciplinary care** models, nurses often take on the role of care coordinators, ensuring that patients receive integrated services that meet their full spectrum of needs. This involves not only coordinating medical care but also connecting patients with social services and community resources. For example, a nurse might work with a social worker to address a patient's housing insecurity or help them access food assistance programs. Housing and food directly affect an individual's quality of life and health status. This collaborative approach is essential for addressing the SDOH, which contribute to disparities.

Future nursing practice will also involve more collaboration with community organizations and public health initiatives. Nurses will partner with local agencies to develop programs that target specific health disparities, such as maternal mortality in Black communities or high rates of diabetes in low-income populations. By working together across disciplines and sectors, nurses can help create comprehensive care systems that prioritize equity and improve outcomes for vulnerable populations.

In summary, nursing's future role in health care will expand across multiple domains, from direct patient care to leadership and policy advocacy. Nurses are key agents in promoting fair, just, and accessible health care for all.

Nursing's Future Role

The pace of change is relentless, and this will continue into the future. Society will maintain the need for the services of nurses, and their demand will be even greater as the future progresses. Nurses are the largest group of health-care providers, and their needed numbers will continue to increase. Nurses' role will continue to expand, and the role of patient advocate will include more patient education and validation of compliance with health regimens (Mahlin, 2010). It is possible nurses' role will involve more consultation as self-care is promoted for patient health maintenance (see Figure 18.2).

Nurses will use their knowledge base to be professional patient partners and consultants for healthcare delivery. Self-care will be promoted through genomics and nanotechnological innovations. Patients will have astute knowledge of potential diseases that they self-monitor and use holistic mechanisms (e.g., nutritional, spiritual, pharmaceutical, psychological, and physiological) of care to manage. Nurses will continue to be primary information managers. They will collect data, transform these data into information for patient management, collaborate to integrate information from individual care providers and other records, analyze information, make

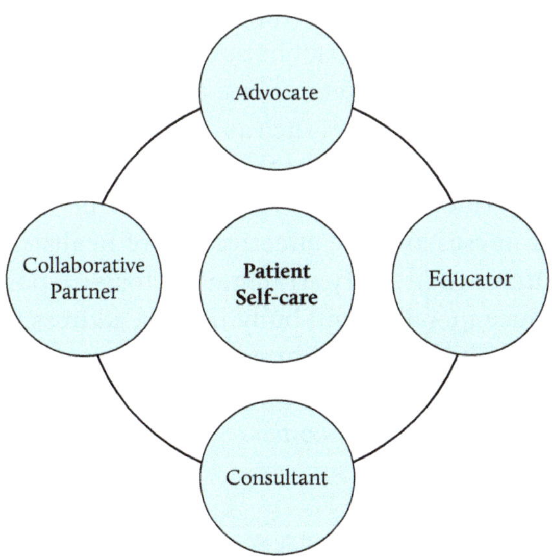

FIGURE 18.2 Nurse Role in Patient Partnership

decisions based on the data collected from technological and nontechnological means (nursing wisdom components), and effectively communicate this information to professional (e.g., other nurses, physicians, therapists) and nonprofessional (e.g., patient and family) care providers.

Health records will be open and readily accessible to patients. Individuals may be able to access their health record from any computer terminal. Health records will be seamless and interactive from any health delivery site. Nursing information placed on individualized records will be available for immediate review by the patient or any other healthcare provider with a need to know. Nurses will be more involved in politics and function in more collaborative healthcare organizational roles. Nursing will be dynamic in how it works in organizations. Research will be an expectation, and evidence-based practice will be the norm.

Nursing will be tested in new and complex ways as health care evolves and increases in complexity (Janzen, 2010; Paton, 2007). The pandemic challenged the nursing profession in ways not imagined years prior to its development. As society grows, the nursing workforce will need to be stronger and more diversified. Graduates will need to be practice-ready, know how to maneuver in a digitally focused environment, and be able to function as an effective member of an interdisciplinary team in order to deliver high-quality, competent, patient-centered care (Hazanov et al., 2020; Ortega-Lapiedra et al., 2023).

Key Future Nursing Challenges

Nurses play a crucial role in delivering high-quality health care, but they may face challenges that can impact both their workforce and patient care. Among these issues is the need to create a positive and supportive work environment and to address issues such as incivility and bullying, which can undermine teamwork and morale. At the same time, the nursing profession is grappling with workforce shortages and burnout, both of which threaten the well-being of nurses and the effectiveness of healthcare delivery. It is important for nurses to identify strategies to foster a positive workforce environment, reduce incivility and bullying, and address key challenges of workforce shortages and burnout. Through awareness and strategies, nurses can develop solutions to support longevity in the nursing workforce and improve personal and patient outcomes.

Workforce Shortages

One of the most significant challenges facing the nursing profession today is the workforce shortage. The aging population, coupled with an increase in chronic diseases, has placed greater demands on healthcare systems, leading to a growing need for nurses. Unfortunately, nursing schools are often unable to keep pace with the demand, and many regions face a shortage of qualified nursing professionals. To address this issue, healthcare organizations and policymakers must invest in strategies that attract and retain nurses. Effective ways to encourage individuals to enter nursing include increasing funding for nursing education programs, offering scholarships, and providing loan forgiveness for nursing students who commit to working in underserved areas. How can you as an individual address workforce shortages? Individual strategies include (a) investing in a multistate nursing license that offers flexibility to work across state lines; (b) promoting activities that encourage longevity in the nursing profession, such as promoting a positive workplace, maintaining work-life balance, and investing in professional growth through certifications and education; (c) engaging in political activism to promote awareness and professional needs; and (d) joining nursing organizations that correlate to specific interests.

Burnout

Nurses often work long hours under high-pressure conditions, which can lead to physical, emotional, and mental exhaustion. This condition is called ***burnout***. It is a significant issue that affects the nursing workforce. Burnout not only affects the well-being of nurses but also compromises patient care and safety. Burnout can impair nurses' cognitive abilities, hampering decision-making skills and negatively affecting interpersonal interactions, which can reduce the ability to provide optimal patient care. According to the World Health Organization (2019), symptoms of burnout include "feelings of energy depletion; increased mental distance from one's job, or feelings of negativism or cynicism related to one's job; or reduced professional efficacy." Awareness of the symptoms is important for nurses to recognize early for intervention. Self-intervention includes promoting work-life balance, prioritizing self, and identifying organizational systems that support one's balance between life situations and the professional job. These can include flexible scheduling and access to mental health resources. Promote a supportive work environment where you and your peers can take breaks, access counseling services, and feel empowered to manage workloads, all of which are important components in preventing burnout.

Resilience is another important aspect of addressing burnout. Resilience is the ability to adapt to difficult situations. Through resilience training programs, one can learn coping strategies to manage stress, maintain emotional well-being, and bounce back from challenging situations. Proactively work to incorporate resilience-building exercises into the workplace

(Anderson et al., 2021). These can include promotion of mindfulness training, stress management workshops, and peer support groups, to develop the mental fortitude needed to navigate the professional demands of nursing care delivery. Growth opportunities can improve job satisfaction. Continuing and formal academic educational endeavors can serve to promote the acquisition of mentorship roles, garner recognition, and allow for leadership role eligibility, which can combat feelings of burnout and disengagement.

Strategies to Create a Positive Workforce

In nursing, creating a **positive workforce environment** is crucial for promoting job satisfaction, retention, and patient safety. A positive environment encourages collaboration, mutual respect, and communication, which are essential for high-quality patient care. One effective strategy for creating such an environment is fostering a culture of open communication. It is important to feel comfortable voicing concerns, sharing ideas, and seeking help from colleagues without fear of retribution. Leadership can encourage open communication by implementing regular team meetings, feedback sessions, and open-door policies. Additionally, fostering interdisciplinary collaboration ensures that nurses work harmoniously with physicians, therapists, and other healthcare professionals, creating a more cohesive and supportive workplace.

Another critical strategy in the workplace is promoting professional development and recognition. Many organizations have nurse awards to address this strategy. Nurses who feel valued and supported in their career growth are more likely to experience job satisfaction and remain committed to their work. Providing opportunities for continuing education, mentorship, and career advancement encourages nurses to develop their skills and expertise. Organizations can establish programs that recognize and reward nursing excellence, whether through financial incentives, public recognition, or promotions. By investing in the growth of nursing staff, healthcare organizations not only improve employee morale but also enhance the quality of care provided to patients.

Strategies to Address Incivility and Bullying

Addressing incivility and bullying in the workplace is essential for maintaining a positive environment. The American Nurses Association (n.d.) defines ***incivility*** as "one or more rude, discourteous, or disrespectful actions that may or may not have a negative intent behind them" and ***bullying*** as "repeated, unwanted, harmful actions intended to humiliate, offend, and cause distress in the recipient." Bullying and incivility can lead to high turnover rates, reduced job satisfaction, and impaired patient outcomes. To combat these issues, healthcare organizations have and implement clear policies that define unacceptable behavior and outline consequences for those who engage in bullying or incivility. These policies are reinforced with training programs that educate staff on how to recognize, report, and prevent bullying (Smith et al., 2020). It is important to be knowledgeable of policies and reporting mechanisms for putting them into action. All nurses should model respectful and professional behavior, setting the workplace tone for collegiality and serving as examples for others in the workforce. Be aware of available organizational conflict resolution resources, such as mediation services or employee assistance programs, which can also help resolve interpersonal issues before they escalate.

Summary

Nursing is a satisfying and rewarding profession. The future of nurses educated at all levels is multifaceted, involving a combination of advocacy, research, leadership, and collaboration based on degree. Nurses will continue to be essential in addressing health disparities by advocating for policy changes, engaging with communities, promoting culturally competent care, and embracing technology to ensure equitable access to health care. Their leadership in promoting technology use for better patient management and creating diverse and inclusive workforces, advancing interdisciplinary care, and driving evidence-based solutions will be crucial in shaping the healthcare landscape. As health care becomes more focused on population health and the SDOH, nurses will remain at the forefront of efforts to ensure that every individual, regardless of background, has access to the care they need to live a healthy life. Nursing challenges include workforce shortages, burnout, incivility, and bullying. These are not insurmountable and can be overcome with individual and organizational interventions. By continuing to prioritize professionalism qualities and addressing challenges, nursing will lead the charge in transforming health care to be the best system it can be for a healthy society. By addressing individual qualities, nurses can maintain a positive professional perspective and sustain engagement in a rewarding profession—nursing.

References

American Nurses Association. (n.d.). *Protect yourselves, protect your patients.* https://www.nursingworld.org/practice-policy/work-environment/end-nurse-abuse/

Andersen, S., Mintz-Binder, R., Sweatt, L., & Song, H. (2021). Building nurse resilience in the workplace. *Applied Nursing Research, 59*, 151433. https://doi.org/10.1016/j.apnr.2021.151433

Douglas, M. K., Rosenkoetter, M., Pacquiao, D. F., Callister, L. C., Hattar-Pollara, M., Lauderdale, J., Milstead, J., Nardi, D., & Purnell, L. (2014). Guidelines for implementing culturally competent nursing care. *Journal of Transcultural Nursing, 25*(2), 109–121. https://doi.org/10.1177/1043659614520998

Hazanov, Y., Gehman, Y., Wilf Miron, R., & Kagan, I. (2020). Nursing work environment, professional self-actualization and marketing of the nursing profession: Cross-sectional study. *Nursing Open, 8*(1), 434–441. https://doi.org/10.1002/nop2.644

Janzen, K. (2010). Alice through the looking glass: The influence of self and student understanding on role actualization among novice clinical nurse educators. *Journal of Continuing Education in Nursing, 41*(11), 517–523. https://doi.org/10.3928/00220124-20100701-07

Mahlin, M. (2010). Individual patient advocacy, collective responsibility and activism within professional nursing associations. *Nursing Ethics, 17*(2), 247–254. https://doi.org/10.1177/0969733009351949

Ortega-Lapiedra, R., Barrado-Narvión, M. J., & Bernués-Oliván, J. (2023). Acquisition of competencies of nurses: Improving the performance of the healthcare system. *International Journal of Environmental Research and Public Health, 20*(5), 4510. https://doi.org/10.3390/ijerph20054510

Paton, B. (2007). Knowing within: Practice wisdom of clinical nurse educators. *Journal of Nursing Education, 46*(11), 488–495. https://doi.org/10.3928/01484834-20071101-03

Scott, S. M., & Scott, P. A. (2021). Nursing, advocacy and public policy. *Nursing Ethics, 28*(5), 723–733. https://doi.org/10.1177/0969733020961823

Smith, C. R., Palazzo, S. J., Grubb, P. L., & Gillespie, G. L. (2020). Standing up against workplace bullying behavior: Recommendations from newly licensed nurses. *Journal of Nursing Education and Practice, 10*(7), 35. https://doi.org/10.5430/jnep.v10n7p35

Spencer, T. D. (2020). Improving diversity of the nursing workforce through evidence-based strategies. *Journal of Nursing Education, 59*(7), 363–364. https://doi.org/10.3928/01484834-20200617-01

World Health Organization. (2019, May 28). *Burn-out an "occupational phenomenon": International classification of diseases.* https://www.who.int/news/item/28-05-2019-burn-out-an-occupational-phenomenon-international-classification-of-diseases

Image Credits

IMG 18.1: Generated using Adobe Firefly.

Index

D

U

V

W

Y